THE PSYCHOANALYTIC WORK OF HANSI KENNEDY

THE PSYCHOANALYTIC WORK OF HANSI KENNEDY
From War Nurseries to the Anna Freud Centre (1940–1993)

Edited by
Jill M. Miller and Carla Neely

Routledge
Taylor & Francis Group
LONDON AND NEW YORK

First published 2008 by Karnac Books Ltd.

2 Park Square, Milton Park, Abingdon, Oxfordshire OX14 4RN
52 Vanderbilt Avenue, New York, NY 10017

Routledge is an imprint of the Taylor & Francis Group, an informa business

First issued in hardback 2019

British Library Cataloguing in Publication Data

A C.I.P. for this book is available from the British Library

ISBN13: 978-1-85575-523-9 (pbk)
ISBN13: 978-0-367-32857-3 (hbk)

Edited, designed, and produced by
Florence Production Ltd, Stoodleigh, Devon
www.florenceproduction.co.uk

CONTENTS

ACKNOWLEDGEMENTS xi

ABOUT THE EDITORS xiii

INTRODUCTION xiv

THE MAKING OF A CHILD ANALYST xix

PART 1: MEMORY **1**

CHAPTER ONE

Cover Memories in Formation 3

CHAPTER TWO

Problems in Reconstruction in Child Analysis 16

CHAPTER THREE

The "Baby at the Breast" Experience: Memory or Fantasy?
Some Further Thoughts on Reconstruction 32

CHAPTER FOUR

Both Sides of the Barrier: Some Reflections on Childhood Fantasy 43
(*with George Moran, Stanley Wiseberg and Clifford Yorke*)

PART 2: INSIGHT **53**

CHAPTER FIVE

The Role of Insight in Child Analysis: A Developmental Viewpoint 57

PART 3: CONFLICT AND DEVELOPMENTAL DISTURBANCES **75**

CHAPTER SIX

Pseudobackwardness in Children: Maternal Attitudes as an Etiological Factor 80
(*Maria Berger and Hansi Kennedy*)

CHAPTER SEVEN

Some Reflections on Infantile Neurosis 107
(*Rose Edgcumbe, Hansi Kennedy, Joseph Sandler and Clifford Yorke*)

CHAPTER EIGHT

Childhood Neurosis vs Developmental Deviations: Two Clinical Case Histories 121
(*with Clifford Yorke*)

CHAPTER NINE

Different Types of Sado-Masochistic Behaviour in Children 142
(*Marion Burgner and Hansi Kennedy*)

CHAPTER TEN

Steps from Outer to Inner Conflict Viewed as Superego Precursors 161
(*with Clifford Yorke*)

CHAPTER ELEVEN

The Developmental Roots of Self-Injury and Response to Pain in a 4-Year-Old Boy 169
(*with George Moran*)

CHAPTER TWELVE

For or Against Child Placement: A Clinical Illustration 187

CHAPTER THIRTEEN

Growing up with a Handicapped Sibling 196

CHAPTER FOURTEEN

Trauma in Childhood: Signs and Sequelae as Seen in the Analysis of an Adolescent 216

CHAPTER FIFTEEN

Reflections on the Aim of Child Analysis 227
(*with George Moran*)

PART 4: ANALYTIC TECHNIQUE WITH PRE-LATENCY CHILDREN 247

CHAPTER SIXTEEN

The Technique of Psychoanalysis with the Pre-Latency Child 249

CHAPTER SEVENTEEN

Psychoanalytic Work with Under-fives: Forty Years' Experience 267
(*Mary Target and Hansi Kennedy*)

COMPLETE BIBLIOGRAPHY OF HANSI KENNEDY'S PUBLICATIONS AND PRESENTATIONS 294

BIBLIOGRAPHY 305

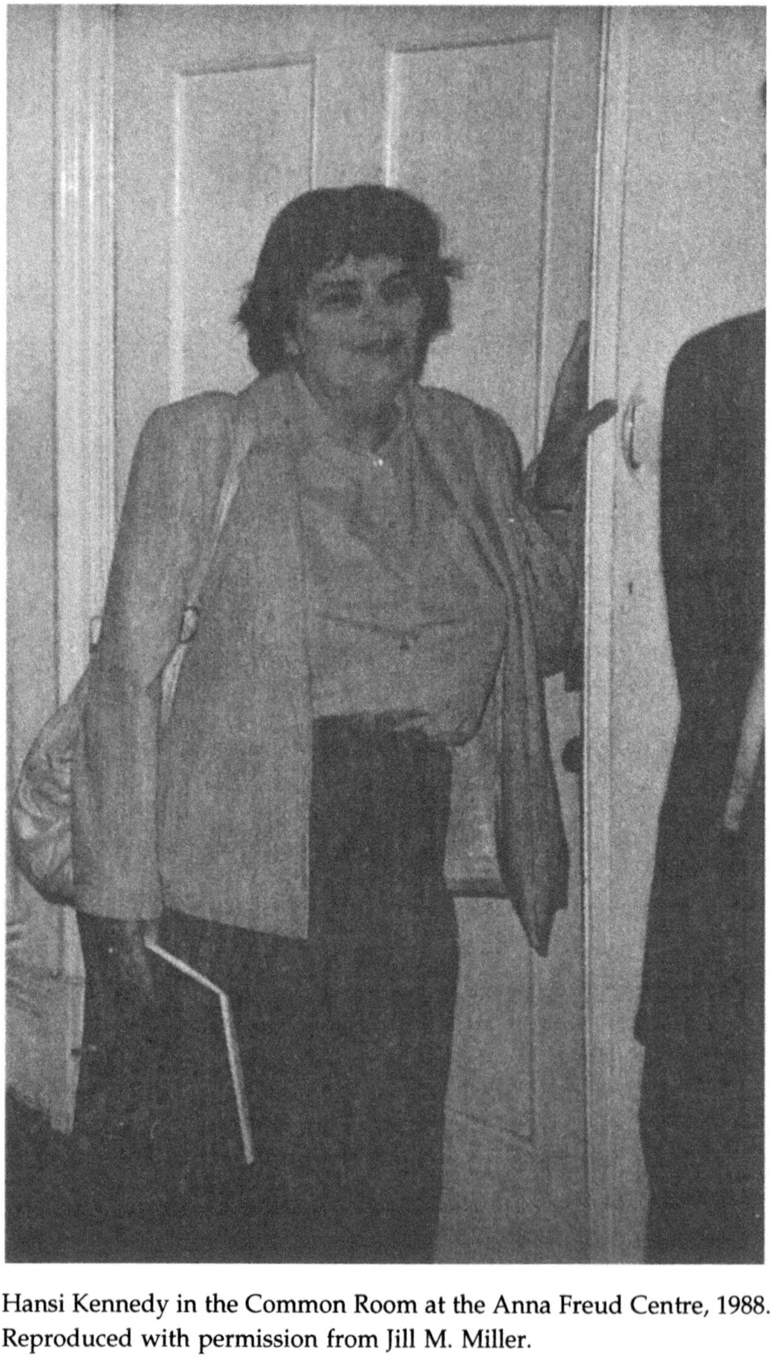

Hansi Kennedy in the Common Room at the Anna Freud Centre, 1988.
Reproduced with permission from Jill M. Miller.

ACKNOWLEDGEMENTS

We are especially indebted to Hansi Kennedy's family. Her sister Suzie Wiener graciously shared her early memories of Hansi. Her son Steven Kennedy, his wife Sue Jessup and daughter Catherine, Hansi's granddaughter, offered their warmth, their home and their recollections. Sue, thankfully, had interviewed Hansi three years before her death as part of a project for her master's degree, and it is from this document that we drew much of our biographical information. Jan Wiener, Hansi's niece, herself a Jungian analyst, was entrusted with Hansi's papers and professional memorabilia. To her we are enormously grateful for her time, thoughtfulness and help. Jan had the good sense to interview her aunt shortly before her death, and thus was able to provide the most detailed account of Hansi's early life, emigration, and young adult years. We would also like to thank Maria Berger and Audrey Gavshon, longtime colleagues of Hansi's at the Anna Freud Centre.

Thanks also goes to Diana Mangels for her valuable assistance with the manuscript, Peter Fonagy who facilitated the publication of this book, and Victoria Hamilton who encouraged us to broaden our scope. To Al and Elizabeth Neely, your constant patience and support is deeply appreciated and not gone unnoticed. Lastly, to Hansi herself for all that she gave to us, to children, and to the field of psychoanalysis, we are forever grateful.

ABOUT THE EDITORS

Jill M. Miller, Phd, and Carla Neely, Phd, are Child, Adolescent and Adult psychoanalysts.

The editors did their child analytic training in different eras at the Anna Freud Centre; Dr Neely when Anna Freud was active and Dr Miller when Hansi Kennedy became Clinical Director. Both were supervised by Hansi Kennedy and participated in numerous clinical activities benefiting significantly from the clarity of Kennedy's thinking. Beyond training Dr Miller and Dr Neely have maintained their involvement with the AFC contributing to the Annual Colloquium which began in 1980 and continues to present day.

INTRODUCTION

Hansi Kennedy was a model of a child psychoanalyst. Having immigrated to London from Vienna as a teen, she found her way to the War Nurseries and to Anna Freud and Dorothy Burlingham where her career began. In the height of World War II, as London was being bombed, her interest in children and psychoanalysis blossomed. As she recalled at the memorial for Sara Rosenfeld, her dear friend and fellow worker in the War Nurseries " . . . what we discovered anew, and what became the most exciting and stimulating experience of those days was our first contact with psychoanalysis and I have the most vivid recollection of hours and hours of discussion with Sara, walking up and down Finchley Road after a 10 hour working shift at the Hampstead Nurseries, and letting all the buses go by. We began to discover the enormous gaps in our knowledge and we began to read more systematically and to discuss what we had read. And this eventually gave impetus to our wish to study and to try and make up for our interrupted education" (Kennedy, 1973, p. 8). These years in the War Nurseries had a profound effect on Kennedy. Looking back on this beginning, she later said: "I have no doubt in my mind that this historical background has been a beneficial influence on our work. Although many of the younger members of staff joined us at later stages of our development, all have undergone a common training and have similar aims and interests to those of us who have been there from the earliest days. Our shared experience of working together over a very considerable period of time has given us stability and continuity . . ." (Kennedy, 1978, p. 7).

Kennedy's thinking was clear, disciplined and sophisticated, with a depth that demonstrated her understanding of development and of the mind of the child. Unburdened by concerns of what was and was not analysis, and whether child analysis was equivalent to adult analysis, she followed the children, first in the War Nurseries, then in the Hampstead Nursery School and the children she and others analyzed at the Hampstead Clinic, later the Anna Freud Centre.

Not surprisingly, her first interest was in memory and its fate through the developmental process. Kennedy had a "personal longstanding interest in the formation of early childhood memories and their developmental and defensive distortions," as well as in "what remnants of the infant's earliest experiences appear in the analytic material" (Kennedy, 1982, p. 1). As we examined her writings, it was evident that this theme appeared again and again as she challenged traditional psychoanalytic thought. Ahead of her time, Kennedy's ideas foreshadowed contemporary psychoanalysis. She was always concerned with how children perceived the world and how they structured their experience, as well as how these processes were faulty (integration and psychosis, separation, narcissism and borderline disorders, sado-masochism). Her curiosity about how the mind worked and ways to understand it was immense (fantasy, conflict, cognition, insight, regression and progression, and children's responses to pain, illness, trauma and environmental failures). And always Kennedy focused on technique in concert with the developmental process, how the analyst listened, understood, intervened, and worked within the relationship (reconstruction, transference, aims and the complicated mixture of techniques applicable to work with children and adolescents). Perhaps due to her early work during the war, but also as a young analyst working with Liselotte Frankl on disturbances of integration and treating highly disturbed children with Ruth Thomas, Sara Rosenfeld, and others, Kennedy explored the pathways of development beyond those of the neuroses.

She expanded the field of child psychoanalysis to include those suffering from developmental disturbances, a focus which dominates psychoanalysis today. Her interest in very young children never faltered; she was always highly involved in the Hampstead Nursery, as she integrated her ideas and those of others to contribute to our understanding of analytic work with this age group.

Kennedy was never one to blow her own horn nor did she enjoy the spotlight; hence, the significance of her work has gone unnoticed by many. She loved thinking about, sharing and debating ideas, was at ease expressing strong opinions and encouraged students and staff to do the same, and as can be seen from her bibliography, enjoyed working with others. She was immersed in Study Groups, which were embedded in the culture at Hampstead. Study Groups, she believed, brought together the clinical, the analytic training, and research. "This continuous exchange of ideas provides an ongoing learning experience for staff and students alike. It makes the Clinic a particularly stimulating and rewarding intellectual environment to work in" (Kennedy, 1978, p. 10).

Kennedy often talked about continuity and its importance in the Centre. At the 30th anniversary of the Anna Freud Centre Nursery School, she looked back at the early days in Vienna, the War Nurseries, and historical changes and noted: "There are, of course, other areas of continuity, development and change we could discuss. But perhaps these themes can be encapsulated in one small item of un-recorded history, in itself of no real significance but which serves to symbolize continuity for me, which is that the breakfast counter in the War Nursery, which originally came from the Jackson Nursery in Vienna, is now used by generations of children to sit on during story time" (Kennedy, 1988, pp. 274–5). She, herself, provided enormous continuity to the field, as one of the last survivors of the War Nursery student workers, one of the first staff members when the Clinic opened in 1952, and eventually becoming a highly valued colleague and confidante of Anna Freud's. When Anna Freud died, it was Kennedy who was entrusted with the Clinic. As she said at the funeral, "Though all of us will greatly miss her, she leaves us with her most precious legacy. It was her wish that her work at the Clinic be continued and extended after her death and perhaps her teaching and expectations have been sufficiently internalized to help us in this endeavor" (Kennedy, 1983, p. 12).

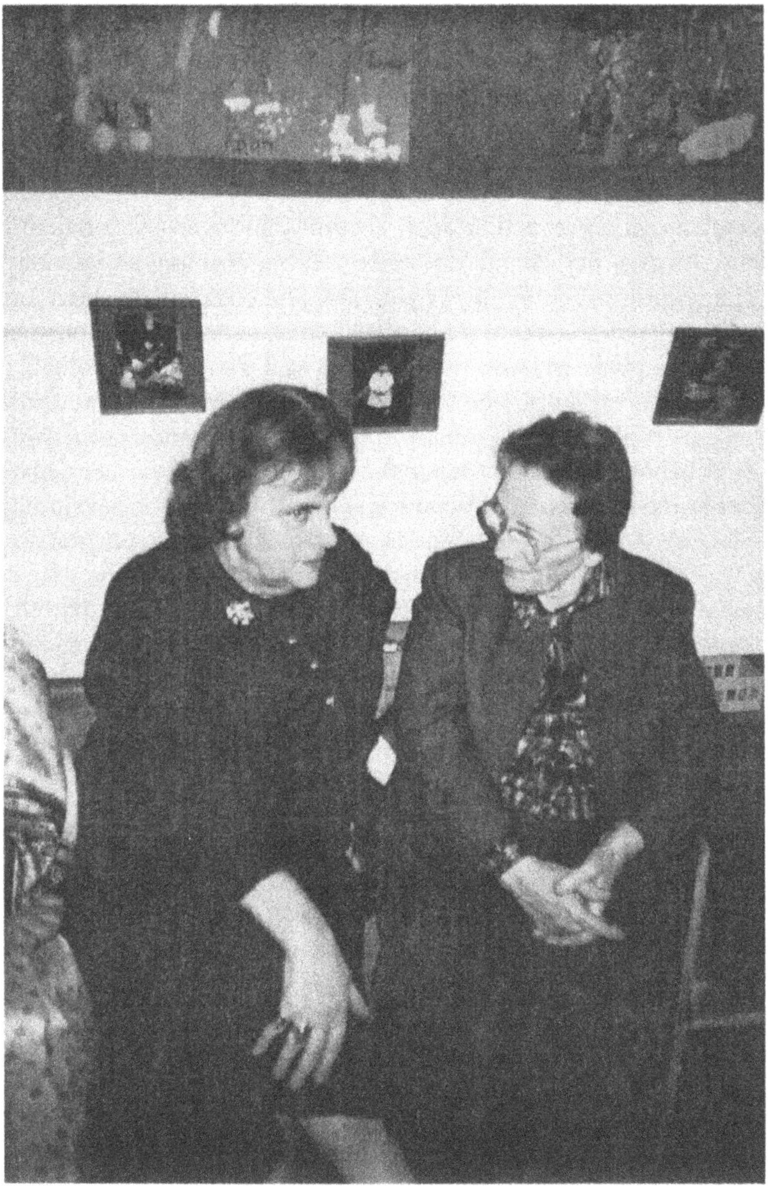

Hansi Kennedy with Manna Friedmann in the Anna Freud Centre Nursery, 1989. Manna Friedmann was the primary teacher in the Nursery from its inception in 1957 until 1978. Reproduced with permission from Jill M. Miller.

Kennedy's family and home life were central to her, yet private as she kept her personal and professional lives somewhat separate. She had a long and loving relationship with her husband Gerald, adored her two sons Tony and Steven, maintained strong ties with her sister Suzie and niece Jan, and was overjoyed with the birth of each of her grandchildren, Catherine, Rebecca and Ben. Kennedy loved music, to play and to laugh, absurdity and even a little naughtiness. As Ava Bry Penman described in her obituary of Kennedy: "Hansi could reach in. She could wait. She could be touched, and a slightly teary shine came to her eyes at certain deeply felt moments. When she made feelings, thoughts and fantasies understandable it felt like a good story, one that brought relief through some truth. And she could patiently persist in thinking about and approaching overwhelming states that made the inchoate bearable . . . She liked people and seemed equally comfortable with colleagues, developing therapists, worried parents, and troubled children . . . In her practical way, Hansi was instructive in her appreciation for both the robustness and delicacy of child analysis as well as work with parents. She loved analytic work and faced, with interest and courage, the inevitable hard times as they came" (2004, p. 189).

With Kennedy's death in 2003 a chapter in child psychoanalysis closed. This book is an attempt to honor her memory and to share her ideas.

THE MAKING OF A CHILD ANALYST

An accurate reflection of the work of Hansi Kennedy requires the placement of her writing in the context of a life lived in the relatively early days of the development of child psychoanalysis. As a witness to and participant in the work of Anna Freud, Kennedy's own perceptions of her early professional life include the pivotal period of the migration of psychoanalysis from Vienna to London. Her role in the Hampstead War Nurseries and later in the Hampstead Child Therapy Course and Clinic included much of significance in the evolution of psychoanalytic thought regarding children and their psychological development.

That which is known about Kennedy's early childhood comes from interviews she gave to her daughter-in-law Sue Jessup in 2000 and to her niece Jan Wiener shortly before her death in 2003. We are fortunate to have their reports of her childhood as told to them by Kennedy herself. The records they provided allow us to consider the events of her childhood, which may bear significantly upon Kennedy's life work.

Hanna Engl Kennedy (Hansi) was born in Vienna in 1923, the younger of two girls, to parents who were of eastern European, Jewish descent. Her father worked in the family hat-making firm, providing a comfortable lifestyle for his wife and daughters. There was a relatively large extended family in Vienna, including both sets of grandparents.

Kennedy attended the local primary school, a mixed school of both Jewish and non-Jewish students from all economic backgrounds. She was particularly aware of peers who suffered anxiety and believed this early experience enabled her to empathize easily with others. Her first contact with psychoanalysts occurred when, at age 10, the Lampl de Groot family, colleagues of Sigmund and Anna Freud, moved into the house next door. Kennedy recalled her curiosity about the children and adults coming for analytic sessions each day. A friendship grew between Kennedy and one of the Lampl de Groot daughters until the daughter fled to Holland to join the Resistance.

During her primary school years, her paternal grandparents died and the family business also began to struggle, as did much of commerce in Vienna in the early 1930s. Economic conditions led Kennedy's father to move the business to London in 1934. Kennedy experienced this time as quite difficult. Not only was she close to her father, his absence also involved the closing of their Vienna home and a move to the home of her maternal grandparents. From age 11 to 15, the family was in a period of transition with her father in London and Kennedy, her sister, and their mother left behind in Vienna.

Life in Vienna began to change, too, as a result of the impending war. As a latency aged child Kennedy was aware of changes in attitudes in her community as anti-Jewish sentiments grew. During her pre-adolescence the situation worsened, Kennedy recalling anti-Semitic comments among her peers and even shooting in the streets. In March of 1938 when she was fifteen, the Anschluss brought troops marching into Vienna. Kennedy was by this time in secondary school, which closed for a month and then reopened to complete the year. When Kennedy returned she found that many of those students who were not Jewish were now wearing the uniform of Hitler's Youth Army. When school reopened in the fall, all Jews were required to attend a Jewish-only school. As she was beyond school-leaving age, Kennedy decided not to return to formal education.

In March of 1939 Kennedy and her family were able to emigrate from Vienna to London where her father had rebuilt the family business. He had worked to obtain visas for them, a desperate and stressful task, although easier to do from London than from Vienna. With visas in hand and by paying the Nazis, the family arrived safely in London, as did their containers of furniture and other household goods. "We were fortunate," said Kennedy, "to get out not only with our skins but our belongings." Grandparents and aunts were also helped to leave and much of Kennedy's extended family settled with them. By August of that year the family had secured a home in Hampstead where Kennedy eventually reared her two sons Steven and Tony, and remained until her death.

Kennedy's sister Suzie expressed a sentiment shared by both girls: that there was no reason to look back, but only to look forward to the future in England. At fifteen Kennedy left childhood behind.

It was at this time, having through family friends learned about the efforts of Anna Freud and Dorothy Burlingham to establish residential care in Hampstead for London children made homeless by the War, that Kennedy sought employment in the Hampstead War Nurseries. There were no openings and work visas were difficult to obtain; however, several months later a new baby home was opened and restrictions on visas lifted due to War needs, and Anna Freud offered Kennedy a position as a student worker. The 16-year-old Kennedy worked 10 to 12 hour days with other young emigrant women. As most were without families, the War Nurseries provided them with housing and pocket money, in addition to the training in childcare, development, and childhood illness. Kennedy remained in the War Nurseries until they dissolved in 1945.

Despite the War and her very full life in the War Nurseries, Kennedy sought formal educational training once again. Upon her arrival in London, she took correspondence courses through Wolsey Hall at Oxford in Maths, Biology, German, and English for foreigners. With this serving as her first degree, and by passing the entrance exam in psychology, she was accepted for post-graduate psychology training in 1942. Kennedy attended classes at Kings College until they were evacuated, then on weekends at Birkbeck College. She graduated with an academic postgraduate diploma in psychology in 1945, just as the war ended. Kennedy was 22 years old.

The following is an excerpt from an unpublished paper by Kennedy entitled "Reminiscences of Anna Freud (1895–1982)" presented at a meeting in Mexico City in 1993. It provides in her own words her experience as a student worker in the War Nurseries.

World War II offered Anna Freud the opportunity to apply psychoanalytic knowledge to enhance the welfare of children who had suffered through bombing, shelter-sleeping, indiscriminate evacuation and the break-up of their families. The Hampstead War Nurseries provided *residential* care for 80 such children, aged from birth to five years, and was located in an area of London of comparative safety from air raids, yet within easy reach of their families for regular (often daily) visits.

At the time Anna Freud formulated four main aims for opening the War Nursery:

1) *To repair* the damage already done caused by their wartime experiences and serve as a convalescent home or home for problem children. (Therapeutic aims)
2) *To prevent* further harm being done to children by providing the security of a stable environment with optimal opportunity to form or maintain the attachment to their parents. (Preventative aims)
3) *To study* the children's reactions to war-time experiences, separation from their families, the influence of community life at an early stage of development and to work out patterns of nursery life which can serve as a model for peace-time education. (Research aims)
4) and *to instruct* people interested in the forms of education based on psycho-analytic knowledge of the child. (Training aims)

It was in this capacity that I became a Trainee, or student worker as we were called, in the War Nursery from 1940–1945. For the trainees, most of them still in their late "teens" and themselves refugees from Austria or Germany, Anna Freud devised an extensive training programme. The highlight of these courses was a weekly Wednesday afternoon meeting with Anna Freud where problems with individual children were discussed, and possible new ways of dealing with the child suggested by her. Anna Freud visited the Nursery every day and often following such a discussion, would spend time specifically observing this child and bring her observations and further thoughts to the next meeting. It stimulated everyone to observe and think about difficulties presented by individual children and to explore better ways of handling them. In due course we were encouraged to write down our observations on index cards and thus a set of observations was compiled on each child recorded by different observers and in different settings, a method that continues to be practiced to the present day in the Nursery School of the Anna Freud Centre. [The Nursery School is now closed.]

Such observations can be used as source material for teaching child development, insofar as one's eyes are opened to elaborate, confirm, or question through subsequent observations the same child, what one has learned. For us War Nursery Trainees who cared for these children on a 24 hour basis it was a way of absorbing psychoanalytic theory in a most natural and meaningful way.

We also learned a great deal from observing Anna Freud's conversations with individual children. She had a wonderful way in responding to children who addressed her with a question or demand. In a room full of other people she could give her full attention to such a child and make the child feel truly special.

This was characteristic also of her contact with staff and trainees. Everyone had ready access to her for discussion or advice regarding work or personal matters and she could usually make helpful suggestions and then at a later stage enquire how things had been resolved. One felt immensely supported, valued and stimulated to try and work out difficulties on one's own. Instead of the usual tensions between workers in a closed hard-working community—it supported a wish in all of us to work out rivalries, and discontents, so that they would not impact on the well-being of children.

In spite of her practical involvement in the life of the children and the staff and the daily problems of running an organization of this kind, Anna Freud never lost sight of her research aims and it was tremendously exciting to play a part in this aspect of her work as well.

Observations of the children in the War Nurseries revealed differences in the chronology of early development and convincingly demonstrated that primal scene and oedipal fantasies appeared with regularity also in children who lived without knowing their fathers and with absence of any kind of oedipal experiences. But the most important lessons learned related to the effects of separation from mother on a young child's development. These facts are so well recognized today that they will hardly impress you at all. Anna Freud referred to these observations afforded during the War as "*an experimental setting provide by fate*". She had, of course, known about the importance of the mother-child relationship for development and had set up the War Nursery to enable mothers to visit regularly so as to establish or maintain the relationship with the child. When she recognized that even regular visits and good substitute care in a well staffed residential setting did not provide the opportunity for the child to establish the quality and depth of attachment to a special object needed to modulate and curb affect and drive development, Anna Freud re-organized the War Nursery into small family groups where the physical and psychological care became the responsibility of one substitute mother. I mothered such a child from the age of 9 months to 5 years. [See Kennedy 1950.] For the trainees these were important years which inspired many of us to go on working with young children in one way or another.

To have worked in the Hampstead War Nurseries gave one life membership in an exclusive club. When Anna Freud talked about children in later years, she would often refer to a telling example of a War Nursery child and cast her eyes around the audience to spot someone who remembered the story as she did . . . (Kennedy, 1993, pp. 2–4).

At the end of the World War II there was a tremendous need to provide services for children who were suffering because of the impact the war had on them. New child guidance clinics were set up throughout England with the assistance of child psychoanalysts. Staff was urgently needed. Kate Friedlander, who had attended Anna Freud's Wednesday seminar for the War Nursery staff, started the West Sussex Child Guidance Service with clinics in Horsham, Chichester and Worthing. She offered Kennedy a job as a psychologist and trainee in child psychotherapy. Kennedy recalled that she was "very green and inexperienced, but it was a wonderful learning process while I started my analysis. She [Friedlander] and I knew more about children than anyone she could find and she would supervise my cases" (Essenhigh, 1995, pp. 350–1).

Kennedy chose Dorothy Burlingham as her analyst, wanting a female who also had children, probably anticipating her own future. For the next four years Kennedy worked at the Chichester clinic. Describing this time in her life Kennedy later said: "It was difficult. I did analysis in the morning, then left for Chichester—saw my patients—stayed over night, worked my session, then returned in the evening for analysis—and then again in reverse" (Essenhigh, 1995, p. 351).

We return to Kennedy's 1993 Mexico City paper remembering Anna Freud as she describes her training in child psychoanalysis and the early years at the Hampstead Clinic:

> Some of the War Nursery trainees had taken academic courses in psychology or social work to prepare for future careers and when the War Nursery closed they were given employment in newly set-up child guidance clinics. They soon became aware that they were inadequately trained to undertake psychotherapies of children. Their wish for a comprehensive training course in psychoanalytic child therapy eventually led Anna Freud and some colleagues to found The Hampstead Child Therapy Course in 1947. Perhaps another reason to embark on this venture stemmed from Anna Freud's longstanding belief that child psychoanalysis should be undertaken by young people with special interest and understanding of children, rather than remain an additional field of specialization for the analysis of adults. Thus, the first five students accepted in the training course were former War Nursery trainees. [Kennedy was one of these.]
>
> The Course began without funds, without a meeting room or library but a great deal of enthusiasm on the part of students and teachers. Then, as now, it involved a personal training analysis, 3 training cases under supervision and courses and seminars. With the growth in the scope of the training and the increase in the number of students, the need

for a Clinic became urgent. Anna Freud found funding and a house, less than a few hundred yards from the site of the former War Nursery and the Hampstead Clinic was opened in 1952. Some of the first graduates of the Training Course were now offered staff positions as child analysts, though Anna Freud continued to refer to them for some years and with some pride as "our former students". [Kennedy, now 29 years old, was one of the first staff members.]

In these early years the clinic operated on a small scale which again provided ideal conditions for learning. A small staff with a limited number of treatment cases can easily share and discuss clinical work. We knew each other's cases almost as well as our own. This became more difficult when the work of the Centre expanded and staff and student numbers increased. Anna Freud now requested that therapists should write weekly reports on each treatment case—a practice which also has continued to the present day. This enabled her, and anyone else interested, to keep herself closely informed of the progress of each case treated in the Clinic even though the Centre's case load soon increased to 40 or 50 cases in analysis at any one time. For some 25 years she received a thick folder of weekly reports every Friday for her week-end reading. She kept this material readily in her mind and therapists often had the experience of hearing her express a thought or comment about the child they were treating when they met Anna Freud in passing. Sometimes these comments revealed no more than an expression of shared interest or reassuring support, but one such instance had a lasting effect on me and remains vividly in my mind.

At the time I treated a severely disturbed 10-year-old boy, whose behaviour often caused general upheaval in the Clinic, and was therefore often discussed. He was one of a group of children, taken on as research cases, and was brought to his daily session by ambulance from a psychiatric in-patient unit. [See Thomas 1966.] The core of his pathology manifested in his severely impaired object relationships and affect disorder. (For example, he talked to everyone about "his therapist" by name but could only recognize me when I entered the waiting room and not in any other place of the Clinic.) This and his excessive anxiety about any kind of change became the initial focus of the treatment. Later oral features began to dominate the transference and fantasy material and his anxiety focused on running out of supplies, starving and being empty and depleted. He became excessively demanding and dissatisfied both in and outside the session and also began to steal and hoard food, especially candy. In the session he battered me with demands for sweets and often brought his own supplies and greedily stuffed himself while worrying all the time that supplies will run out. All sorts of attempts were made to interpret this material.

We knew from his history that he had been exposed to a sudden weaning experience at 4 months, when his mother lost her milk quite suddenly, following a physical abuse by her husband. This was followed by prolonged feeding difficulties and a total refusal to eat solid food until he was two years old. There was also a reported second trauma at 4 and one half when his mother left him for two weeks in the care of grandparents, while giving birth to a sibling, and he nearly starved to death.

When he also began to blame his mother for his current and past distress and misery, I attempted to link his current anxiety of running out of supplies to his past childhood experiences. I had considered this "reconstruction" for quite some time and felt quite satisfied with myself for making this interpretative link, perhaps because I had temporarily diverted the effects of being battered by his unremitting demands to his mother. A few days later I had a brief encounter with Anna Freud on the stairs of the Clinic. She expressed special interest in my patient's treatment material and then asked with a serious questioning expression "*Do you really think that telling him about his traumatic weaning is going to make him less demanding?*"

Of course it did not. Even the following day he came to his session saying "I know my mother did not give me enough milk when I was a baby but could I have a biscuit now because I am starving." However, Anna Freud's question occupied me for days and I began to think hard about the purpose and function of reconstructing the patient's past which some years later led me to write a paper on the subject. [See Kennedy 1971.] While Anna Freud encouraged autonomy, she was an indefatigable source of inspiration. The fact that one knew that she read all weekly reports did not undermine one's clinical self-confidence, but probably spurned one on to attain greater expertise. For Anna Freud following all those treatment cases meant gaining access to a far greater number of cases than any individual psychoanalyst can ever treat in his or her own lifetime. [Kennedy continued this practice after Anna Freud's death.]

Over the years nearly 800 cases of children and adolescents have received psychoanalytic treatment at the Centre and a greater number still have been seen for assessment. The Centre was established as a charity so that these services can be provided for any child in need of them, irrespective of their parents' ability to pay for the analysis. Under Anna Freud's leadership study groups were established for the refinement of clinical and theoretical concepts, and, for example, to investigate the implications of blindness, deafness and chronic illness on early development.

Her interest in applied psychoanalysis found fresh expression in the establishment of the Centre's Educational Unit consisting of a Well Baby Clinic, a Mother-Toddler Group and a Nursery School. These did not only provide preventative care but also gave staff and students and Anna Freud herself the opportunity for observation (Kennedy, 1993, pp. 4–6).

The preceding report gives the reader a glimpse into both the War Nurseries and the later training course but also tells a story of the powerful influence Anna Freud came to have in Kennedy's professional life. Less known is the impact Kennedy had on Anna Freud's work. In a collection of tributes paid to Sara Rosenfeld, another student and close friend of Kennedy's in the War Nurseries, upon Rosenfeld's death in 1973, Anna Freud made the following statement: "It is a fact that our Training Course might never have been started if there had not been, among others, two girls, Sara and Hansi, who had proved their worth in the Hampstead War Nurseries to an extent to make it quite impossible for us not to offer them further training and a further career. Our first efforts at training were built up around them and, I suppose, we learned as much from teaching them as they learned from being taught by us" (A. Freud, 1973, p. 1). Kennedy remained a close colleague of Anna Freud until Miss Freud's death in 1982.

Kennedy was the Co-Director of the Centre with Anna Freud from 1978. When Miss Freud died, the name of the Hampstead Clinic changed to the Anna Freud Centre, and Clifford Yorke, who was also the Medical Director, became Kennedy's Co-Director. They remained in this position for the next five years until George Moran took over this post in 1987. Kennedy then became the Centre's Principal Child Therapist. Throughout her career Kennedy was highly sought after as an analyst, a supervisor and a teacher. She was an editorial advisor for *The Bulletin of the Hampstead Clinic*, later *The Bulletin of the Anna Freud Centre*, from its inception in 1978 until she retired in 1993, and on the editorial board of the *Psychoanalytic Study of the Child* from 1984 through 2002. She co-authored, along with Joseph Sandler and Robert Tyson, the now classic book on analytic technique *The Technique of Child Psychoanalysis: Discussions with Anna Freud* (1980). The long list of presentations found in Kennedy's bibliography serve as testament to her worldwide reputation as a valued speaker and teacher. In 1984 the Association for Child Psychoanalysis, where she was one of the original members, honored her with the Marianne Kris Award. At her retirement on 31st August 1993, Kennedy became Honorary Principal Child Therapist at the Centre until her death on 30th October 2003 at the age of 80.

PART ONE

MEMORY

Introduction

Kennedy's first publication "Cover memories in formation" (1950) grew out of her experience as a caregiver in the Hampstead War Nurseries. There she collected extensive documentation on the development of memories in a child Bridget who was in her primary care from her entry to the Nursery at age nine months until her return to her family just before her fifth birthday. Kennedy then followed Bridget's development through home visits from age six to seven and one-half years. The longitudinal nature of the relationship allowed Kennedy to observe the mechanisms by which Bridget's memories were altered over time. She provided examples of cover memories in formation via changes in content, affect, and displacement.

The developmental fate of memory continued to be of interest to Kennedy. The second paper in this section, "Problems in reconstruction in child analysis" (1971), focused on the technical aspects of reconstruction. She took this pathway from Freud's notion that the work of analysis is a search for a complete picture of the patient's forgotten years. Reconstruction was thought by Freud to facilitate the recovery of forgotten memories. In contrast Kennedy believed that reconstruction in child psychoanalysis and the recovery of childhood memories were not so closely linked. Her previous work on cover memories encouraged the view that childhood experience could not be remembered in its original form. Her understanding of the impact of ongoing development on the content and structure of memory led Kennedy to highlight the analyst's focus on patterns of experience, rather than on the attempt to uncover specific veridical memories. The very process of remembering was said to create a reorganization of memory, and Kennedy added the idea that the analyst's reconstructive interpretation is part of that reorganization. This paper anticipated Kennedy's further work on the concept of insight in psychoanalysis.

In her paper "The 'baby at the breast' experience: Memory or fantasy? Some further thoughts on reconstruction" (1984), Kennedy considered what had been learned to date from developmental research and applied it to the psychoanalytic understanding of children. She used extensive observational material of a child from infancy to four years of age, looking at memory and experience. In the preverbal child she suggested that experience is not formed into memory structures with content and fantasies attached. Rather, she thought that developmental tendencies were created from experience, taking the form of somatic memories, modes of functioning, and attitudes. Over time such memories are absorbed into the new memory structures of the verbal child. As suggested in her previous paper on reconstruction, with further development these memories are reorganized and restructured in different contexts.

Kennedy used her knowledge of memory to distinguish it from fantasy in a paper written with Moran, Wiseberg, and Yorke and given at the 1983 International Scientific Colloquium on the Role of Fantasy in the Adaptive Process ("Both sides of the barrier: Some reflections on childhood fantasy", 1985). Here they described the nature and function of fantasy and its alteration with the onset of the repression barrier. Like memory, fantasy also alters with the developmental process.

CHAPTER ONE

Cover Memories in Formation

Hanna Engl Kennedy 1950

In the following pages I would like to discuss some early childhood memories, as they were told to me by a child at the beginning of the latency period. The opportunity for this study was rather unique as Bridget was under my care from the age of nine months, when she was admitted to the Hampstead Nurseries. She returned home shortly before her fifth birthday. I was thus responsible for most of her early upbringing, could make first-hand observations on her development, and as her "substitute-family-mother," was an important early love object.

The development of this child is interesting for various reasons, but in this paper I want to concern myself chiefly with her present memories of her experiences at the nursery, as they seem to me of interest for the study of the formation of cover memories.

Early development

Bridget is an attractive, vivacious, dark-haired girl of mixed parentage, an Indian father and an Irish mother. She was born in July, 1940, and is the second youngest of five children, of whom two boys and two girls are living at home now. She came from and returned to an extremely good and harmonious working-class home, which had to be broken up during the War because of bombing and the parents' War work. There is no financial stress or material need in the family, but living conditions are crammed. Her mother especially is an emotionally warm woman, demonstrative and outspoken in her affection for the family. Most of this affection was concentrated on Bridget during the early months of the War, as the only child living at home at that time. She is said to have been a happy, contented and very good baby, normal, if not advanced in her physical development. She was never breast-fed, always a good eater, eager for her food and at three months she took to a mixed diet without difficulty. It appears that her first object relationship was an excellent one, and satisfactory for both mother and child. Sudden separation from her mother at the age of nine months was followed three months later by the birth of a baby boy. This made visiting during the first period at the nursery almost impossible for the mother, and undoubtedly increased the traumatic effect of the separation.

She was unhappy and could not settle down for several weeks, and soon afterwards began to show many problems concerning her daily handling and upbringing, which manifested themselves in various forms in the different phases of development, but persisted throughout her stay with us. These difficulties showed themselves first in the feeding situation where her intense greed and inability to stand even a minimum of waiting periods, often made eating impossible. Temper tantrums became a usual occurrence at meal-times, and her complete refusal to be comforted in the real despair that followed, was typical. Her greed greatly exceeded her appetite and our gradual, persistent attempts at helping her to gain control were doomed to failure until she was nearly three. She then became rather faddy with her food and concentrated her greed on puddings, sweets and chocolates.

Parallel to this craving for food was her direct craving for love and affection. With the exception of the first few months Bridget's parents visited regularly once a week. Later when she was older and the air raids less frequent, she occasionally spent a day, a weekend or even a few days' holidays at home. She had a good relationship throughout to both parents, showing preference for her mother at first, and for her father during the oedipal phase. She showed no sign of attachment to any member of the staff until eighteen months old, and disliked the handling involved in the routine physical care. Later she formed a strong relationship to me, which for various reasons proved exceptionally difficult to use for her character development, and instinct modification. In all respects Bridget was exceedingly passionate and demanding, and determined to gain satisfaction for her insatiable craving for love. She continually wanted to be fondled and reassured, and took every attempt at restriction as an indication of complete loss of love. She was very possessive and unable to separate from her love objects, especially jealous of all rivals (brothers and sisters as well as other nursery children), and quite unable to get any satisfaction and contentment from these relationships. She was clinging and exaggeratedly friendly to visitors and new workers, always wanted their exclusive attention. From about three years onwards she showed particular interest in male visitors, but nursery life provided little opportunity to show clear signs of oedipal wishes. It is evident that Bridget suffered greatly from her inability to get satisfaction through her inability to bear frustration.

Perhaps the most serious difficulties in her upbringing were encountered in her training for cleanliness. Lenient training was started at home with occasional successes, and continued in the nursery on much the same lines until she was fourteen months old. The following four or five months she refused the pot completely, and every attempt caused a temper tantrum. After a few weeks interruption, training was started anew, and she would then remain on the pot for a few minutes if sufficiently entertained, only to get up just in time to wet the floor or her knickers. She gained bowel control at two and a half years, but took considerably longer to achieve control of the bladder. In fact, her habit training was an almost classical example of our theoretical knowledge concerning the various stages of superego formation which are necessary before success is permanent. Some of these examples have been published elsewhere. Bridget reacted to every slight emotional upset with incontinence, and was not reliably dry during the daytime before the age of four and a half. She suffered from nocturnal enuresis until several months after her return home.

There were similar though not such severe problems regarding her aggression. Between thirteen and eighteen months she had several temper tantrums daily, and for several years occasionally reverted to such outbursts. At about the same time she became very aggressive toward other children, which of course is normal at that age, but again she was quite unable to check her impulses. She used biting as her main form of aggression. At times she was stubborn and very easily offended.

Bridget's exhibitionism was as pronounced as all her other manifestations of instinctive urges. She proudly showed off her body when undressed and wanted to be admired both by the staff and the other children, especially the boys. She was easily excitable at such times and used to invite other children to sexual games. She was very particular about her clothes, always wanted new and clean things, and usually found fault with the garments she was expected to wear. Occasionally she tried to draw attention to herself by good behavior or some achievement, but more frequently chose to show off with provocative and disruptive attitudes in the group.

She went through a very marked and prolonged phase of openly showing her penis envy. First she denied being a girl, then pretended ignorance in regard to sex differences, and referred to all boys as "she." Next followed a period where she imitated boys: e.g., by urinating in a standing position, by trying to join their games or herself initiating boyish activities. At about the same time she developed acute fear of dogs which, for a short time, disturbed her sleep. For many months she complained of pains or hurts which were either purely imaginary or exaggerations of minor ailments.

It was most interesting to observe the fate of her strong exhibitionistic tendencies when they clashed with the manifestations of her penis envy. She ceased to exhibit her body, often did not want to undress, or only do so in seclusion, and was tearful and unhappy in every situation that aroused in her a feeling of inferiority. She also became unable to perform tasks which required physical strength or skill, the very same activities that she formerly used for showing off. Her exhibitionism thus was not modified but temporarily overshadowed by instinctive urges in the service of her penis envy.

It is noteworthy that there was neither noticeable thumbsucking nor masturbation. This is probably due to the fact that she had established a very early and intense object relationship to her mother, and therefore before entering the nursery had reached a stage of development where gratification is expected from the love object and can no longer be attained by autoerotic activities. We can assume that the mother's loud and demonstrative affection had enabled her to reach this phase earlier than we commonly find in children, and that part of her great unhappiness and lack of satisfaction at the nursery was due to her inability to gain pleasure autoerotically.

Later development

I was able to follow up Bridget's development during the last two and a half years since she returned home. She has developed into a very normal, well-adjusted child in the latency period. She appears secure and satisfied and evidently has been able to deal with her instinctive urges effectively. Her relationships to the family are excellent, she has strongly identified with her mother and elder sister and takes delight in typically feminine activities. She is protective and tolerant towards her younger brother, but chooses the company of girls in preference to boys who, she thinks, are too rough. Her social contacts with children and adults are very good, she is popular and not at all shy, yet does not cling to strangers as she did formerly. She still enjoys loud, frank signs of affection, cuddling, kissing and fondling, and is herself demonstrative in her love but her mother seems to satisfy her completely in this respect. She is no longer demanding, receives presents with pleasure but is very ready to share, and her former possessiveness has been successfully turned into generosity. There is evidence of other reaction formations and she shows definite signs of pity and shame. She is a good eater, neither faddy nor greedy about her food. She takes keen interest in school and is said to be a good scholar. Her enuresis has cleared up, she has no special fears and creates no difficulties in management.

Memories

Since her return home in June 1945, I have visited the family on many occasions; the first time after one year and subsequently at two or three monthly intervals. It was possible to arrange to see Bridget, both in her own home with the family, and alone on various outings and walks. It is from these visits that the following material has been collected.

To begin with there was an almost complete amnesia for all that happened before her return home. When asked about her memories she would recite one or the other incident she had been told by her mother, or else make vague statements like "we had lots of toys there" etc. From the beginning, however, she felt some kind of familiarity with the names and occurrences I discussed, an indistinct form of recollection without being able to recall. This perhaps was brought out clearest in her first reactions to me, when we met after one year's separation. She had been looking forward with considerable excitement and expectancy to my announced visit, and then received me with a completely estranged stare and the words: "You have changed—your face has changed." Later on a walk, she held my hand most of the time, gazed at me intently, and gradually brought a few memories chiefly regarding my clothes. She made correct statements about articles of clothing which she had seen before and those that were "different."

On this first visit when she was still unable to verbalize her memories, she acted them out. On our walk in the neighborhood of her home she had a continual urge to urinate. At this time, bladder control was no longer a problem to her, and there has never been a recurrence of a similar situation since. It is likely that some children might never go beyond this stage of acting out their early childhood memories in this manner, at this age.

Bridget, I think, found links to her early experiences again through her relationship to me. These memories are preconscious and come up by very definite associations, many interestingly enough through familiarity of locality.

Looking at the material as a whole, it is easy to distinguish between incidents she only knows from reports but does not actually remember herself; a few isolated facts (for instance a swing in the garden), and such memories which appear clear and vivid at the time of remembering and which have undergone some definite distortion. The first group are hearsay memories which are common in both children and adults, the second group may or may not contain important early material. For instance the memory of the swing may represent the pleasure she experienced in this activity, but we have no possibility of further investigation. It is the last-mentioned group which most specifically deserves the name of potential cover memories.

These memories have a few common characteristics. They strike one as insignificant, isolated pieces, outstandingly clear and colorful in intensity. Bridget is invariably the central figure in them, and I am almost always the object. They are distorted in different ways and varying degrees, most of them make use of the specific mechanism of condensation (e.g. frequently repeated everyday occurrences are remembered as single incidents). They have thus most of the special characteristics of screen memories that Freud described in his early paper on "Screen Memories" (2). In this paper he also first suggested a grouping of screen memories based on the temporal relation between the screen memory and the memory it screens. He found that there were three possibilities: 1) Retroactive or regressive (*rückläufige*) cover memories, where the content of the screen memory belonged to the first years of childhood, while the thoughts represented by it belonged to a later period in life; 2) Encroaching or interposing (vorgreifende) cover memories, where the content of the screened memory lies chronologically beyond the screen memory; and 3) Contemporaneous or contiguous (gleichzeitige) cover memories, where the connection of the screened and the screen memory is not only through content but also through contiguity of time.

While it is possible to group all adult cover memories in this manner it will be self-evident by the nature of the material that this cannot be done in our investigation.

We can assume that the formation of regressive cover memories belongs to a later period in life, and that probably most of our material will belong in the third group, the contemporaneous or contiguous. In order to prove this, however, we would have to obtain the associations necessary to analyze each memory fully. We know that this cannot be done, but, I think, the detailed knowledge of the early development that I have tried to outline briefly above, should enable us to understand much of the now unconscious content of the memories. They are, as yet, much nearer the surface and distortions much less elaborate and complicated than in the case of an adult. We also no longer need proof of accepted psychoanalytic findings, and our interest therefore will be directed more to the mechanisms used in the formation of cover memories than their actual content.

On closer examination it became clear that Bridget's memories can be grouped into three categories according to the modification they have undergone.

1. Memories with minor changes in content and reversal in affect due to hallucinatory wish fulfillment

Example 1: On a walk in the neighborhood of the nursery, at the other end of London from her home, she suddenly remembered that she had been here before and remarked, "A lady once talked to us here and gave us sweets." Our children had won the heart of a few elderly people who used to meet them frequently on their walks and sometimes gave them sweets.

Example 2: On another walk she recognized a baker's shop and remembered, "Once you brought me here on a walk and bought me a bun." Many different members of the staff had taken the bigger children to this and other shops and had bought them buns on their walk.

Example 3: On one of my recent visits she practically greeted me with the announcement: "I told my big brother yesterday that in the nursery you always used to have tea in the kitchen, and that you sometimes took me along and gave me a cup of tea and cake." This again was a frequent occurrence but not invariably connected with me. Usually this privilege for Bridget ended up in a scene because she could not have all the available food for herself.

Example 4: The first memory that Bridget ever told me was given as proof that she recognized me, and was, "Once you took me to a restaurant and bought me ice cream and lots of cakes." On a few special occasions during her stay at the nursery, I had taken her out for tea. This particular memory, however, was so clear and vivid that I am almost certain it referred to the farewell outing, the day before she returned home.

I have tried to emphasize in my description of Bridget's early development that this child has had an unusually unhappy and frustrating early childhood, that her craving for love and open affection could not be satisfied by any other person than her mother from whom she was separated at a time when the need for her was greatest. I have also tried to describe all the manifestations of this intense need for love, her demands for special and preferential treatment and material tokens, especially food. All these memories point to original experiences where she should have gained satisfaction, but where the intensity of her greed made this impossible. It now appears as a pleasant memory and entails a strong element of personal gratitude to me, which becomes even more apparent in the tone of voice and manner of talking than the actual memory.

The manifest content of the memory thus has certain characteristics in common with fantasies and dreams, an element of hallucinatory wish-fulfillment. This mechanism might readily serve as an explanation for the myth of happy childhood.

The first example given above is perhaps most clearly a potential screen memory, the incident is insignificant and isolated from any emotionally charged content, and the object removed from the original love object (i.e., a strange lady). Yet it is essentially similar in content to the second memory described, which is already nearer to the true material contained. The manifest content in all the memories in this group is centered around being given food, and thus clearly represents her oral greed which I have discussed before. We know that underneath this craving for food was her craving for love which was so very pronounced in Bridget. The first two memories date back to a time of her later childhood when she had already joined the nursery-school group, which we must recognize as a pointer. They also clearly contain a strong desire or wish which she had wanted me to satisfy, and we may assume, on the basis of our theoretical knowledge and our specific observations on this child, that these memories represent her former strong penis envy. The third and fourth example quoted point really in the same direction but are more ambiguous. Being allowed to have tea with the staff was a special privilege which was a sign of being loved, for Bridget. It invariably aroused a conflict in her because she expected her love object to gratify her instinctive desires. These of course were manifold and differed in accordance with the relevant phases of development. Thus it may represent on one level the frustrating experiences in general which she encountered with all her instinctive urges, or it may represent the more specific frustration she met with regard to her wish to be a boy. Similarly, I think, that the memory of her last outing with me, before her return home, might easily contain the whole of her early relationship to me, in a nutshell as it were, and distorted as "in all these years you gave me all I wanted, and lots of it" (i.e., lots of cake). It is obvious that on a deeper layer it may again represent her penis envy.

2. Memories with minor changes in content and reversal in affect due to ego development

I have tried to point out that the process of socialization was particularly slow in Bridget. Her instinctive urges evidently could not be controlled by the ego, and the first signs of instinct modification were interrupted by long phases where the instinct broke through in its original form. I have described that since her return home, which roughly coincided with the beginning of the latency period, she shows satisfactory reaction formations and sublimations. Her former greed, possessiveness, jealousy and envy have now become enjoyment in sharing and giving away her belongings.

The memories that I propose to put in this group show very definitely a distortion of the original affect in the light of her newly acquired modification of instinct. It is, I think, the most common mechanism of distortion that we will find in latency-period children.

Example 5: Bridget's mother arranged a birthday party for her seventh birthday. She was particularly happy on this day and a perfect hostess to her guests. She urged them to eat, allowed them to play with her new presents, in short she saw to it that everyone should have a good time. On that day she told me the following memory: "Once I had a birthday in Netherhall and my mummy came with a big cake and gave a slice to every child." She indicated that she had greatly enjoyed sharing her cake at that time, and that it had been a very pleasurable experience. Again the facts are correct, every year on her birthday her mother brought a cake to share out amongst children and staff. Bridget never verbalized a complaint, but her resentment for not being given the whole cake for herself was always very open in her behavior and repeated itself every year.

Example 6: Another time when I gave her some sweets she suddenly remembered, "Once my mummy came and brought me sweets and gave one sweet to a little girl who was crying." Bridget's mother always was very sympathetic with children who had no Sunday visitors and often gave them sweets. As a young toddler an incident like this caused an outburst of anger against the mother. Later there were instances where she first refused to share her sweets, but the pressure of mother's demand made her give in unwillingly in the end. She of course often consented to share in her mother's presence but then made return claims on the children at a later time.

In both these examples the present affect in situations of this kind has been imposed on experiences of the past. This is not a general mechanism for all her early experiences.

3. Memories with displacement of affect to a different content

Example 7: On one of our walks, again in the neighborhood of the former nursery, we came to a footpath which has railings in the middle. Bridget remembered that on top of the hill was the school that a few of our children had attended, and then told the following story: "You took me here sometimes to fetch the school children home. Once we chased each other under the railings, you told me to stop but I went on and on, and you got angry." Our nursery children knew that the school teacher used to punish her pupils for climbing these railings, but our staff did not object strongly to such harmless pleasures as chasing around the railings.

Example 8: Soon after, she remarked that she was too small then to go to school but as far as she remembered they went to a kind of school (nursery school) and there was a piano. "Once I kept on playing the piano and you told me to stop, but I continued and you got very angry with me." There really was a piano in our nursery school and the children were not supposed to play it. The rule however was never rigidly enforced.

It will hardly be necessary to expand here on the methods in upbringing used in the Hampstead Nurseries. We did not believe in giving the child "complete freedom" in the sense of "modern" education. There were rules and regulations intended to maintain the order and routine so necessary for the children's welfare, and such restrictions as would help them to strengthen their ego and build up their personality. We did not enforce these rules but made gradual, persistent demands, and expected a slow progress rather than complete obedience.

This, I think, we must bear in mind when investigating the last-mentioned memories. The two incidents would not have roused real anger in any member of the staff, and we can immediately recognize the displacement. The type of behavior it describes was not unusual for Bridget, it was one of her ways of showing off and getting attention, and has thus remained undistorted. In my account of Bridget's early development I have stressed the difficulties we encountered with her instinct modification. There was an all-out battle with every single instinctive urge, and a particularly strong and prolonged one over her training in cleanliness. It is this that I believe to be the screened memory. We do not know of any masturbation conflict in this child, but otherwise would probably assume that such a conflict is contained in these memories. They do represent the original objects with their correctly attributed affects, the frustrating adult, and the child who experiences pleasure as well as guilt feelings, for not conforming to the demands.

Conclusions

We will be in agreement that these memories are not formed cover memories but cover memories in formation. We have found that, although they have certain characteristics in common with the screen memories of adults, they cannot be grouped in the same manner. The material presented in this paper was divided into three categories according to the chief mechanism of distortion. We cannot conclude that these are the only or the most common mechanisms used in the formation of cover memories, nor can we say with certainty that they are specific for this individual child or her early experiences. We will expect further distortion and modification in the manifest content, but we cannot predict any particular development. We do not know if the three mechanisms are different stages in the same process of distortion, or if certain early experiences show definite tendencies to be distorted more readily by means of any one of the mechanisms described. It is more likely, however, that the mechanisms used in the formation of cover memories depend on the personality of the individual. We generally expect to find definite defense mechanisms suitable to certain types of personalities, in accordance with their constitutional make-up and their acquired character.

We know that childhood memories do not give a true picture of early experiences as they have actually occurred. They are built up at a later time, when, for one reason or another, an early experience is reactivated. It is likely that the renewed contact with me revived these memories in Bridget, and it is probable that they were built up partly on the occasion of the visit, and partly in the interval between visits.

The particular situation in which this material was collected seems very favorable, her emotions now are far removed from me, and I represent for her a part of the past with which I bring her in contact on every visit. In cases where the relationship to the mother has been continuous and uninterrupted, it will be more difficult to get this type of memory verbalized.

References

Freud, A. & Burlingham, D. (1944). *Infants Without Families: The Case For and Against Residential Nurseries*. London: Allen & Unwin Ltd. New York: Int. Univ. Press.

Freud, S. (1899). Screen memories. *Collected Papers V*.

CHAPTER TWO

Problems in Reconstruction in Child Analysis*

Hanna Kennedy 1971

In his paper "Constructions in Analysis" (1937), interestingly enough published in the same year as "Analysis Terminable and Interminable," Freud describes the work of analysis as a search for a "trustworthy and in all essential respects complete picture of the patient's forgotten years." The work of analysis consists of "two quite different portions" and "involves two people, to each of whom a distinct task is assigned . . . the person who is being analysed has to be induced to remember something that has been experienced by him and repressed; and the dynamic determinants of the process are so interesting that the other portion of the work, the task performed by the analyst, has been pushed into the background . . . His task is to make out what has been forgotten from the traces which it has left behind or, more correctly, to construct it. The time and manner in which he conveys his constructions to the person who is being analysed . . . constitute the link between the two portions of the work of analysis, between his own part and that of the patient" (p. 258f.).

Thus Freud used the term "construction" or "reconstruction" in two senses, namely, *reconstruction as a process in the mind of the analyst, and reconstruction as a type of verbal intervention.* He also introduced the notion that the analyst's reconstructions of aspects of the patient's forgotten past facilitate the recovery of childhood memories. Obviously, this topic is a wide and complicated one, encompassing, in addition to many other aspects, the cognitive and technical facets of Freud's use of the term as well as the processes involved in the recovery of childhood memories.

The main focus of this paper will be on the technical aspects of reconstruction. I intend to emphasize the point that the technique of *reconstruction in child analysis and the recovery of memories in the course of psychoanalytic treatment*, although intimately related, are not as close as might be assumed.

We know that some previously forgotten memories arise spontaneously during the work of analysis, some emerge following transference interpretation of what is currently going on in the analytic situation. Indeed, we expect, ideally, that the interpretation of a transference resistance, for example, will be followed by a freeing of material, much of which might include or otherwise relate to past memories. Conversely, some reconstructions are not followed by the recovery of confirmatory memories, but they *do* have an effect on the course of the analysis, as is evident in the material brought subsequently by the patient. It is the problems involved in phenomena such as these, especially as they manifest themselves in child analysis, which I intend to discuss and clarify.

Analysts have generally attributed great significance to the actual recall of forgotten or repressed memories, and even used "recall" as an index of progress in the evaluation of therapeutic results. These notions are deeply rooted in the history of psychoanalytic theory and practice, and can be traced back to the first phase of Freud's thinking when he worked with the traumatogenic theory of hysteria (1893–1895). These ideas still influence our thinking, even though changes in psychoanalysis have occurred with the introduction of the structural theory, advances in ego psychology, and the increasing role played by studies of child development. With these advances in mind, I shall question the tradition-bound importance attached to recall.

Even if we no longer see the recovery of childhood memories as a *sine qua non* of successful treatment, the recovery of memories still has a special significance for both patient and analyst, and we need to re-examine the reasons for this.

It must be obvious to all of us that we are constantly searching for supporting evidence for our reconstructions, in the hope of refining both theory and technique. This too has its historical roots because it was from reconstructions in the analysis of adults that Freud arrived at his discoveries of infantile sexuality and the important part played by childhood development in the neurotic disorders of later life. These reconstructions could later be corroborated and refined through psychoanalytic childhood observation and child analysis, for example, in the Little Hans case.

It is also obvious that in analytic work with our patients, we feel gratified when our reconstructions appear to be validated by the recovery of childhood memories, but as we know this does not always occur.

It seems to me that our search for confirmatory evidence is based upon our equating the effectiveness of our interventions, especially in the realm of reconstruction, with an assumption that what is reconstructed is an exact reflection of what actually occurred. However, there appear to be grounds for questioning this in the light of our knowledge that childhood experience cannot be recovered in the exact original form. This point has been emphasized by Ernst Kris in his illuminating paper on "The Recovery of Childhood Memories in Psychoanalysis" (1956), on which I shall draw substantially. Kris pointed out that we are misled in believing that we are, except in rare circumstances, able to find "the 'events' of the afternoon on the staircase when the seduction happened" (p. 73). He stressed that in analysis we are dealing with a whole period in which a seduction may have played a role *and that the distortions of later developmental conflicts* became superimposed on the original situation.

Whereas reconstructions from the analysis of adults has led to an understanding of the role of "screen" or "cover" memories, direct work with children has focused on the multiplicity of the pathogenic happenings, and the complex distortions and ramifications that occur during development. Anna Freud (1951) pointed out that the analyst's search for *the* traumatic event or experience has led him to underestimate the extent of the "telescopic" nature of memory until he was reminded of it by the results of direct childhood observation. "One traumatic prohibition or punishment, remembered or reconstructed, becomes the representative of hundreds of frustrations which had been imposed on the child; one longer separation from the mother takes over the combined effect of innumerable times when the infant has been left alone in his cot, his room, at bedtime etc." (p. 27).

There is a further complicating aspect with regard to memories, namely, that later events may add special significance to earlier experiences, which may then be recalled as *if* they themselves had been traumatic or of particular psychopathological significance.

Much has been learned about these processes by comparing data obtained from children who were first observed in longitudinal studies and later in analysis. Such studies have opened up a variety of different areas of research. Heinicke (1970) has recently described how this approach can be utilized in the attempt to devise a methodology to validate psychoanalytic reconstruction in child analysis.

I believe that it is important to keep in mind the distinction between what one might call the genetic-reconstructive approach in psychoanalysis and the developmental approach. These have been implicitly equated by child analysts for many years, but we need to consider whether in fact the two are identical. The genetic-reconstructive approach is concerned with the analyst's reconstruction of the patient's past, on the basis of the analytic material brought by the patient. The developmental approach, on the other hand, is much more concerned with internal and external influences in actual ongoing childhood development, especially those leading to a failure to make the crucial transition from one developmental phase to another. We would all like to believe that what we reconstruct in the work of child analysis is identical with the actual developmental processes which have taken place, but Ernst Kris offers much evidence, as does our own clinical experience at Hampstead, that this is not so. We must also keep in mind that in analysis we are dealing with the world as the child sees it—that is, not only the internal world of the child's drives and fantasies, but his own unique perception of the external world. The case reported by Mary Bergen (1958), to take just one example, illustrates this point with particular clarity.

Thus the developmental approach may lean more heavily on child observation and external sources for evidence of what went on, for example, in the child-parent relationship, whereas the genetic-reconstructive approach leans heavily on what the child brings to the analysis. The reconstructions based on what is brought by the child at different points in his analysis may therefore differ from what a psychoanalytic observer may have seen at a specific point in development. The two approaches to the child are not contradictory; rather, I believe they are different but complementary standpoints from which to view the child. It will be evident that in child analysis we constantly move from the developmental approach to the genetic-reconstructive and from the genetic-reconstructive to the developmental, but the assumption that the two points of view are the same may contribute to unclarity in our thinking.

Not all of our child patients have been observed longitudinally; but we usually obtain a detailed developmental history from the parents, the school, the pediatrician, and other sources, and these fragments of information undoubtedly influence our view of the material. In addition, throughout the course of the child's treatment, we frequently obtain external information about both his past and his present. A crucial question is the extent to which we permit such information, often biased, to prompt the formulation of a reconstructive interpretation, without it always being adequately substantiated by the analytic material brought by the child. While we may at times have to rely on such information in child analysis, we may occasionally focus too much on the genetic-reconstructive approach in our thinking. This is particularly evident when we make the assumption that what the child brings or enacts in the present is an exact repetition of what occurred or was experienced in the past. This may lead us at times into analyzing what the child is experiencing predominantly in terms of his defenses, and his projections of wishes, fantasies, and conflicts, without acknowledging sufficiently that, in certain cases, what the child brings is shaped by the fact that he lived in a "crazy world" which has become internalized.

With regard to the function of memories in the course of development, we have the notion of, so to speak, a "two-way traffic"; i.e., early experiences may color and distort later ones, just as later events sometimes add special *significance* to *earlier experiences*. The child analyst is confronted by the additional problem of distinguishing between the developmental and the genetic-reconstructive view of the material, a distinction he must keep in mind when he considers how past experiences enter into the analytic process and what part *reconstruction* plays in it.

The developmental age at which a crucial event takes place is of great importance. Events which occur very early in life and give rise to strong affective, experiences and somatic reactions are, as we all know, of the highest significance for later development. They have a profound influence on the child's personality development by determining his modes of functioning and by coloring his attitudes and response patterns.

To take a simplified example, experiences of physical overstimulation in the first year may show up in later life in a variety of ways. We may see a child with a heightened excitability which manifests itself in all phases of libidinal development. We may recognize in such a child a tendency to search over and over again for similar exciting experiences, and these general features may or may not become secondarily involved in later psychopathology, as Anna Freud has stressed recently (1971). What we see is a complicated style of approach to the world, spelled out so beautifully by Erikson (1950), in what he calls the "modality of social life." This is determined originally, for instance, by somatic experiences, and can show itself as a characteristic in all developmental phases, even though the child may reach phase dominance in the various phases through which he passes.

It is important to keep in mind that what is created by such early experiences are not conflict situations but attitudes which may not have specific fantasy or memory content attached to them. This is often lost sight of in clinical work.

Let me give a brief clinical illustration of a 10-year-old patient who was excessively demanding, yet permanently dissatisfied and always anticipating loss. Oral features dominated the transference and fantasy material and also found expression in behavioral manifestations. We know from his history that he had been exposed to a sudden weaning experience followed by prolonged feeding difficulties which persisted in one form or another through all the developmental phases. Feeding difficulties still played an important part in his present symptomatology. The core of his pathology, however, was in his inappropriate affective responses and severely impaired object relationships, and these were the areas focused on by the analytic work and explored from the very beginning of the analysis. It is natural for the *analyst to assume that the unsatisfactory early feeding situation contributed to the disturbances in the mother-child* interactions. Having made this obvious assumption, we may have some differences of opinion with regard to specific details: some analysts will attach more importance to the sudden so-called "loss of the breast"; others, to the infant's inability to make adaptive moves and to accept whatever substitute was offered at the time. We may not agree on the significance of such developmental reactions; some will regard them merely as signs that all is not going well now; others will view these experiences as inevitably laying the ground for *later disturbances*. We may differ in our emphasis on whether the major contribution to these mutually unsatisfactory experiences comes from the mother or from the infant. But despite these differences, all of us will naturally construct some sort of mental bridge from the present pathology to these early experiences. Here a knowledge of the developmental history will certainly color our view of the child.

The questions we really have to examine are *when* and *why* we reconstruct such early experiences for the patient, and *how* they become meaningful for him. First, with regard to the timing of a reconstruction, I want to quote Ernst Kris (1956), "the analyst watches a reorganization of forces in the patient's behavior and guides this reorganization by his interpretations . . . In the course of this process the past emerges into the present, and a readiness, a 'need' for reconstructive interpretation may be noticed" (p. 58f.). These comments refer predominantly to the analysis of adults and older children and are crucial in that context. Although they also apply to child analysis, we may find that there is less "readiness and need" for reconstruction, especially with younger children.

The child patient may *follow us* or *lead us* along the path from the present to the past experiences. Even children who show little interest in their past will begin to do so when they become involved in the analysis because they are responding, step by step, to those of our interventions which lead them in this direction. Others, and these are more often the more disturbed children, lead us directly to the past via their material. But which past?

The 10-year-old borderline patient mentioned earlier came to analysis with a firmly established conviction that the roots of his current problems were to be found in his distressing childhood experiences. This enabled him covertly to blame his parents for causing his distress and misery. There were several early experiences, all on a similar theme, which we may call "childhood memories" and which were constantly reiterated.

A typical memory of this sort related to sitting behind the bars of a cot, panic-stricken and helplessly immobilized while watching a fight between his parents, who threw crockery at each other. The feelings the patient ascribed to this experience afforded the bridge from the present to the past because the patient could see that they were identical to the panic states he frequently experienced in his current life. He constantly referred to experiences in his daily life which "paralyze me with fear" or made him feel "frozen on the spot," and interpretation could serve to make the link with the past.

From the developmental history we know that violent scenes between the parents prevailed throughout his infancy and early childhood, often leading to prolonged periods during which the parents were separated. In analysis we are, of course, not concerned with whose "fault" it was. What we are concerned with is that the patient re-experienced something which he remembered from the past; and that the reconstruction, which in this case was not difficult, afforded considerable relief to the patient because it enabled him to gain a perspective on his difficulties and this he previously had not had.

While this example illustrates the bridge from the present to the past, the enactments in the transference displayed the past in the present. He re-created a situation in which his unremitting demands could never be satisfied or modified, and which inevitably had to evoke feelings of hopelessness, despair, utter isolation and emptiness. The analytic exploration and interpretation of the patient's current feeling states and defensive maneuvers, and the attempt to understand his current conflicts in terms of the early experiences he remembered, did not diminish his misery and dissatisfaction. Nor did this analytic work lessen the pressure of his demands for supplies from the analyst, but interpretations involving the patient's feeling states helped to crystallize his demands into oral cravings for unlimited and "continuously flowing" supplies of orange juice and sweets (candy).

At this point in treatment an attempt was made to reconstruct the unsatisfactory early feeding situation and the sudden weaning experience. It should be noted that in this reconstruction the therapist avoided focusing on the specific traumatic event, i.e., sudden loss of milk or breast, but attempted to catch and verbalize the affective significance and atmosphere of this whole period in his life. This is in keeping with Kris's and Anna Freud's views that experiences are molded into patterns and that the analyst deals with these patterns rather than with specific events.

Before examining the function of reconstructive interpretation in general, I wish to insert some brief comments on the special problems posed by so-called primary repression in relation to the reconstruction of *preverbal* experiences. Discussions of experiences of the preverbal stage always present particular problems because, as Hartmann (1958) has pointed out, the structure of the mental apparatus and the laws governing it are less familiar to us and we do not have enough experiential checks available for verification.

We assume that a child exposed to a traumatic experience will at a later stage in development have formed a memory structure with ideational and affective content, which can (at least theoretically) become "recoverable" as a memory of an experience. According to our classical theory, the recovery of such early forgotten memories mobilizes affects and creates the possibility of assimilating the experience in a different way. The "traumatic" experience which has hitherto found expression in a pathological reaction can now find new solutions. But can similar alterations be achieved with regard to preverbal experiences?

There are analysts (for example, Winnicott, M. Little) who claim to have devised techniques which reach the individual's earliest experiences. It is their belief that by encouraging regressive transference relationships they enable their patients to relive early affective experiences which can then be "corrected." They argue that the regression not only leads to a repetition of the past, but also affords the opportunity to relive the past in a more satisfactory way.

Anna Freud has often pointed out, in discussions of this kind, that classical psychoanalytic technique was devised not to *undo* experiences but to help the individual understand and deal with them internally. At Hampstead we maintain that we cannot change the problems, we can only change the solutions of the problem.

When we consider the aftereffects of an experience which the child had, or is having (and this applies to preverbal experiences as well), we must also take into account the effects that interpretations have on the mental apparatus of the child in the present, because interpretations which reconstruct the past are, after all, also new experiences.

While theoretically every subjective experience (in the sense of the German *Erlebnis*) leaves a memory trace which is in some way recoverable, one might with equal justification say that nothing is recoverable in its original form. The trace itself is, of course, never recoverable. What can be recovered is another experience structured by that memory trace. The recovery of a memory is in a sense like a perception, so that remembering something from the past is like *perceiving it anew*, in exactly the same way as an external perception of the same sort of event is perceived anew by the child when he is older. *Even ordinary remembering is thus a reconstruction of the past rather than a simple reproduction of the past.* In the same way as every percept is a construction, every memory is intrinsically a reconstruction—an achievement of the mental apparatus of the child. This is also in line with the views of Ernst Kris.

It follows from this that in the process of remembering in any form, the material of past experience is reorganized in a new way, albeit slightly. The new memory structures that are created will reflect the maturational and developmental level of the child's mental apparatus. Interpretations and reconstructions by the analyst inevitably enter into this reorganization as well, so that the child, by establishing causal relations in connection with the memory, *changes the content* and *structure of the memory*. He will be seeing it in a new way. This may be different from cases of traumatic war neuroses in adults, who, when they are treated by abreaction or catharsis, relive essentially the same traumatic experience. From this viewpoint we can say that reconstructions allow a drive derivative or other derivative (e.g., an omnipotent wish) to find new pathways in the form of a thought or a fantasy which acts as an organizer of experience. These new formations will in turn, through being subjected to the analytic process, lead to the emergence of less and less distorted derivatives and will facilitate unconscious content becoming conscious. But, and I want to stress this, repressed memories can never return entirely or exactly in their *original* form. Freud referred to this progressive aspect the analytic process when he said (1937, p. 260f): "The analyst finishes a piece of construction and communicates it to the subject of the analysis so that it may work upon him; he then constructs a further piece out of the fresh material pouring in upon him, deals with it in the same way and proceeds in this alternating fashion until the end."

This brings us to another conceptual problem, namely, whether "reconstructions" viewed in this way can be differentiated from other interpretations, except in a descriptive way. Freud (1937) commented that, if in accounts of analytic technique, little is said about "constructions," it is because "interpretations" and their effects are spoken of instead. He then proceeded to suggest a distinction on the basis that "interpretation" applies to something one does to single element in the material (such as an association or a parapraxis), whereas in "constructions" one lays before the patient a whole piece of his forgotten past. Hartmann (1958) makes a similar distinction between an interpretation which aims at establishing connections and "another level of cognitive interpretation [where] a great number of data ... and a considerable amount of hypothetical thinking have to be introduced in order to come to a conclusion" (p. 135). Loewenstein (1951) speaks of dynamic and genetic interpretation, as does Kris (1956), who suggests that genetic Interpretations should be depicted as a continuum ranging from archaic impulses related to preverbal and nonverbal ideations embedded in unconscious fantasies to those which establish a historical context and are based on inferences drawn from many sources in the analytic material (e.g., screen memories or recovered memories).

The distinction between interpretations and reconstructions may, as I have suggested, be useful from a descriptive point of view, but all interpretations are essentially reconstructions. Interpretations may be conceptualized as reconstructions of the present, in analogy to "constructions" or "reconstructions" of the past. Kris expresses a similar view when he says, "even the yesterday is part of the past" (p. 56). I would add that even the child's last unexpressed thought is part of the past. Even our interpretation of what is happening in the present session, however exact it may be, structures a previously unorganized experience, aspects of which have usually been unconscious.

The role of verbalization in the efficacy of interpretation and its contribution to the ego's method of adaptation have been much discussed in the psychoanalytic literature. Its importance for childhood development, especially its function in promoting secondary process thinking, has been emphasized by Anny Katan (1961).

Anna Freud (1965) has stressed the special significance of verbalization for children who enter analysis at an early age and for those who have severe delays, arrests or defects of ego development. We may focus here especially on the role that verbalization plays in organizing preverbal experiences into more comprehensible and meaningful ones. *In analysis, the putting of words to unorganized sensations, which might be part of early memories, creates new memory structures that replace the old ones. This is equally true for postverbal experiences.*

Loewald (1960) has given a beautiful description of the organizing role of the analyst's interpretations, which aptly applies to the problems I am discussing. He says:

> . . . the analyst structures and articulates . . . the material and the productions offered by the patient. If an interpretation of unconscious meanings is timely, the words by which this meaning is expressed are recognizable to the patient as expressions of what he experiences. They organize for him what was previously less organized and thus give him the "distance" from himself which enables him to understand to see, to put into words and to "handle" what was previously not visible, understandable, speakable, tangible . . . The analyst functions as a representative of a higher stage of organization and mediates this to the patient, in so far as the analyst's understanding is attuned to what is, and the way in which it is, in need of organization. [p. 24]

Enactments or references to primitive bodily sensations and experiences that appear in the analytic material of children may often indicate to the analyst that such experiences are in need of organization through reconstruction of preverbal experiences.

I have previously stated that no reconstruction corresponds exactly to an experience the child has had, but I have not yet discussed the problem implicit in this statement: whether for this reason our "incorrect" or inexact reconstructions are therapeutically less useful or effective.

A reconstruction may be inexact, but, provided it satisfies certain criteria, it will have a therapeutic effect and further the analysis. In order to examine this problem we must look at the patient's responses to the reconstructions, not so much in terms of their being immediately accepted or rejected or ignored, but in the way in which they affect the subsequent analytic material and the subsequent course of the patient's development, including the resolution of conflicts.

For example, my 10-year-old patient "used" the reconstruction of his unsatisfactory early feeding experiences in a variety of ways: as a sign of my rejection (he brought his own supplies of candy the next day); as a challenge to me that implied his mother was a bad mother; as an excuse to become even more demanding. But more important than any of these defensive responses was the one significant word he added to my reconstruction. In my attempt to get hold of his affective experiences I had linked his excessive demandingness with his feeling hungry and empty inside, to which he responded with: "You mean all deserted." This ushered in a wealth of material about the more recent past when he felt "all deserted" while waiting for his mother, always convinced that she would never return.

While he was working through this material in the transference and in current experiences outside the treatment, he periodically returned to his childhood memories of watching his parents quarreling and fighting, in a position of helpless panic. One gained the impression that these memories still carried the full impact of the "traumatic experiences" and were therefore constantly impinging on his current experience. This impression, stemming from the developmental approach, temporarily impeded the analyst's understanding of *the new significance* that now emerged in relation to this memory. As soon as his feeling of being "all deserted" by his fighting parents (and of being frightened and immobilized as a result of it) could be reconstructed, the memories decreased in importance and were subsequently only rarely referred to. The analysis entered a new phase.

What I am trying to demonstrate is that reconstructions must have an "intrapsychic fit" at any given point in the analytic work, and this can be achieved by picking up the affective elements (especially anxiety) in the material, so that the child can get a new perspective on something which previously had psychic reality him.

By drawing the child's attention to previously unconscious feelings and ideas and by establishing links between his present concerns and these feelings or ideas that may have been conscious but isolated, we give the child insight, that is enlarge his self-awareness. Thus reconstruction in child analysis functions primarily as a means of providing a conceptual framework to the child whereby he can understand his present experiences and dilemmas. Reconstruction also leads to a release of dammed-up impulses and affects and to their abreaction, but this function is relatively less important in children. This may be so because in children dammed-up impulses and affects can find expression in enactment or in some other mode that represents an adaptation the child has made to what has been defended against.

It follows from this that the interpretative work with children is much more effective when it deals with the child's current interaction with his parents, his peers, and his feelings about himself. *Although in the transference past object relationships and experiences may be relived in some form, the interpretation of the transference aims at showing the child why he tends to function in a particular manner at the moment, and not at the reconstruction of the past,* but this may be brought in for purposes of adding conviction.

In the face of conflict the child's mental apparatus finds it very difficult to maintain its controls as well as its functioning at the highest level of maturity reached, as Anna Freud (1952) has stressed. She pointed out that in the immature personality the ego often does not stand firm under the pressure of instinctual regression, but regresses simultaneously. The regressed ego then becomes compliant toward the regressed id demands. Anna Freud emphasizes that this compliance mitigates the intensity of the child's internal conflict, but it produces instead arrests in development, infantilisms, failures in adaptation, and so forth.

The "compliant" aspects of the child's ego development may also facilitate a tendency to absorb the affects aroused by traumatic experiences and by other situations as well. Thus we may in child analysis be very much concerned with dissecting the child's adaptation to the pressures which he feels operate on him. The whole of this approach relates to the aim of child analysis, which at the Hampstead Clinic is to restore the child to the path of normal development. We see the child's difficulty and his symptoms as being a present adaptive solution which prevents his taking the next step in development, and the aim of our work is to allow him to take this step.

This approach may give us a basis for taking a pragmatic view of our interpretative interventions, which are aimed at enabling the child to resolve conflicts holding his development back, rather than aimed at giving him a complete and "true" insight into everything that happened in the past. This point is perhaps particularly underscored by the fact that young children, after they have completed their analysis, tend very quickly to forget what insights they have had, even though they have moved forward developmentally in a satisfactory way, and pathological conflicts have disappeared sufficiently for the move forward to take place.

As a final comment I should like to say that although the reader may not agree with what has been said, which I know is to some extent controversial and provocative, the main purpose of the paper really is to encourage us as child analysts to take a new look at the meaning of our technical interventions and the things we have previously taken for granted. I hope that, in spite of all that was said, we will all continue to get that feeling of satisfaction that usually follows a "good" reconstructive interpretation.

Note

* This paper was presented at the Sixth Annual Scientific Meetings of the American Association for Child Psychoanalysis at Williamsburg, Virginia, on March 20, 1971.

References

Bergen, M. E. (1958). The effect of severe trauma on a four-year-old child. *Psychoanalytic Study of the Child, 13*: 407–29.

Breur, J., & Freud, S. (1893–1895). Studies on hysteria. *Standard Edition* 2.

Erikson, E. H. (1950). *Childhood and Society*. New York: Norton.

Freud, A. (1951). Observations on child development. *Psychoanalytic Study of the Child, 6*: 18–30.

Freud, A. (1952). The mutual influences in the development of ego and id: Introduction to the discussion. Psychoanalytic *Study of the Child, 7*: 42–50.

Freud, A. (1965). *Normality and Pathology in Childhood*. New York: Int. Univ. Press.

Freud, A. (1971). The infantile neurosis: Genetic and dynamic considerations. *Psychoanalytic Study of the Child, 26*: 79–90.

Freud, S. (1937). Constructions in analysis. *Standard Edition, 23.*

Hartmann, H. (1958). Comments on the scientific aspects of psychoanalysis. *Psychoanalytic Study of the Child, 13*: 127–46.

Heinicke, C. (1970). In search of supporting evidence for reconstructions formulated during a child psychoanalysis. *Reiss-Davis Clinical Bulletin, 7*: 92–110.

Katan, A. (1961). Some thoughts about the role of verbalization in early childhood. *Psychoanalytic Study of the Child, 16*: 184–8.

Kris, E. (1956). The recovery of childhood memories in psychoanalysis. *Psychoanalytic Study of the Child, 11*: 54–88.

Loewald, H. W. (1960). On the therapeutic action of psycho-analysis. *International Journal of Psychoanalysis, 41*: 16–33.

Loewenstein, R. M. (1951). The problem of interpretation. *Psychoanalytic Quarterly, 20*: 1–14.

CHAPTER THREE

The "Baby at the Breast" Experience: Memory or Fantasy? Some Further Thoughts on Reconstruction*

Hansi Kennedy 1984

By highlighting the complex early interactions between infant and mother, experimental psychologists and researchers have provided important new information about the behavioural potentialities of infants. This information has significant bearing on our understanding of "sensitive periods" for "bonding" and for establishing early modes of communication, which may lead to changes in the handling of infants.

We must, however, seriously question whether these complex interactions between infant and mother can be designated "object relationships" in spite of the experimental evidence which suggests that distinct perceptual schemata of "self and other" begin to form in the earliest months of life. Experimental proof of the infant's sensory and motor capacities, and a predisposition to make self-other differentiation from birth tells us nothing new about the infant's *subjective* experiences of self and object. It does *not* suggest that the infant has meaningful awareness of his "interactions with other" *qua* other, or that he has intentionality. It tells us that the infant is biologically "programmed" to interact in those specific ways which may facilitate and influence the development of the psychological relationship. However, the processes involved in the building up of the psychological relationship, with the differentiation of self and object that this implies, requires considerable ego maturation and structuralization.

W.W. Meissner (1979) suggests that we use the term "*object relatedness*" to describe the *real* and *external* interaction with objects, and that we reserve the term "*object relations*" more specifically for the intrapsychic dimension of the subject's experience of objects. Such a distinction will help us examine more closely the intricate developmental advances which accompany what Stern (1983) has described as a shift of locus from "external reality" to "in the mind" over the course of the infant's early life.

The delineation of self and object representation can only come about gradually with maturation and experience. Sandler and Rosenblatt (1962) see the building up of a representational world as a *sine qua non* for ego development and a prerequisite for progressive adaptation. They assume that initially the infant's subjective experiences register as sensations and global feeling-states of pleasure and un-pleasure. Primitive perceptual and memory structures gradually lead to the building up of inner representations which then act as a basis for the ongoing organization experiences and motor activities. Eventually a "Representational World" is created which enables the child to begin to perceive different sources of his experiences and to organize them in more meaningful ways. Sandler and Rosenblatt conceptualized representations as a kind of mental furniture and likened the representational world to a theatre stage set for the ego's perceptual structuring of sensory data, for imagination and fantasy, for direct and modified action, for language, for symbols and for trial action in thought. In this analogy the characters on the stage correspond to self and object representations. In a later joint paper (1978) the Sandlers described an object relationship as "an intrapsychic relationship depicted via mental representations and forming an intrinsic part of a wish". They developed the idea that external relationships can be considered to be derivatives of underlying wishful fantasy role relationships which occur intrapsychically and are "actualised".

These distinctions between "biological" and "psychological relating", or between "object relatedness" and "object relations" (Meissner, 1979) have clinical relevance. They affect our understanding of patients' material, pertaining to early experiences and the technique of reconstruction.

Let me illustrate these points with some clinical material[1] from the opening phase of the treatment of a four-year-old boy.

At the time of referral the parents were concerned about John's extremely aggressive and destructive behaviour. Mother described repeated battles with her son, who confronted her on every issue and did not seem to want to please her. John also had frequent fights with his younger brother (2 years, 3 months), often hitting him without any provocation. John was described as so aggressive towards other children that their mothers did not want him to play with them. He had an easier relationship with his father who would spend a whole hour alone with him each morning, when he would read to him, to their mutual enjoyment.

The parents described John as a troubled and unhappy child who also had many fears. He was frightened of the dark and of being alone in a room, and he had recently begun to come into the parents' bedroom at night, asking to sleep between them.

He was seen for assessment in the usual way and the following Diagnostic formulations were arrived at:

> John's relationship to his mother seems to have been fraught with difficulties from his birth. He was born at a particularly stressful period of his mother's life. At birth John was bruised, severely jaundiced and required a blood transfusion. These are some of the known factors which interfered with the mother's cathexis of her firstborn baby. There are many indications in the developmental history that she never felt quite "in tune" with him; and *his* experiences of her may have been of a frustrating object who was insensitive to his needs.
>
> By the time John was six months old the environmental stress on the mother had lessened and she found it easier to comfort and care for him; but this relationship deteriorated again when she became pregnant with her second child. John was 21 months old when his brother was born and was moving into the anal–sadistic phase during which aggression reaches a normal peak. The birth of his brother probably increased his dissatisfaction with his mother and fuelled his aggression, thus increasing his difficulty in negotiating his

> rapprochement crisis. These experiences must be seen as the developmental underpinnings of John's present conflicts and anxieties which now interfere with his progressive development. As ongoing attempts at mother guidance work have not proved adequate in helping John to better adaptation, analytic help is recommended.

It is to these assumptions about developmental underpinnings and their significance in our understanding of the analytic material and our analytic interventions that I wish to address myself.

John insisted that mother stay in the room for the first two sessions. His noisy and self-assertive behaviour was much in evidence and his play revealed fantasies of fighting, biting and devouring crocodiles and of soldiers shooting with big guns. In contrast to this was his much calmer mood in the third and subsequent sessions when he was able to remain on his own with the analyst. He now wanted to paint and through this activity began to introduce his conflicts over messing. The therapist's initial verbalization of her understanding that he sometimes wished to make a big mess and that it was hard for him to be a big boy all the time, seemingly acted as a licence to regress. The fantasy of being a well-cared-for, gratified baby, began to dominate the material for the next few weeks. It was ushered in when John found a toy baby-bottle in the treatment room and at once began to suck it. He commented that little babies drank from mummy's breast and that he had done so when he was a baby. In the following session he wanted to create absolute quiet in the room and complained about the intrusive noises of other children. He closed the curtains and lay on the couch for a long time, just sucking his thumb and watching his therapist in silence. This became a daily occurrence with only minor variations; sometimes he filled the bottle with water and drank from it, sometimes he pretended to sleep, and at other times he kicked his legs in the air while lying on his back. He also began to assign the role of the caring mother to the analyst. She had to check how much he had drunk from the bottle; she had to pick up the bottle when he dropped it on the floor. Occasionally he would make remarks such as "babies drink from mummies' breasts, big boys don't"; or, while chewing the bottle-teat, "my mummy had to give up breastfeeding me when my teeth started to grow". Mostly John enjoyed his analytic hour and it seemed that his therapist had become an important person for him in a very short time.

We can now pose a number of questions about the nature of John's relationship to his therapist and why he took to analysis as a duck to water.

Was it the one-to-one relationship in the analytic session in which the child can feel special and have the analyst's exclusive attention for an hour a day?

Did this special setting provide him with an opportunity to escape from his anger with mother and brother and enact current wishful fantasies of being loved and cared for, as he felt his envied brother was when he was a baby?

Did the therapist become important because she was able to "tune in" to John's feelings and the things about which he was in conflict, and because she could talk to him about his regressive wishes and convey her uncritical acceptance of him?

Or do we view John's relationship as a transference relationship based on the revival of wishes from earliest infancy?

Can we in fact make any direct link between the kind of material enacted by John in these first few sessions and his experiences as an infant sucking at the breast? Are the wishes and longings to have been a happy and contented baby who received caring ministrations from mother, *memories of his infancy or memories of his brother feeding at the breast*; and how do we see these as linked?

The assumption in the analyst's mind that the unsatisfactory or very satisfactory early feeding situation plays a part in the mother-child interaction is obvious. From an historical viewpoint, in which the memory of an experience is traced to its ultimate source, we must assume that *some element* of the infant's experience at the breast has to be contained in whatever John now knows and feels and fantasizes about babies and mothers and the breast. Although we do not know much about the structure of the mental apparatus during the preverbal phase of development, we generally assume that what are initially created by these earliest experiences are somatic memories, modes of functioning, and attitudes—that is, developmental tendencies rather than memory structures with specific contents and fantasies attached to them. We think that these experiences become absorbed, in a continuous process, in new memory structures created in keeping with maturation and the development of the mental apparatus. This I now hope to demonstrate through material taken from infant observations on John whose development was followed by various members of this Clinic from the time he was one month old (through Baby Observation, the Mother-Toddler Group and our Nursery School). Those who had been in contact with him had expressed concern about his relationship with mother from early days.

Breastfeeding was the one area of mutual enjoyment for mother and baby. It was easily established and John was fed on demand. He was a vigorous feeder and mother put him to the breast whenever he was restless. At eight weeks mother commented to the pediatrician that he was not really happy unless he was either being fed or asleep and characterized him as an "uncuddly" baby. It was noted that he was a baby who was difficult to soothe and who did not mould comfortably when held. When he was four months old the observer noted that for John contact with mother and others *through vision* seemed more important and more satisfying than physical contact. At about this time solids were introduced and mother linked this with broken nights. John was finally weaned at nine months with no problems. When he was one year old the observer described him as competent at feeding himself, and at that time he started walking. Soon after this mother became pregnant.

At 17 months John began to attend our Mother-Toddler Group. Mother was five months pregnant and had begun to talk to him about the baby. They continued to attend regularly after the birth of John's brother, Martin, who was brought along and often slept in his carry-cot.

His first attendance with mother and the new baby at 21 months was marked by his apprehensive and brooding appearance, his anxious clinging to his mother and complete refusal to engage with the familiar adults in the group. This continued for some weeks. Quite often Martin awoke from a nap crying and mother breastfed him in the group session. At these times John either stayed very close to mother and baby or made persistent attempts to gain mother's exclusive attention by clutching her hand and trying to drag her to the opposite side of the room. It was observed that when he could not get space on mother's lap because of the baby he filled every available inch with his toys. On one occasion, following weeks of watching mother's attentiveness to the baby, John arrived curled up in mother's arms, sound asleep. He remained sleeping and cuddling in her lap throughout almost the entire group session. The observer noted that it was rather ironic that John's thirst for physical closeness with mother, a form of relating to her which he had rejected in his infancy, had now become so important.

Two further observations are of particular relevance in connection with the creation of new memory structures which presumably absorb earlier ones. While mother was feeding Martin, John tentatively touched the feeding baby's head and wistfully burrowed his head into mother's lap right next to the baby. On another feeding occasion, John stood next to them with thumb in mouth and stared absently into space away from the mother-baby couple, while his free hand rested gently on baby's head, as if sharing in the feeding experience.

These examples help us to draw some inferences in regard to John's feelings about "the brother at the breast" experience. He clearly wanted the baby's place on mother's lap, in her arms and at the breast, and seemed able almost to become the baby in fantasy. But these observations soon after the birth of his brother cannot be viewed in isolation. During the next five months other feelings must have been aroused relating to "the brother at the breast" experience. John's confusion about sucking, eating and biting must have become interwoven with wishes, fantasies and experiences drawn from other aspects of his life: his toilet training, for example, which had then begun. And the considerable advances in ego development during this period must have helped to reorganize and create new memory structures of his and his brother's "baby at the breast" experience. He became a very verbal and articulate child and mother valued and enjoyed his advanced language development and was inclined to offer lengthy and sophisticated explanations about everything.

We must also look at John's relationship with mother before Martin's birth, in relation to his aggressiveness. Mother began to worry about this in his first year of life when she found it difficult to accept his very determined grabbing, clambering and yelling when he wanted something. Later she was troubled when he was rough with the cat, pushed over towers of bricks as well as other children. In fact, mother was intolerant of any aggressive, vigorous toddler activity, though John may have shown more such behaviour than is usual. With evident guilt feelings the mother wondered if she herself might have caused John's aggression by her rough handling of him, both in a playful and also not so playful manner. And yet she decided consciously not to pick John up when he tumbled over or hurt himself unless he made a great fuss. In the Toddler Group it was noted that she sometimes carried this to extremes, leaving him when he had a bad fall. Indeed, he had evidently given up crying on such occasions. John was aggressive to other children who visited his home and occasionally also to the children in the Toddler Group when they had something he wanted. His later aggression to his baby brother when he was present in the Toddler Group was much more object directed. He would hit or poke his head surreptitiously while he was lying peacefully in his cot away from mother. This, of course, occurred frequently at home and at such times mother became very punitive, scolding or spanking him and locking him in his room.

In examining the antecedents of his heightened aggressiveness in the second year of life, we have to consider the contributions of his endowment, of mother's relationship to him, and how these affected the earliest interactions between mother and child. We have to consider how John's active assertiveness, which mother experienced as aggression, and mother's so-called "aggressive" handling, interacted and what part these features played in mother's inability to help John curb his aggressive impulses. We must take into account how his aggressiveness was fuelled by mother's punitive responses, and by her pregnancy and the arrival of the baby at a period in John's development when mastering ambivalence and individuation were major developmental tasks.

Let us now return to the question we asked earlier about the contents of John's opening phase of analysis. Could the baby-mother enactments be understood as revived memories of his own "baby at the breast" experiences?

I would postulate that the infantile experience was a prototype of what later, at 21 months, became organized, i.e. acquired its meaning, by becoming integrated with the experiences, wishes and fantasies he had when he watched his brother at the breast. These memories subsequently became further reorganized, and restructured in different contexts, and in accordance with ongoing maturation and development. Indeed we could say, following the Sandlers (1978), that John, at the age of four, "actualised" in his sessions a *then* current wishful fantasy role-relationship, where he was the idealized baby and the therapist the idealized mother. Enacting or "actualizing" this wish helped him to attain some measure of wish fulfillment.

This formulation would in no way contradict the suggestion that the treatment setting provided John with the opportunity to get away from his conflict and anger with mother, and that the fantasy enactments served defensive purposes as well.

The opportunity to establish a one-to-one relationship with an adult who was exclusively available to him, and for whom he was special, also met a current need. This was underscored by the fact that John enquired from mother whether the therapist had a little boy, even before he was taken to his first interview. In the interview he asked his therapist directly whether she saw other children in her room. His persisting need for exclusive possession of the object could also be seen in the Nursery School. He related warmly to the teachers when they were able to give him special attention, but became noisy and disruptive in the group when this did not happen. His calm enjoyment of the reading time with father also pointed to this need and was in sharp contrast to his wild and noisy behaviour at home during the rest of the day.

These conceptualizations will contribute to the clarity of the therapist's thinking and to her understanding of the child's material, but they may not have a direct bearing on the way she will interpret to a young child. John talked about his own feeding at the breast while he was sucking the bottle. Although we can safely assume that he obtained this information from mother, this will not mean that it will need to be clarified for John.

Interpretations must "fit" intrapsychically, rather than be "objectively" correct. The therapist may then want to take up John's wishes to recapture the fantasised bliss of his infancy even if she knows that these wishes are likely to relate to identifications with baby brother or are connected with his envy of him. Four-year-olds lack the full capacity to place experiences in a reality-orientated time-sequence. The detailed tracing of historical links to specific experiences in the past, via reconstruction, is in any case not as Ernest Kris (1956) and others have pointed out. For the under-five it is even developmentally inappropriate. Analytic work is aimed at fostering self-knowledge but with under-fives this goes hand in hand with the developmental process itself. The analytic work fosters the child's ability to contain and verbalize wishes and feelings, and to reflect. In terms of the conceptual model we are discussing, this implies "experiencing in a new way".

I now wish to return briefly to another question asked in relation to the therapist's first intervention. Did the fact that she had verbalized John's wish to be messy and that it was hard for him to be a big boy all the time, lead to the therapist becoming important because she was able to "tune in" and understand what John was feeling at that moment?

I believe that feeling understood is an important ingredient of transference, giving impetus in the therapy to doing analytic work and contributing to the acquisition of self-awareness and self-understanding. I want to make a link here and suggest that the infantile prototype of the later feeling of being understood by the analyst originates in the infant's affective experience of his mother responding appropriately, with her more sophisticated understanding, to his needs. This analogy can be taken further; just as mother understood what the infant needed before the infant could do so, so the child-analyst's insights into his patient's wishes, fantasies or motivations usually precede the patient's insights. This suggests that the genesis of affective awareness and self-understanding has to be sought in the experience of being and feeling understood. "Feeling understood" is not necessarily a response to the therapist's verbalizations and interpretations but can also be communicated non-verbally. This is especially important with children who experience interpretations as criticizing, or as attacking, or as humiliating, and who literally cover their ears or insist that the therapist stop talking. It is also illustrated by those who do not necessarily reject the therapist's words *per se*, but who do not hear them, or have taken them in but have perceived them only as "friendly noises". Technical problems of this kind often highlight the experiential components in the analytic situation and alert us to the fact that a considerable number of our child patients need the affective experience of "feeling understood" before they can feel safe enough to participate in the often painful endeavour to increase self-understanding. In this sense the recapturing of early affective components of "being understood" may represent the affective quest for self-understanding.

This underlines what is perhaps a central point for us: that it is the elaboration and refinement of affective experience, as this occurs in development, which is inseparable from the development of structures. There is no doubt that connections exist between the external relations of infant and mother and the complex and multifaceted developmental processes which enable the child to form object relationships, but they are not simple shifts in location.

Notes

* An earlier version of the paper was given as a panel contribution at the 1982 Annual Meeting of the Association for Child Psycoanalysis in Denver, Colorado.

1. I am indebted to Geraldine Fitzpatrick, Jill Hodges, Claudia Lament and Nancy Brenner, on whose clinical records I have drawn.

References

Kris, E. (1956). On some vicissitudes of insight in psychoanalysis. In *The Selected Papers of Ernst Kris* (pp. 252–71). New Haven: Yale Univ. Press, 1975.

Meissner, W.W. (1979). Internalization and object relations. *Journal of the American Psychoanalytic* Association, *27*: 345–60.

Sandler, J. & Sandler, A-M. (1978). On the development of object relationship and affects. *International Journal of Psychoanalysis, 59*: 285–96.

Sandler, J. & Rosenblatt, B. (1962). The concept of the representational world. *Psychoanalytic Study of the Child, 17*: 128–45.

Stern, D. (1983). The early development of schemas of self, of other, and of various experiences of "self with other". In: J. Lichtenberg & S. Kaplan (Eds.), *Reflections on Self Psychology* (pp. 49–84). Hillsdale: Analytic Press.

CHAPTER FOUR

Both Sides of the Barrier: Some Reflections on Childhood Fantasy*

Hansi Kennedy, George Moran, Stanley Wiseberg and Clifford Yorke 1985

In the psychoanalytic view, fantasy brings together diverse mental content, in the service of wish fulfillment, in constructions which do not correspond with either a past or a present reality. Fantasy is thereby distinguished from memories and percepts, although memories and percepts, distorted or not, may be used as material for fantasy formation. Indeed, affect, percept, and all other forms of mental content provide the psychic bricks with which fantasies are constructed, whether drawn together by primary-process ideation or variously disciplined by secondary-process thinking. Fantasy may relieve drive pressure and thereby have an economic function; in this respect, it is internally adaptive, although, if it arouses too much anxiety or interferes with certain aspects of ego functioning, it may jeopardize adequate adaptations to the external world. We are, however, very familiar with many of the ways in which fantasy fosters adaptation to reality: Hartmann (1939) has laid particular stress on this aspect of fantasy functioning.

Two further points need to be added. First, in its wish-fulfilling function, fantasy is by no means exclusively a representative of the id. In its function as an internal regulator, fantasy may reconcile or bring into contiguity *conflicting* wishes. Second, the view that fantasy can fulfill manifold functions is linked with the concept of transmogrification—that is to say, the change in form and function over the course of development, sometimes in the most surprising manner. A brief vignette illustrates these points.

A woman whose childhood sexuality was characterized by beating fantasies experienced, in adulthood, masturbation fantasies in which she imagined the stages of her trial and sentence for a violent crime. She would mount the scaffold to be beheaded, and orgasm would occur with the fall of the executioner's sword. In addition to id derivatives, a fantasy of this kind includes a powerful superego component. This could not have been established when beating fantasies began, in early childhood, since it would have preceded the formation of the superego as a comparatively stable internal structure. From the standpoint of the topographical model, the beating fantasies existed *before* the repression barrier[1] was established, while the retributive elements in the execution fantasy were provided *after* it had been laid down. Stable internalization is crucial for the consolidation of the repression barrier and the suppression of infantile sexuality by infantile amnesia.

It is our intention to provide clinical illustrations relating to periods before and after the repression barrier is fully formed. We shall, however, concern ourselves with the *internal* rather than the *external* adaptive function of fantasy.

In the preverbal period of childhood, a wide range of activity organizes and expresses drives and conflicts in an action mode. Many of the play activities in the first and second year of life operate in the service of mastery and ego development and provide pleasure, though some would argue that these activities do not fully qualify as illustrations of fantasy. Examples include reversal of the feeding situation in the first year of life when a child attempts, with evident pleasure, to put a spoon or a biscuit into his mother's mouth, gives his unwanted food to the dog, or, somewhat later, prepares, eats, or serves "pretend food." Another typical sequence, in this case in the service of mastering separation, begins with peek-a-boo games, and proceeds to more complex activities in which the child leaves the mother and waves good-bye, plays games of hide-and-seek, or pretends to leave for the office or factory or to set out on a long journey. Defenses against feelings of helplessness and passive capitulation to mother's control, as well as a simple wish to be grown up, find expression in the wearing of mother's shoes, the carrying of father's briefcase or mother's shopping bag, and extend to more elaborate games involving dolls, props, and playing at mommies and daddies.

Such action-based behavior suspends, in some degree, reality appraisal. In the case of a 2-year-old, the dividing line between fantasy and reality is fluid and easily transcended, while in a 3-year-old reality appraisal is more firmly established and the distinction between current reality, past reality, and fantasy is more easily made. The boundaries will of course be repeatedly blurred and often be ill defined. Hand in hand with these developments, however, fantasy increases in complexity. In the example which follows, we see how fantasy copes with both impulse and defense in a way which serves internal adaptation, but which seeks the cooperation of the real world for its reinforcement.

Susie, a bright 3-year-old, was well aware of her mother's pregnancy and frequently spoke of "our baby" in either the mother's tummy or her own. Following the mother's miscarriage in the fifth month of pregnancy, Susie had difficulty in sleeping through the night without joining the parents in their room. She also began to insist that she was not Susie but "Katie," a 12-year-old "big girl." After battles with her mother, Katie would return to her, commiserate, and agree that Susie was "such a naughty girl." She would become very upset and protest when her parents did not address her as Katie. In her fantasy Susie did not go to nursery school but went to "big school" instead. She demanded that her classmates and nursery school teacher, as well as her parents, comply with her insistence that she was Katie. She introduced herself to strangers and friends as Katie and, when questioned about Susie's whereabouts, explained that Susie lived up the road or was buying flowers. Her father recalled that, just before he took Susie to visit her mother in the hospital, they had bought flowers "because Mommy was feeling sad." Katie confided to her parents that Susie's daddy had died, but the next day she reported that he was alive again.

Susie's death wishes were scarcely disguised. Although they were clearly conflictual, her development was not yet sufficiently advanced to make effective use of repression. Instead she tried to rid herself of the conflict by dividing herself into a "good" and a "bad" girl. While both remained in consciousness, she repudiated Susie's role, and gave herself the maturity, and hence the instinctual controls, of an older girl. This reflected her wish to avoid criticism and loss of love. We may even postulate that she had a primitive self-ideal and an emerging self-critical faculty. But the death wishes could not be repressed; and she probably knew that Katie was an invention.

Susie, then, attempted to deal with her death wishes and fears through a defensive fantasy. The threatened arrival of a new baby had fostered the need to be more grown up; and the strength of her destructive wishes demanded a greater degree of control than this little girl was able to mobilize. By changing her identity, she could also disown responsibility for Susie's actions, while at the same time continuing to express them. In this instance, the fantasy attempted to reconcile opposing wishes.

Some children of Susie's age are capable of expressing their anxieties and conflicts in more symbolic forms which do not require a comparable degree of manipulation of reality, of their objects, or of their self representation. James, a 3¾ year-old boy, was preoccupied with phallic competitive wishes toward his father and concomitant castration anxiety. On a visit to his aunt, he challenged his father for the attention of his hostess. He told his aunt about the film *Star Wars*, and drew her attention to a small stick. This, he said, was his "life force," like that of Luke Sky Walker and Darth Vader. James said that he was Luke and that he was only just learning how to use the life force, i.e., the stick. He put on a "pretend" helmet so that he could not see what he was doing while he learned to use his life force. This was necessary because otherwise he might touch his leg with his life force and cause it to fall off. He stood with his eyes tightly shut, slashing at the air and turning scarlet with the effort and excitement. He asked his aunt if she could see Darth Vader and if she could see whether his leg was all right. When he was reassured, he said that he would take off the helmet and announced: "I have learned how to do it. My leg will be all right as I won't touch it now that I can see . . . Do you know the story of *Star Wars*? Darth Vader dies. Wasn't that sad? But Luke had the life force then." James at once became quite placating to his father, whose attention was suitably distracted from the aunt by these goings-on. The boy then reassuringly told his father to put the helmet on James/Luke again, because he had not quite learned how to use the life force and keep his leg safe.

James had reached a stage at which he revealed castration anxiety. He expressed this in a crude symbolization. A stick with a "life force" was not very far removed from the part of the body it represented. James utilized the ready-made fantasy of Star Wars which afforded him the protective omnipotence of its heroes. He compensated for his vulnerability through identification with a figure representing masculine prowess. For all his adopted strength and power, the fear of losing a part of his body remained in consciousness, even though he shut his eyes in a vain attempt to exclude it.

John, an articulate and intelligent boy of 6½, chose to express himself, both in analysis and at home, through dramatized play enactments. He was not much interested in formal learning but was very well aware of his surroundings and had a large fund of knowledge. Fantasy play gave him pleasure and served him defensively. Conflicting wishes were kept at a distance because he strenuously held on to the idea that he was *only* playing.

During the second year of analysis the content of his fantasy games focused on family romances and suggested attempts to resolve his oedipus complex which had featured prominently in the material. For example, he introduced a game in which two brothers, Fred and George, ran off to find a new home. In one variation, one brother was rescued by a nice man. (John had a male therapist.) In another, the boys heard their father coming; Fred told George that he hated his father, and the brothers ran off together. In another version, both parents went to the hospital, Fred and George ran away, became assistant managing directors of a supermarket, and lived with a nice shopkeeper.

John also created a wide range of royal family fantasies. He pretended that he and the therapist were artists living in poverty who were nevertheless invited to the palace and later became King and Queen. On another occasion he became Prince Charles and turned his therapist into Prince Andrew. In this he reversed his real relationship to his older sibling. Later, John played a "Prince game" in which the royalty bestowed on him tremendous privileges and authority and compensated for his lowly school performance. In this way he raised his self-esteem and gave the clear impression of one "born to be King." He knew that his father could trace kinship to Queen Victoria.

John utilized his store of knowledge to create stories which matched his conflictual wishes and sought to resolve them through dramatic transformations which were acceptable and even a source of pleasure, as long as he could insist that he was "only playing." The links with the oedipal constellation remained evident to the analyst, however, in spite of John's creative disguise. Attempts at interpretation were met with dismissive rebuttal and an urgent demand to continue the play. The royal robes were diaphanous, but John had no more than one foot across the repression barrier.

We set out from the long established position that repression proper can scarcely be said to operate before the establishment of the repression barrier and the onset of infantile amnesia with the resolution of the oedipus complex. Indeed, neither James nor Susie shows evidence of repression proper. Both children display their current conflicts, disguised rather than repressed, while John appears to be at the threshold of this developmental achievement.

The masturbation fantasies of children in the latency period are evidence of repression proper and are not nearly so transparent as the fantasies we have cited above. They also serve subsidiary aims of compensating for a large variety of frustrations, deprivations, and disappointments.

Lucy, who was 9 when she began analytic treatment, was very fond of horses. She said she did not ride because it was too expensive and "anyway there was no room in the front garden for a horse." For several months she had kept an imaginary horse called Black Beauty who lived in her bedroom and to whom she talked. The mother tolerated the child's fantasy companion, and regretted the fact that the family could not pay for riding lessons. Lucy claimed that her father was getting fed up with the horse, but "he should not be angry as it might upset Black Beauty."

At school, among her peer group, horse games provided an outlet for fantasy. It was after such a game that Lucy lost her voice. On this occasion her friend had designated Black Beauty's brother, Prince, as Lucy's horse. Although Lucy herself denied any angry feelings about this, she said she would have to leave her friend time to "simmer down." She needed this dominating friend, who was full of ideas, but resented her control. She eventually confided that although she outwardly complied with her friend's directive and called her horse Prince, she took secret pleasure in pretending that it was really she and not the friend who was the rider of Black Beauty. In the *shared symbolic* fantasy with the friend, she could accept the friend's domination; in the *private* fantasy, the situation was reversed in a secret triumph.

Black Beauty played an important part in the course of Lucy's treatment. She brought him to the Clinic and tied him up in the waiting room, and her references to him indicated the nature of her conflicts. If she was feeling tired and lazy and her mother had pressured her, she claimed she rode him on the way. She reported on the "naughty things" of which Black Beauty was capable, such as knocking over her mother's favorite vase and eating the flowers. Black Beauty could also be obstinate and, once dressed, he wouldn't open his mouth to eat his breakfast, and once fed, he wouldn't go out.

The unconscious conflicts behind Lucy's use of, and fantasies about, Black Beauty are more difficult to establish than in the three younger children. Psychoanalysts will infer a good deal from the material, but its meaning was much more effectively hidden from Lucy herself. The overall inference is that Lucy has an established repression barrier.

In the examples we have cited, we can see a healthy use of imagination to solve problems and ensure gratification in fantasy. This is not to say that fantasy cannot be indulged at the cost of object relationships and achievements. To some extent we have equated the young child's play with fantasy: indeed, actionplay is the principal mode in which small children can express and communicate what goes on in their minds.

The development of the capacity to play is subject to a variety of influences from early infancy onward. As Winnicott (1971) has so well described, it is in the first instance rooted in the interaction of mother and child. In certain cases studied at the Clinic, playful interactions between mother and small child were absent. Explanations for this state of affairs varied. Sometimes a mother expected her young child to play with toys, by himself, and to stay quiet and occupied. Sometimes the mother failed to respect her child's pleasure and absorption in play activity, and intruded or interrupted him. Sometimes a child's play was directed by the mother to a point at which her own fantasies or externalizations were imposed on him, so that he was not allowed to express his own wishes in his own spontaneous way. Yet again, play was sometimes directly denigrated on account of its "childish" and unrealistic content. Such attitudes may interfere with the child's capacity to enjoy his or her fantasies-in-action and even lead to their total inhibition. Fantasy play then becomes a source of disapproval, danger, and shame.

We have tried to illustrate some of the ways in which fantasy undergoes change in the course of development, becomes subject to increasingly sophisticated defense activity and censorship, and thereby plays an important role in internal adaptation. It is well known that when the psychoanalyst attempts to undermine tenuous defenses, the very young child's only recourse may be to obliterate the therapist's voice by shouting or by covering his ears. In this way he seeks to keep at bay the words that threaten to call attention to unwanted or disowned mental content. Although the child increasingly builds up internal controls and defensive maneuvers against the eruption of primitive wishes, the repression barrier remains relatively permeable until superego structuralization, drive diminution, and the other changes which usher in latency have brought about its consolidation. Henceforth preconscious and unconscious systems compartmentalize the mind, but the degree of permeability remains of vital importance. Some measure of this capacity remains essential for imagination and creativity. Excessive impermeability leads to mental woodenness, inhibition, excessive personal constraint, and intolerance of id derivatives in self and others. The extent to which the individual can fantasize and control his fantasy depends, not only on the permeability of the various censorships, but also on the developmentally acquired characteristics of his ability to play and imagine.

Notes

* This work is part of a Study entitled "A Project to Study Variations of Normality and Pathology in Relation to Personality Development". In collaboration with P. Cohen, S. Marans, and P. Radford. This is an amended version of a paper presented at the 5th Annual International Scientific Colloquium entitled "The Role of Fantasy in the Adaptive Process", the proceedings of which are published in the *Bulletin of the Hampstead Clinic*, *7*: 149–212, 1984.

1. The term "repression barrier" is widely used at the Anna Freud Centre and bears the meaning allotted to it by a number of previous analysts, in particular Edward Glover (1949, pp. 53, 57, 71, 90, 126). We refer to the point at which the division betweedn id and ego has become structuralized and sufficiently stable to play a major part in determinining the onset of childhood amnesia and in facilitating the onset of latency.

References

Glover, E. (1949). *Psycho-analysis*. London: Staples Press.

Hartmann H. (1939). *Ego Psychology and the Problem of Adaptation*. New York: Int. Univ. Press, 1958.

Winnicott, D. W. (1971). *Playing and Reality*. London: Tavistock.

PART TWO

INSIGHT

Introduction

Insight as a concept relevant to child psychoanalysis was of interest to Kennedy as early as 1971 when she wrote on reconstruction. The publication of her papers specifically on insight should, however, be set in the context of the Hampstead Clinic's general interest in therapeutic action. Insight was viewed as a central concept to be addressed in the examination of methods of therapeutic action, and Kennedy's first paper on insight was presented at the Anna Freud-Hampstead Center Symposium at the Michigan Psychoanalytic Society. The year of its publication was also the occasion of the first annual International Scientific Colloquium at the Hampstead Clinic where the topic was insight in child psychoanalysis.

This paper, "The role of insight in child analysis: A developmental viewpoint" (1979), examined the kinds of insights children acquire in analytic treatment and the relative capacities for insight at various stages of development. Kennedy's conclusions were drawn from the material gathered from cases treated at the Hampstead Clinic over twenty-five years. In collaboration with colleagues there, she proposed a developmental line of insight beginning with the infant's awareness of pleasure and pain to the adult's capacity for objective intrapsychic self-observation.

Kennedy then joined with Clifford Yorke and Stanley Wiseberg (1980), who had already delineated a developmental line of anxiety (1976), to discuss the intertwining of the two lines throughout each phase of the lifespan. Unfortunately we are unable to reprint Kennedy's second paper on insight, "Some clinical and theoretical aspects of two developmental lines"; however it represents a significant contribution not only to the subject of insight per se, but it also demonstrates Kennedy's ability to integrate various lines of development into a cohesive picture.

In this paper the authors make a distinction between those lines of development which have readily identifiable outward manifestations (e.g. the line from ego-centricity to companionship) and those that are not so easily viewed through behavior. The lines of anxiety and the capacity for insight fall into the latter category. In other words, all lines are reflective of the development of internal psychic agencies, but some are less readily observed. Insight, particularly, is a capacity noted most clearly only in the psychotherapeutic process.

The article summarizes previous work done by the authors on the lines of anxiety and the capacity for insight and then proceeds to address the interaction of these two lines in their support of each other over the lifespan. Development is described chronologically and divided into five stages.

The initial stage occurs in the first year of life wherein the infant progresses from relatively primitive states of vegetative excitation to the first indication of mentalized anxiety at around eight months. The second phase involves the growth of secondary process thinking with its associated capacity for delay of action. This second period reaches its climax with the so-called resolution of the Oedipus Complex and the concomitant structuralization of the superego. Superego anxiety (guilt) signals a further differentiation of and control over affect. The third stage of life, latency, is represented by a fairly stable capacity for signal anxiety with its anticipation of internal and external danger. This ability to anticipate allows the latency child to institute defensive measures, thus avoiding traumatic anxiety states. In latency, however, children are still reliant upon the support of adults in order to contain anxiety adequately. The fourth stage, adolescence, involves considerable upheaval of various lines of development with the result of instability on the anxiety line. A major task of adolescence is the enduring re-stabilization of the anxiety line, and the chaotic regressions of this period actually prompt the further consolidation of signal anxiety. Adulthood, the fifth stage, heralds an increased stability of the anxiety line, although even here there are certain conditions in which reversion occurs.

The authors further describe a progression of the line of the capacity for insight that leads from infantile awareness to a wish for self-understanding. The initial stage of this line involves no more than the infant's subjective experiential awareness, while the second stage is represented by a variable and fluctuating self-awareness and reflection. Self-observation grows as parental expectation and approval are internalized. Latency brings fully internalized conflict with relatively stable defensive maneuvers to ward off unacceptable impulse. Superego structuralization adds to the security of the capacity for self-observation and self-reflection, and the operation of latency defenses allows the child to turn away from internal conflict to the outside world. The latency child, focused outward, looks for external solution to conflict, rather than self-understanding. Adolescence, the fourth stage, brings a renewed turn inward; introspection and self-reflection are heightened but the intensity of sexual and aggressive wishes heightens anxiety dramatically. These new dangers require strong defenses which limit the capacity for insight. The authors view adulthood as the first stage in which the degree of objective self-observation is high enough to encourage the wish for self-understanding. Here self-observation is autonomous, and successful analysis will create the capacity for insight at its highest level. When anxiety is poorly controlled, just as when in earlier stages it must be defended against, the capacity for insight is limited. When signal anxiety functions well, it clears a path for the development of insight. Insight itself then can aid in the maintenance of internal and external harmony.

Despite the fact we reprint only one of Kennedy's papers in this section, we believe the subject of insight was a building block in her thinking. She questioned the psychoanalytic theory where insight was central and the aim of the analysis. An analysis, Kennedy believed, could not be evaluated by the degree of insight attained, and perhaps insight wasn't even necessary. This conceptual reconsideration followed on her challenging another central analytic concept, that of reconstruction. Rather than reconstruction of experiences based on the recovery of the past, Kennedy proposed that what was most important was the construction of the affective significance of patterns of experience which influenced the child's ability to function in the here and now.

Kennedy's ideas about insight and reconstruction, as well as memory, laid the groundwork for her later conceptualization of psychopathology, analytic aims and technique, and the examination, with her Hampstead colleagues, of other key analytic concepts like conflict and infantile neurosis. The next section lays out some of these ideas from a developmental point of view, and outlines Kennedy's delineation of developmental disturbances from conflict and the differences in technique dependent on the type of disturbance.

CHAPTER FIVE

The Role of Insight in Child Analysis: A Developmental Viewpoint*

Hansi Kennedy 1979

Some time ago I concluded a short paper on "Problems in Reconstruction in Child Analysis" (1971) by suggesting that our interpretive interventions are aimed at enabling the child to resolve conflicts impeding his development, rather than at giving the child insights into what happened to him in the past. My argument emphasized the fact that young children usually forget whatever insights they acquire during their analysis, even though their developmental progress is satisfactory. Since that time it has been increasingly clear to me that I omitted to explore the kind of insights children acquire during analysis and their capacities for doing so during different developmental stages.

This realization provided the motivation for starting, some eighteen months ago, a small study group whose purpose was to closely scrutinize the role of insight in child analysis. Our findings form the basis of this paper, and I gratefully acknowledge my indebtedness to all the participants on whose contributions and clinical material I have freely drawn. Nevertheless, the views expressed are my own and are not necessarily shared by other members of the group.

The initial question presenting itself concerned the meaning of the concept of insight. While some children are described in clinical discussion as having "good insight," it was not at all clear whether this referred to children who were in touch with their own feelings, were especially aware of their problems, or even had insight into their own unconscious motivations. Nor was it clear at what stage in treatment this "good insight" manifested itself. Was it present initially at the time of referral, or did it develop during or at the termination of treatment? Furthermore, did "good insight" correlate with analyzability (as one might expect) and, conversely, did "lack of insight" tend to lead to negative treatment results?

Throughout the development of psychoanalysis, "conscious awareness" and "self-understanding" have, *inter alia*, been considered important as "currative factors."[1] In the extensive literature exploring how, when, and under what conditions therapeutic changes occur, few papers deal specifically with the role of insight in psychoanalytic therapy, though exceptions include articles by Kris (1956), Meyerson (1965), Richfield (1954), and Hatcher (1973). These papers share the following points of view. First, "awareness of one's feelings", "self-knowledge," and "insight" are related phenomena which play an important part in the therapeutic process, but are of course also in evidence in people who are not undergoing analysis. Second, self-observation is a prerequisite for the acquisition of insight, but does not necessarily lead to it. Self-observation can be utilized for gaining gratification; it can be at the service of a critical superego; it can be used defensively; or, for that matter, it can even signify a pathological split in the ego. Hatcher (1973), for example, points out that self-observation is not necessarily connected with *conscious awareness* as it occurs in dreams. Third, insight can be purely "intellectual"—an early recognition by Freud (1913) when he spoke of patients "knowing and not knowing." In later papers, this kind of intellectual insight is often contrasted with emotional insight. Richfield (1954) suggests a connection between these and the two types of knowledge described by Bertrand Russell as knowledge by description and knowledge by acquaintance. The latter involved experiential contact with the subject. The importance of "experiential insight," as contrasted with intellectual understanding, has often been stressed, particularly by those authors who believe that reliving in the transference is the one crucial element leading to psychic change (Strachey, 1934).

Kris (1956) defined insight as a *process* which makes use of the ego function of self-observation in both "experiential" and "reflective" form. The former provides material for understanding, the latter the active effort to understand. Miller et al. (1965) distinguish four forms of self-observation: consciousness of self, as in early infantile self-awareness; cognition of self; critical self-evaluation, and integrative self-observation as an autonomous ego function. This list serves as a useful starting point for a developmental scrutiny of insight. Let us start by examining the concept of "infantile self-awareness."

We must assume that, in the infant, whatever penetrates the stimulus barrier provides "experiential material." But what kind of "experiential awareness" can we assume in someone entirely under the impact of primary-process functioning? Such experiences can only have the most tenuous associations, and, initially, experiential awareness can only amount to transitory feeling-states. Because of the pleasure-seeking quality of the drives, the most primitive differentiation of experiences probably occurs around those associated with pleasure.

Gradually some ego functions will evolve due to the continued *interaction between* drives and the impingement of the external world, and on the basis of the constitutional and maturational aspects of ego development. This will enable the infant to build, little by little, rudimentary representations of his experiences and, on the basis of this further differentiation between them, to begin to establish body boundaries and to distinguish between inside and outside, the "me" and the "not me."

We may now speak of infantile experiential awareness if this means that some integration can occur of experiences that are intrapsychically, though not yet objectively, meaningful. It is important to keep in mind that these first differentiations are probably made on a purely subjective basis; that is, that pleasurable experiences are assigned to the "me" and unpleasurable ones to the "not me" (Freud, 1915); Sandler and Rosenblatt, 1962). But can we see this as a primitive form of self-observation?

The infant will by now have some capacity to differentiate between feelings, but will have minimal ability to contain and control them. Instinctual wishes seek satisfaction, and the infant has little capacity to delay their gratification, whatever the demands of reality.

Some scanning of experiential content arising from instinctual wishes, perceptions, and especially the feeling states to which they give rise, will now occur, and this function may well be an antecedent of the "inner" eye that is needed for self-observation. Because of the infant's limited capacity to tolerate painful feeling states, the inner eye will need to become increasingly more selective in its perceptions—painful experiential awareness has to be denied or externalized, that is, intrapsychically shifted from the self to the object representation, however rudimentary these will be.

In so far as the child has established trust in the object, he will increasingly expect the object to provide satisfaction and to remove painful feelings. The location of "bad feelings" in, and the expectation of good feelings from, the "outside" is quite in keeping with the young child's mode of functioning. Contradictory contents, feelings, and wishes can exist side by side, for there is very little causality, very little notion of time, very little reality appraisal, and very little reality testing.

The development described extends through the preverbal phase. With the gradual acquisition of language, cognitive development is significantly accelerated. Word representations create new possibilities for integration of experiences (Yorke, 1965). Verbalization is also an important tool in learning to contain and control feelings and actions (Katan, 1961).

With this degree of structuralization in the mental apparatus, the child can begin to make some limited sense of his experiences. This is the earliest stage at which we would consider accepting children for analytic treatment. Whatever rudimentary capacity for self-observation the child has now acquired will be in the service of maintaining his current states of well-being rather than subserving an active effort to understand himself. Even when self- and object representations are more consolidated and he has the capacity to sustain a special relationship to his love objects, the full achievement of object constancy—which requires recognition of the object's own needs and feelings—is likely to be beyond his capacities. Until the age of six or seven years the child is cognitively egocentric and his understanding of others is limited to subjective experiences (Rees, 1978).

According to Kris (1956), insight depends on the "integrated, sequential operation of several ego functions." Because control over affective discharge is needed, affects must be accessible, must not be overwhelming, and must not be acted out. Tolerance of painful affects is necessary, as well as the capacity for controlled ego regression. According to Hatcher (1973), detached, objective self-observation must have an "intrapsychic focus" and the ego's integrative function must "bring insight into useful contexts." *Quite obviously the use an adult patient is expected to make of his "experiential insight" is quite beyond the capacities of an under-five or a latency child.*

Let me try to illustrate these points with clinical examples. Young children express their wishes, feelings, and fantasies freely; and while this makes the analyst's task of understanding the material easier, the child's inadequate defenses, his tendency to enact, and his cognitive immaturity make analytic work more difficult. Our youngest patients are constantly threatened and often overwhelmed by their feelings and wishes because they lack adequate controls. Child analysts know only too well that they are liable to be hit and hugged or kicked and kissed, often within a few moments. Contradictory wishes and feelings can still exist side by side. Under the immediate impact of strong feelings the young child will be quite unable to reflect; and he will often need to be controlled. The analyst's constant endeavor to put the child's wishes and feelings into words aims at channeling action into thought and verbal expression.

Carol, only two years, nine months when she began treatment, was referred because of her unremitting jealousy of her eighteen-months-younger sister, whom she openly attacked at every opportunity. In her very first session she crawled and talked baby language. She readily agreed with her therapist's view that she wished to be a baby. She followed this by talking about her sister, who was "a nuisance, always taking away my things and disturbing me." On many subsequent occasions Carol played at being a baby with great enjoyment, commenting gleefully: "Look at me, I am a baby," thereby inviting the therapist to become the admiring and approving mother. This wish continued to be similarly enacted at home, although her mother disapproved of such behavior. Carol was looking for ways of gratifying her wishes and not for understanding. Like most young children, she often protested when her therapist discontinued participation in play to offer explanations. She imperiously demanded that the therapist "stop talking and play" or "stop talking and cry" when the latter tried to step out of the role assigned her in a fantasy enactment and made interpretations. These protests continued throughout her treatment.

Carol's wish to be a baby was not conflictual. To avoid conflict over anger with her mother and to avoid painful feelings of rejection, her ego complied with her regressive wishes. But this readiness for regression also created technical difficulties in the analysis. She often took verbalization of her barely defended regressive wishes as license to regress; and this, too, is typical of young children. For example, Carol messed with pools of water, which she repeatedly and deliberately made on the floor. When the therapist commented that she must be reminded of her former wishes to play with her urine puddles, Carol at once wanted to urinate on the floor. Quite apart from any pleasure gain that might have been achieved in this way, she probably lacked adequate orientation in time to make an appropriate appraisal of what were past and what were current wishes.

The acquisition of insight is further impeded by the child's inability to tolerate painful feelings and the almost universal readiness to "externalize" everything painful and conflictual. At the beginning of treatment, Carol attributed everything that made her feel bad to her baby sister. Later, she came to refer to her so-called symptoms as "hurts." Externalizations such as these continue well into latency and beyond.

Carol's precocious ego development and unusual verbal capacity frequently enabled her to report on events that had occurred at home or nursery school and even to put her fantasies into words. Early in her analysis she confided: "I get cross with the baby and shove her down the hole, and she comes out again, and I get cross." On other occasions she got excited when attacking a doll in the treatment room and suggested the analyst should join her in "flushing the baby down the lavatory." Once, after ten months of treatment, she listed the "hurts" she wanted to get rid of as "monsters, bugs, things that make me sad and naughty." Then she cheerfully suggested, "Let's throw all the hurts out of the window," and proceeded to enact this with much satisfaction.

This acknowledgment of "things" that made her anxious and unhappy demonstrates a capacity for self-observation of both an "experiential" and a "reflective" kind. Her wish to get rid of these "things" could even form a basis for establishing a rudimentary treatment alliance. However, her understanding of the treatment process was limited by her "cognitive style," in which early patterns of externalizing unwanted experiences went hand in hand with the impingement of pleasurable anal-aggressive fantasies. Carol was only capable of finding concrete solutions in keeping with her conceptual and intellectual functioning.

A similar example is taken from the treatment of a four-year-old little girl. Rosmarie was very deprived and excessively demanding when she was brought to the Clinic because of her mother's alarm at the child's request to suck at her breast. Indeed, there was a good deal of oral fantasy content. In this connection, it is of interest that she attempted to rid herself of her fear of monsters by suggesting that they be locked into a cupboard in the treatment room "so they will starve and be dead."

The child analysts' interventions repeatedly introduce a sequence of cause and effect and suggest the need to look for motivation. To some extent the child will try to identify with the analyst's reasoning at his higher level. Carol's therapist had explained that talking might help to get rid of the "hurts." In a subsequent session Carol remarked impatiently: "We are talking now—why don't they go away?" Once, when she had a bad knee during a holiday, she told her mother that her therapist would make it better.

None of this implies an objective understanding of the treatment process or of the role of the therapist. It is simply in keeping with the child's perception of the adult as possessor of magical powers. This, too, impedes work as a joint endeavor between patient and analyst in an attempt to reach insightful understanding. The very young child assumes that the adult is all-knowing and all-powerful and therefore sees failure to meet his needs and wishes as deliberate refusal to help. This will mobilize anger and hostility. With the gradual internalization of a self-critical attitude (the precursors of superego development) the child will feel increasingly threatened by the omniscient therapist who may at any moment retaliate and punish him. Repercussions of this affect the relationship with the analyst even in children of latency age. If the child's conceptual ability is still tied to magical thinking, this will influence his understanding of the treatment process. For example, Nancy, age 9, said of her therapist; "If he was really clever he would do magic."

Young children see the world in terms of their own wishes and feelings and are tied to their current experiences. They understand other people mainly from a subjective point of view, which also precludes the possibility of gaining "objective" insight. Even after a great deal of working through of many aspects of his castration anxiety, a four-year-old boy could not conceive that his therapist did not want a penis. He generalized his own intense concerns with phallic pride and oedipal rivalry. At the end of his analysis he brought his therapist a present of a box "so that you can catch a snake to put in it."

Transference interpretations are particularly difficult for young children to comprehend. The oedipal child usually has intense transference involvements with the analyst. This is not only because the one-to-one contact in the analytic situation lends itself to oedipal fantasy enactments or because such fantasies are less conflictual in displacement, but also because there is an affective overspill. The child's ego is simply not strong enough to sustain itself adequately in the face of id pressures. The child cannot easily contain the intensity of his feelings. He finds it hard to distinguish reality from fantasy and to recognize the "unreality" of transference feelings. His sense of the continuum of past, present, and future is still relatively undeveloped and contributes to this difficulty. Real insight of how the past affects current experience will be extremely rare in the under-five.

Although psychological development proceeds with forward and backward moves, entry into latency marks the attainment of significant emotional, social, and cognitive development. How does this affect the latency child's capacity and wish for insight? Self-observation, now strongly under the influence of superego strictures and high self-ideals, exposes the latency child to the experience of further inner conflicts from which he wants to escape. His newly acquired controls over his wishes and feelings strongly resist regression, and he now has a greater and more effective range of defenses available. Still battle-scarred from oedipal disappointments, he tries increasingly to turn away from adults and toward peer relationships, and away from conflictual situations. There is fresh impetus for his interests and curiosity to turn toward the external world. He will endeavor to externalize defensively his internalized conflicts and to look for environmental solutions in preference to internal changes (A. Freud, 1965). All this will strongly work against introspection and sustained and active participation in analytic work, in spite of the new cognitive capacities for insight which should now be available. Secondary-process functioning is much more firmly established. The latency child can use thought and language as efficient tools for dealing with experiential content. His reality testing, time sense, and verbal/conceptual memory organization and reasoning are well established. In other words, the latency child has the capacity for insight, but will fight strongly against it.

Latency children who readily acknowledge and verbalize their problems and wish for help at the beginning of treatment are often referred to as "insightful," but this can be misleading. In talking openly about their symptoms and reasons for referral, they may simply reiterate what they have learned from others or manifest their overcompliance by saying what they feel is expected of them. Other children, who may possibly have a greater awareness of difficulties and a more pressing wish for help, may be unable to verbalize because they feel too anxious, too ashamed, or too guilty. This can lead to the conscious withholding of material or even the deliberate distortion of the truth for a considerable time. Rachel, for example, was seven when she was referred for treatment after she had developed a "touching" symptom which strongly suggested links with masturbation conflicts. At the beginning of treatment she completely denied awareness of the symptom or any worries about masturbation; and, indeed, the symptom completely disappeared for several months. When her masturbation conflicts eventually emerged in analysis, she seemed relieved and spontaneously admitted that she had not told the truth in the initial interviews. She confessed that she had deliberately stopped herself from touching the knuckle of her left hand whenever she felt the temptation to do so because she had felt too ashamed.

Children's responses to interpretations may be misleading as indicators of insightful understanding. Interpretations may be rejected or ignored, yet lead to changes in the analytic material without any indication of whether such changes occurred in response to fresh understanding or to a defensive strategy. An overready acceptance of interpretations may show the child's need for compliance rather than indicate real understanding. Pseudo-insights are used defensively to gain approval and are frequently also utilized to gain gratification; for example: "I know I want things because I am jealous of the baby, but let me have a new toy just today and then we can talk." The search for gratification and intolerance of pain remains operative, too, in latency children, and with some analytic patients it reaches such a pitch that they cannot bear to hear the therapist speak. They run out of the treatment room, cover their ears, or make silence a condition of attendance. To her therapist's suggestion that a current separation might be especially painful because it reminded her of past losses, Nancy, age six, responded with a worried, "Don't talk about it—I might remember." Her remark indicated that considerable analytic progress had been made in Nancy's treatment, inasmuch as, for many weeks, she had insisted that the therapist only read stories to her and had literally tried to shout him down whenever he tried to speak to her directly. This may be an extreme example of "counterinsight," but we found only one latency child among the cases we examined who could be said to have actively and consistently participated in the analytic work throughout his treatment. At first, this child, David, explained that he wanted "to help the analyst to understand his feelings better," but later he evidently wanted to gain better understanding of his difficulties, which he recognized as inner problems.

David was eight years, nine months at referral. He already showed at the Diagnostic Interview that he had an awareness of his difficulties, a capacity for self-observation, an ability to reflect, and unusual verbal facility. His ability to use metaphors poignantly was evident when he described himself in the first treatment session as "feeling shipwrecked and in need of help." Much later in treatment he described the analytic process as "taking the fizz out of the bottle," which he explained by observing that one had to let feelings out slowly so that they didn't explode when "bottled up." More indicative of his wish for insight was his continued attempt to work out the reasons for his actions, feelings, and thoughts. Early in the treatment David spontaneously reported a dream—many children do—but when his therapist remarked that dreams sometimes helped in understanding hidden reasons, he made efforts to remember his dreams and to bring associations. He often reported on changes he perceived in the relative pressures from conflictual forces and showed how he was integrating insights gained from interpretations by bringing them back in different contexts. Of course, even in this analysis there were long periods of resistance. When he was overwhelmed by intense transference feelings, he could not use any of these capacities.

It is not uncommon for latency children to identify with the therapist's analyzing function, but then to apply it only in relation to others. Michael, age nine, told his mother to stop shouting because she frightened him and because it would make her feel bad afterward. This was his way of searching for external solutions; if his mother could change, he would not have to. Child patients also often start to interpret their own behavior or conflicts by attributing the understanding to the analyst. A child may say: "You will say I am doing this to punish myself." This is also a way of "disowning" insight or, at best, an indication of lack of conviction—knowing without believing. Although these examples suggest some degree of budding insights, they show even more clearly how the inner eye is attempting to look in a different direction.

In contrast, adolescents become very introspective and spend much time thinking about themselves. In the effort to establish their identity, they repeatedly compare themselves with others, wish to be different from their parents, and need to prove their independence. They feel confused and overwhelmed by the intensity of their wishes, feelings, and conflicts, and desperately attempt to use their intellect to find solutions. Michael, for example, age fourteen, said: "Germs and genes are really similar. Genes decide what character you have and germs decide what illnesses you have. Like my father, I am passive until someone pushes me all the way. I am very observant, but I can be very ignorant like my mother when I do not want to understand something. I must have got my nervousness from my mother. It is my nervousness that I want to change." Adolescents with obsessional defenses are especially prone to ruminate and intellectualize about themselves, while those with inhibitions and low self-esteem often have difficulties in communicating their self-reflections. Usa, fifteen, showed awareness of feelings and ability to reflect, but at the beginning of treatment she communicated in a "telegraphic" style which pointed to conflicts over talking about herself. Later she only reverted to this after frequent and long silences, which were very painful for her. At such times she also stared at a rug in the treatment room as though to avoid looking at her therapist. The suggestion was eventually made that the use of the couch might facilitate talking. Lisa rejected this outright and said that she needed to watch the analyst's facial expressions for clues. As she gradually became more actively involved in the analytic work, she tried to explain the continuing periods of prolonged silence as "feeling empty" or "blanking out." Eventually, in the 34th week of treatment, she said: "I know I am silent, but before I will be able to use the couch—I feel there is an in-between step. I must be able to ask myself, when I am silent, what am I feeling? Not just I feel empty, but why am I empty, and that will take a long time yet."

The adolescent, certainly the younger adolescent, has a capacity to comprehend what is involved in the analytic work, is introspective, and seeks better self-knowledge, but he cannot permit himself to relinquish ego control, even temporarily, and to lose himself in his transferences and associations. This fear of passive surrender will clearly have different genetic roots in different individuals, but at this developmental level generally relates to the adolescent's terror of the intensity of id pressures and the emotional turmoil of his inner world.

Adolescents can establish a good treatment alliance, but their conflicts over dependency often interfere. Malcolm, seventeen, read Freud so that he could be self-sufficient and analyze himself. Defensive reasons were not far to seek. Transference revival of oedipal longings were ushered in with an attack on Freud's paper on Little Hans and followed by a weekend when he experienced "a flash of insight." He reported that he had suddenly become aware that his transference longings, intensely experienced in the present during the weekend break, were revivals of childhood feelings and that his response to reading Freud's paper was a defensive intellectualization.

Quite a number of our older adolescents use the couch and are prepared to try to free associate. Richard, age sixteen, referred himself in fear that he might mess up his school-leaving exams. He also felt depressed and extremely isolated. From the beginning of analysis he showed a good propensity for forming a treatment alliance. He reacted to initial clarifications by expansion of relevant material, he continued working between sessions, and he frequently made links with material that had previously emerged. He came to his sessions when he did not want to, recognizing that to stay away would be his loss. The analytic material centered primarily on the urgent problem of suicidal wishes, defenses against aggression, and the wish for and fear of closeness. But he remained cut off from his past and very much involved with current difficulties. When work on oedipal problems began, it was initially guilt-provoking rather than guilt-relieving, and, for the first time, genuine resistance set in. After much working through of oedipal material, he began to allow himself much more "freely floating thought" both within the session and by himself. He also began to remember dreams and to bring memories of his childhood. His main interest and concern, however, remained with his current difficulties and with the future, rather than with the reconstruction of the past.

Let me sum up briefly what has emerged from this attempt to construct a developmental line for the capacity for insight: from the infant's transitory awareness of pleasurable and painful feeling states to the adult's detached and objective self-observation with an intrapsychic focus which, together with the ego's integrative functions, bring insight into useful psychic contexts. And let me, then, try to answer some of the questions posed at the beginning.

Under-fives have a limited capacity for the kind of self-observation that leads to awareness of wishes, feelings, and, quite often, to some awareness of their difficulties. It is not easy to mobilize this into a treatment alliance because of the divergent aims of the child and the analyst; the former seeks gratification, the latter understanding. Although the child's capacity to reflect will be accelerated and his self-knowledge widened as a result of the analytic work, the young child lacks the necessary cognitive skills to gain "objective" insight.

The impetus of *latency development* turns curiosity and interest toward the external world. Although the cognitive capacities for insight are more readily available, the latency child's participation in the analytic work will fluctuate. He will resist introspection and insight into inner conflicts and will look for environmental solutions and external changes.

Adolescents are introspective, think about themselves, and use their intellectual capacities to gain fuller understanding; and they have the potential for gaining objective insight into unconscious motivation and conflict solutions. But they are less interested than adults in piecing together their past because their current difficulties and apprehensions about the future absorb them so completely.

We can see that the thrust of developmental and maturational forces, which promote progressive development will, all along, determine and influence the child's greater involvement with his *present and immediate* concerns than with *his past*. This must be an important reason why, generally, we do not aim, in child analysis, to reconstruct for the child a true and "objective" picture of his past, but focus on dissecting his adaptations to the pressures he feels operate on him now. This focus, of course, includes tracing past experiences which determined particular modes of his present functioning, but this will serve mainly to provide a conceptual framework whereby he can understand his present difficulties better. We have to keep in mind that, for the *under-fives*, past and present are often merged, not just because of the restricted time span between past and present, but, more important, because of the forward and backward movement of development, the relative ease of regression, the lack of adequate orientation in time-which alone can place experiences in sequence—and the lack of a reality-orientated conceptual memory organization. In fact, the young child lacks an adequate concept of the past. The *latency child* has acquired a concept of the past but emotionally turns away from *his* past. He is involved with his current life and looks for here-and-now solutions to his problems. Even transference feelings, as I mentioned before, are difficult for him to recognize as stemming from the past. In the *preadolescent*, the past is often so vividly revived in the present that the distinction becomes blurred once more; whereas the adolescent is so concerned and overwhelmed by the intensity of current feelings and conflictual wishes that there is no real chance of cathecting the past.

We see the child's difficulties and symptoms as current maladaptations which prevent his taking the next step in development, and our precise treatment aim is to enable him to take this step. What level of insightful understanding is needed for this to occur?

The analytic situation provides opportunities for the child to relive current as well as regressively reactivated past experiences in a new way. On the most primitive level the interaction between child and analyst represents the situation of the infant whose mother can contain, meet, and anticipate her child's needs. When the child analyst understands the child's symbolic play but responds to it in an indirect way (either through play or verbalization), the child will feel understood, although he will not gain conscious awareness of what he is expressing. His feeling understood may represent his past infantile experience of his mother's responding appropriately, with her more sophisticated understanding, to his needs. Much of this "understanding" the child has to take on trust—mother understood what he needed before he could.

Kris (1956) speaks of id aspects of insight or "infantile prototypes," which, he suggests, are more often an oral interchange than an anal one. I want to suggest that the infantile prototype of experiencing the analyst as an expressor of insights relates to the kind of interchange where mother's responses to the child's needs were adequate and led to his feeling safe and understood. I would call this, not an *"oral interchange,"* but an *"oral-phase" experience*. The revival of such experiences in the analytic situation, albeit on a higher level of organization, may make it possible for the child to feel supported and safe enough to become increasingly able to tolerate his painful feelings, a prerequisite of analytic work.

Our work with children is aimed at fostering self-awareness and self-knowledge. With under-fives this usually goes hand in hand with the developmental process itself. The analytic work fosters the child's ability to contain and verbalize wishes and feelings, and to reflect. Indeed, the way in which parents have helped the child deal with his feelings during his early development may have influenced his capacity for self-awareness and insight. "I know you are angry, but hitting the baby hurts him" may enhance his self-knowledge more than a command "not to be naughty." It also introduces a sequence of cause and effect and the notion of looking for motivation, it is certainly a technique we use widely in our therapeutic work with under-fives.

The analyst's interventions organize and articulate what the child is experiencing. Whenever the analyst interprets and expresses "his insights" in terms that the child is capable of understanding, some new integration will take place. However, as I have tried to show, children are not actively motivated to seek insight, and very often even defend against its acquisition. The need to be compliant, the wish to please the therapist and to get approval, will help reinforce a wish for understanding, and this wish will ultimately contribute to the treatment outcome.

However successful the outcome of treatment may be in terms of making new adaptations and progressive moves, children do not usually fully internalize the analyzing function, nor do they acquire a full dynamic and genetic understanding of their unconscious conflicts. The insights gained usually permit a better grasp of current conflict situations and lead to new ways of meeting them; but such insights will not necessarily help the child deal with conflicts at later developmental stages. As part of the infantile amnesia, the pre-latency child will usually repress much of the "analytic insights" gained during treatment, and older children often cannot recall much of what transpired in their analysis. We must assume that their "analytic understanding" becomes absorbed into the general experiential matrix. This, perhaps, is what happened to Little Hans who, when interviewed years later, had no apparent recollection of his famous and apparently successful childhood therapeutic experience.

Summary

I have traced a developmental line for the capacity for insight. The conclusions reached are based on psychoanalytic material gathered from treatment cases at the Hampstead Clinic over the past 25 years. I have elaborated on the relevance these conclusions have to techniques employed in the analysis of children.

Notes

* Presented at the Anna Freud-Hampstead Center Symposium held by the Michigan Psychoanalytic Society, November 11, 1978. The members at various times were: Maurice Apprey, Pauline Cohen, Audrey Gavshon, Ann Hurry, Hansi Kennedy (Chairman), Dr Edhud Koch, Laurie Levinson, Stephanie Smith, Helge Staby, Robin Turner, Catherine Weinmann, Marie Zaphiriou.

1. For an excellent historical review of Freud's views, see Bush (1978).

References

Bush, M. (1978). Preliminary consideration for a psychoanalytic theory of insight: Historical perspective. *International Review of Psycho-analysis*, *5*: 1–13.

Freud, A. (1965). *Normality and Pathology in Childhood.* New York: Int. Univ. Press.

Freud, S. (1913). On beginning the treatment (Further recommendations on the technique of psycho-analysis, I). *Standard Edition, 12.*

Freud, S. (1915). Instincts and their vicissitudes. *Standard Edition, 14.*

Hatcher, R. (1973). Insight and self-observation. *Journal of the American Psychoanalytic Association, 21*: 377–98.

Katan, A. (1961). Some thoughts about the role of verbalization in early childhood. *The Psychoanalytic Study of the Child, 16*: 184–8.

Kennedy, H. (1971). Problems in reconstruction in child analysis. *The Psychoanalytic Study of the Child, 26*: 386–402.

Kris, E. (1956). On some vicissitudes of insight in psychoanalysis. In *The Selected Papers of Ernst Kris* (pp. 252–71). New Haven: Yale Univ. Press, 1975.

Meyerson, P. (1965). Modes of insight. *Journal of the American Psychoanalytic Association, 13*: 771–92.

Miller, A., Isaacs, K., & Haggard, E. (1965). On the nature of the observing function of the ego. *British Journal of Medical Psychology, 38*: 161–9.

Rees, K. (1978). The child's understanding of his past. *The Psychoanalytic Study of the Child, 33*: 237–59.

Richfield, J. (1954). An analysis of the concept of insight. *Psychoanalytic Quarterly, 23*: 390–408.

Sandler, J. & Rosenblatt, B. (1962). The concept of the representational world. *The Psychoanalytic. Study of the Child, 17*: 128–45.

Strachey, J. (1934). The nature of the therapeutic action of psychoanalysis. Reprinted in *International Journal of Psychoanalysis*, 1969, *15*: 127–59.

Yorke, C. (1965). Some metapsychological aspects of interpretation. *British Journal of Medical Psychology, 38*: 27–42.

PART THREE

CONFLICT AND DEVELOPMENTAL DISTURBANCES

Introduction

In 1981 Kennedy formed a study group on Developmental Disturbance with the aim of clarifying the concept. The intent was to look at the way a child coped, or failed to cope with developmental tasks, to locate where and when development deviated and began to give rise to pathology, and to identify the contribution of constitutional, maturational and environmental factors. Clarifying the technical concept of "developmental help" also became part of the task. A number of these papers foreshadowed this work, while others came after the formation of the study group.

In 1975, Kennedy co-authored a paper with her colleague at the Hampstead Clinic, Maria Berger, entitled "Pseudobackwardness in children: Maternal attitudes as an etiological factor". Here they began to make a distinction between disturbances resulting from neurotic conflict and those arising from faulty development. As members of a Hampstead Index Research Group, Kennedy and Berger examined fifty cases of children with difficulties. Most of these learning problems were the result of deficits in the children's basic equipment; however, in seven children there was clearly the potential for normal development. In these seven children, normal developmental progression was compromised by conflict or environmental inadequacy. While there were many differences in these children's backgrounds, the commonality between them was the mother's attitude toward them, which influenced developmental processes. While conflicts were evident in all of these children, what accounted for their learning difficulties ameliorated by analysis was the development of a distorted self-representation as opposed to neurotic conflict.

In another paper, published in 1978 with colleagues Rose Edgcumbe, Joseph Sandler and Clifford Yorke at the Hampstead Clinic, Kennedy examined the analyses of three children from the viewpoint of psychopathology ("Some reflections on infantile neurosis"). Taking the notion of infantile neurosis as internalized conflict occurring at the oedipal phase of development with consequent drive regression to earlier fixation points, they considered contrasting ways the past influences the development of psychopathology. The authors emphasized the importance of differentiating the contribution of pre-oedipal anxieties that are carried forward into the oedipal phase from their regressive revival. From an object relations perspective, they suggested that early modes of relating develop a degree of autonomy and influence the way later conflicts are managed. Implied is the idea that developmental psychopathology is a fertile breeding ground for later structuralization.

In 1980 Kennedy joined again with Clifford Yorke to write "Childhood neurosis vs. developmental deviation: Two clinical case histories". This paper provided relatively detailed clinical examples of the two kinds of psychopathology wherein the contrast is made between a regression to previous developmental phases that is sought defensively and the distorted developmental process that ensues when a faulty early object tie impedes normal progression.

In the same year Kennedy and Marion Burgner produced a paper on types of sado-masochistic behavior in children, an effort that was the culmination of a Research Group on Sado-Masochism conducted at the Hampstead Clinic ("Different types of sado-masochistic behaviour in children"). Sado-masochism had been addressed previously in the psychoanalytic literature, but Kennedy and Burgner were interested in approaching the concept from a developmental perspective. This point of view led them to structure yet another developmental line, this one grounded in psychopathology and a disturbed mother-child relationship which thus affected the normal process of separation and individuation. The normative anal-aggressive phase was distinguished from a pervasive sado-masochistic pattern, a distinction highly relevant to treatment technique.

In "Steps from outer to inner conflict viewed as superego precursors" (1982), Kennedy, along with Yorke, continued her study of conflict and structure formation. The authors detailed the developmental steps required for external prohibitions to become internal restrictions, and in interaction with other developmental advances, contribute to a structuralized superego.

A Study Group at the Hampstead Clinic was chaired by Kennedy beginning in 1981 with the intent of clarifying the concept "developmental disturbance" and the technique of "developmental help". The paper "The developmental roots of self-injury and response to pain in a four-year-old boy" authored by Kennedy and George Moran arose from this research. The clinical material presented illustrated Anna Freud's idea that personality formation relates to the progression of developmental lines and their interaction. The relative harmony of this interaction was said to predict for adaptive or maladaptive development. It was not only the analyst's interpretations that helped this child, but these in combination with the actual relationship with a benign and trusted object who provided words for difficult feelings, thus presenting himself for containment of affects and as an object for identification.

Kennedy's interest in cases of developmental pathology in contrast to neurotic pathology was continued in a number of papers over the remainder of her career. In "For and against child placement: A clinical illustration" (1985) she departed from her usual pattern of exploration of intrapsychic development to describe the case of a child in the Anna Freud Centre Nursery School whose development reached a crisis point due to significant, ongoing disturbances in the home environment. While a strong tie to her unstable mother had been a source of good ego development for this child, it was also at the root of the child's incipient pathology. Kennedy was interested here not only in the roots of developmental pathology but also in the value of efforts by a team of care-giving professionals to help maintain the positive aspects of the relationship with her disturbed parents despite the negative influence her life at home had on her personality.

Another of Kennedy's papers describing developmental pathology involved the case of a young boy whose older brother died of a chronic neurological illness when the patient was eight years old ("Growing up with a handicapped sibling", 1985). This young boy had grown up in an environment where the primary focus of concern was on the ill sibling, and Kennedy's analysis of the surviving child conveyed the consequent distortion of development, particularly in the area of management of aggression. Again, one sees her careful clinical characterization of the difficulties of progression when the environment cannot support or foster adequate development.

The paper "Trauma in childhood: Signs and sequelae as seen in the analysis of an adolescent", published in 1986, stands as a superb culmination of Kennedy's thinking about memory, insight, reconstruction, and developmental psychopathology. She returned to the case of Peter, the adolescent about whom she had written with Clifford Yorke in 1980, to exemplify the role of trauma as a catalyst for developmental disharmony and distorted structuralization. Trauma in pre-latency had cemented an already troubled primary object-tie and precipitated the consolidation of the development of anal-aggression into perverse sado-masochistic modes of relating in a young boy. He defended against profound depression via violent, torturous masturbation fantasy. The analysis raised many of the technical considerations about which Kennedy had previously written, including Peter's tendency to use reconstructive interpretation to gratify his sado-masochism rather than as insight for productive adaptation. The idea of trauma as the seed of extensive developmental disharmony was given credence in the analytic work, as all avenues pursued in the analysis led inevitably to experiences surrounding the early traumatic event. Regarding the technique of reconstruction, Kennedy found it useful to organize her interventions around the early trauma as well, as they appeared to provide the best intrapsychic fit for the patient.

The final paper in this section on conflict and developmental disturbance is one published with her colleague George Moran in 1991 ("Reflections on the aims of child analysis"). It is an extended and revised version of a paper presented at the International Scientific Colloquium on "The Impact of Developmental Considerations on the Aim of Child and Adult Psychoanalysis" held at the Anna Freud Centre, October 1989. In this paper Kennedy integrated a number of ideas about psychopathology and technique derived from her work and that of her colleagues. Taking a developmental approach, the authors described both intermediary and outcome aims in child psychoanalysis, noting that intermediary aims change as the analysis progresses, affecting technique. These aims are governed by phase-specific developmental capacities, delays, and deficits, as well as conflict and defense. Outcome aims were considered in terms of structural change, influenced by a change in pathological solutions to conflict or ongoing deficient structure formation.

CHAPTER SIX

Pseudobackwardness in Children: Maternal Attitudes as an Etiological Factor*

Maria Berger and Hansi Kennedy 1975

Foreword by Anna Freud

The successful negotiation of developmental sequences needs in every child's case a happy combination of internal and external circumstances. Where cognitive development and mastery of the inner and outer world are concerned, the indispensable elements include a large number of factors such as: the intactness of organic and sensory equipment; its environmental stimulation at appropriate periods; on the ego side, the smooth progress from primary to secondary functioning, i.e., from the pleasure principle to the reality principle; on the side of the drives, the transfer of energy from sexual curiosity and scoptophilia to neutralized pursuits; on the superego side, the absence of inhibiting and limiting prohibitions; on the parental side, the presence of positive response to every forward step. The very multiplicity of factors needed to ensure progress is reflected in the multiplicity of disorders affecting orientation, active mastery, intellectual growth, including the various learning disturbances and school failures. We regard as genuinely backward those cases in which the causes for the defect are located in the basic equipment of the mental apparatus, and we use the diagnostic label of pseudobackwardness when the primary potential for normal development is present, but is interfered with secondarily either by internal conflict or by inadequate and detrimental environmental responses.

The case histories which follow are meant to illustrate the last-mentioned of these possibilities. The life stories and analytic explorations of these children show that at birth and during their first year of life, they did not significantly differ from other infants, i.e., that constitutionally they were well within the norm, with their drive and ego potentialities intact. Moreover, with regard to parental handling, they were neither abandoned, neglected, nor maltreated. There was only one factor missing in their lives and this due to their mothers' own personality difficulties: there was no parental pride and pleasure in the child; accordingly, there was a complete lack of the admiring approval from the parents' side which acts simultaneously as a reward for achievement and as a powerful spur and encouragement toward further efforts in the same progressive direction.

It is a sobering thought that within the complex mesh of influences which shape the life of any individual child, the presence or absence as well as the quality of any single ingredient should have such power to determine the developmental result.

The phenomenon of "pseudobackwardness," referred to in the literature as "pseudodebility," "pseudoimbecility," and "pseudostupidity," has attracted the attention of analysts for a great many years. As long ago as 1910, Ernest Jones wrote of "Simulated Foolishness in Hysteria." In the '30s and '40s several analysts, among them Landauer (1929), Bornstein (1930), Oberndort (1939), and Mahler (1942), described their clinical experiences with such children and their understanding of the relevant pathology. Subsequently Heliman (1954) described her observations of mothers of children with intellectual inhibitions, and Stayer (19530, Buxbaum (1964), and Sprince (1967) discussed the part played by parents in certain learning disorders.

These writers are basically in agreement with each other in their main conclusions:

1. These children do not wish to understand, to know, to see; and this defensive "ignorance" pertains especially to sexual matters.

2. These sexual matters formed part of a family secret, mostly a guilty secret, concerning the sexual lives of parents (either as a couple or as individuals), or of close relatives. They involved the child, more or less directly, as an observer or participant (Mahler, Sprince).
3. The parents unconsciously needed the particular child to be "stupid" or "ignorant."
4. The child responded by conforming to his parents' need in order to preserve their love.

Heliman, Buxbaum, and Stayer discussed the effects of the mothers' personalities on the functioning of the pseudoimbecile patients. Hellman stressed the effects of the mothers' extensive use of denial and lying on the pathology of these children.

The emphasis in all these papers is on the impairment of the childrens' ego functions and on the inhibition of curiosity and scoptophilia which result from the children's unconscious collusion with their mothers in the need not to know the parental secrets.

In the course of examining cases of learning disturbances recorded in the Hampstead Index we came upon another etiological factor that was striking enough to merit investigation. There were about fifty such cases which varied in their severity and spread. Some were children who had specific difficulties, e.g., with reading or arithmetic; others had a more general learning inhibition. At the extreme end of the scale we found a group of seven children who were considered by their parents, or their teachers, as backward, but who, on testing, proved to have at least average intelligence and who lost their "backward" mode of functioning as a result of analysis. Our attention was caught by the fact that in all these cases one could discern specific maternal attitudes which appeared to have had an adverse influence on the children's development from the start. This study is focused on these children.

For the purpose of this paper, however, we have selected only four cases out of the seven, since these four children were especially well known to us. All four had undergone long analyses. Two of them were observed from their infancy or early childhood onward. In addition, the mothers of two children also underwent analyses with members of the Clinic staff.

Case presentations

Case 1

Jane was referred to the well-baby clinic when she was only a few weeks old. From the age of 3 to 5 she attended the Clinic's nursery school. At 5 years of age she was referred for a diagnostic investigation and subsequently went into analysis for four years.

Jane's birth was uncomplicated. Breast feeding was established during the mother's two-weeks' stay in the hospital. However, as soon as Mrs J. returned home and took over the care of her baby, major problems over feeding began. Jane usually fell asleep after taking a few gulps of milk, only to awake screaming as soon as she was put in her cot. Mrs J. became depressed, physically exhausted, and quite unable to take care of her child. The doctor arranged for both mother and daughter to be readmitted to the hospital so that care could be taken of both. Jane is said to have thrived on feedings supervised or offered by the nurses, and the mother was advised to supplement breast feeding with the bottle. Mother and baby appeared to settle down and a more satisfactory feeding routine was established. As soon as they returned home, however, and the mother was again unsupported in the care of her daughter, the struggle over feeding was revived; gradual improvement occurred only after weaning and the introduction of solids. Mrs J. spoke of Jane "refusing" breast and bottle as if she experienced these difficulties as an act of aggression or deliberate withholding. Later she referred back to the early feeding problems by saying, "I tried to do all the right things but could not stand this thing making demands on me."

The mother always complained to the well-baby clinic staff about Jane. For instance, she spoke of Jane's "shyness," calling it a "symptom" she found "difficult to tolerate and hurtful to my pride." There are many references in the baby clinic records to the mother's unfavorable comparisons of Jane with other children, often boys, and to Mrs J.'s derogatory remarks. She described the baby at 14 months as "unintelligent," and readily expressed a strong wish to get away from Jane. Whenever there was an overt sign of physical hurt, Mrs J. seemed especially unable to deal with Jane's needs.

From early on the well-baby clinic staff was concerned about Jane's slow development and immaturity, which they linked with inadequate mothering and lack of stimulation. All along, the staff tried to find ways in which to stimulate Jane's physical and psychological development, but somehow the manner in which the mother carried out their suggestions precluded any positive outcome. The mother's inability to answer Jane's emotional needs was striking. While the mother complained of Jane's lack of contact with her, she was not aware of her own lack of contact with her baby.

Jane was late in sitting up as well as in starting to walk and was found to be generally poorly coordinated. She suffered from frequent ear, nose, and throat infections. For the mother, these were signs that there was always something wrong with Jane's body. When Jane was 17 months old, toilet training was initiated. The mother was alternately strict and indulgent, and Jane was late in gaining bowel and bladder control. Her early refusal to feed later changed to excessive greediness and grasping for food, and she developed particularly messy eating habits, all of which irritated the mother.

When Jane was 3 years old, the well-baby clinic recommended that she attend the Clinic nursery school in the hope that this would counteract some of the adverse environmental influences and offer the child opportunities for new experiences to further her development. Entry into the nursery school coincided roughly with the birth of Dan. The mother, unlike her early reactions to Jane, took great pleasure in her baby son. Dan thrived and was an outgoing, active, and friendly baby. There were no feeding difficulties with him.

Jane reacted to her brother's arrival with a massive regression. Not only did she lose her recently acquired bladder control, but she started to eat and smear feces. The mother reported that while she was feeding Dan, Jane often wandered off, sometimes even outside the house. Mrs J. did not understand Jane's behavior as a reaction to her breast feeding Dan, but saw Jane's wandering away as clear evidence of her daughter's lack of attachment to her. It seemed that at this time Jane turned to her father and attempted to elicit mothering from him, but he found her too demanding and became irritated by her attempts to cling to him.

Nursery school observations of Jane's play, object relationships, and excessive autoerotic activity confirmed her immaturity and slow development. She was preoccupied with messy sand-and-water play that was not considered age-adequate. She was described as possessive and bossy with her friends; she often withdrew into a corner to suck her thumb or masturbate. Most of the time she appeared clumsy, vacant, drooling, and smelled of urine; occasionally she soiled. She was miserable, unhappy, and unlikable.

There was no significant change in the child's behavior and she did not appear to benefit from the educational opportunities offered by the nursery school during her two years' attendance. The staff became increasingly convinced that Jane was intellectually backward and she was referred for psychological testing. She was found to have a high-average intelligence (on the Merrill-Palmer Test). This unexpected test result led to her referral for analysis.

Although Jane was potentially pretty, at the beginning of treatment her appearance and demeanor clearly reflected her self image of a dirty, messy, stupid, unwanted little girl.

Transference manifestations and fantasies during analysis strongly suggested that Jane had complied with the mother's image of her and that this devalued self image was later reinforced by conflicts centering on penis envy. It is not surprising that penis envy became the focus of her developmental problems, because her entry into the phallic phase largely coincided with the birth of her brother.

Many of Jane's fantasies expressed her intense wish to be a boy. There was evidence in the analytic material that she had experienced a tonsillectomy, at the age of 4, as castration. For example, Jane would play with a doll which she said was a boy. This boy was then punished for being naughty by the doctor, who did something to his mouth and turned him into a little girl. Jane's wish to be a boy was reinforced when her mother displayed her obvious affection for and pleasure in her newborn son. The fact that the father also was an unsatisfactory oedipal object for Jane further contributed to her inability to make developmental progress. It was not until after one year of analysis, when a great deal of work had been done on tracing the various sources of her intense penis envy, that Jane became established in the positive oedipal phase.

After about two years of treatment the first signs of a more benign image of herself slowly emerged. Jane expressed the fantasy of once having been "a pretty baby in blue socks." She progressively began to refer to herself as a nice and good girl. She expressed genuine surprise when she discovered that she was able to accomplish something without assistance. Until then, in the transference, Jane had often seen the therapist as the mother for whom she had to enact the role of the retarded child. It would seem that only as a result of a great deal of working through in the analysis, Jane could develop a self image that was not a direct replica of her mother's image of her.

The arrival of a second brother during the last year of analysis briefly reactivated some of Jane's earlier conflicts, but did not unduly disturb her. By the end of the treatment this clumsy, late-developer found particular pleasure in such physical activities as skipping, ball games, cycling, skating, swimming. She discovered many other interests: she greatly enjoyed learning to play the recorder; she liked cooking and "making things" and talked about wanting to become a mother. Her achievements in primary and secondary school were average to good. At present Jane is preparing for a career as a social worker.

Jane's case was clearly one of pseudobackwardness in which the interferences with development stemmed initially from the mother's attitude toward her, and only secondarily from the child's own conflicts.

With regard to the question of etiology, it is important to note that when Jane was a baby, the well-baby clinic observers never noticed any sign of protest from her. This degree of resignation could suggest that Jane was a particularly placid baby. It could also point to an early acceptance by the child of the role assigned her by the mother. Such an acceptance may have been the only way open to Jane to retain contact with her mother, who was otherwise "unavailable." Conversely, to protest against this imposed role may have been felt by Jane as a threat to whatever feelings of safety she had, inviting a total rejection, or even abandonment, by the mother. Her security and safety in her environment probably depended on compliance with the mother's unconscious need to perceive her as damaged. But any feelings of safety maintained in this way would be achieved at the cost of developmental progress. We assume that a well-functioning child wishes to please his parents by his success in learning and developing. Jane seemed to have had little experience of being praised and admired, and the effects of her mother's customary disparagement in the face of any achievement could hardly have spurred her development.

The mother's unconscious need to see Jane as inadequate and damaged constantly impinged on her ability to make more realistic appraisals of her baby. Moreover, she saw this firstborn infant as rejecting and attributed hostile intentions to her baby from the very beginning. We suggest that the mother's defensive externalizations made it impossible for her to pick up cues and respond appropriately to her baby. The baby's slow development later confirmed to the mother her view of the child as damaged.

Jane's acceptance of, and identification with, her mother's view of her may have been intensified by the fact that there was no one in Jane's life—prior to her entry into analysis—who had a different image of her. Gradually her own developmental conflicts enhanced this imposed image of herself. Analysis revealed, among other things, how her intense penis envy was bound up with her parents' preference for her brother and constantly reinforced her already vulnerable self-esteem.

Case 2

Yetta was well known to us from the age of 3 when she was first referred to the Clinic. From then on she and her mother were in contact with the Clinic and were visited at regular intervals by the social worker. From the age of 12 to 18 Yetta was in analysis. Her main referral symptoms were bed wetting, sleep disturbance, excessive clinging to mother, and temper outbursts. Questions about the level of her intelligence, however, had been raised from her first referral at the age of 3.

Yetta was tested on three occasions. (1) At 3 ½ her IQ on the Binet (Form L) was 88, and the psychologist commented that she was "a dull little girl, cooperative but never gave the impression of being any brighter." (2) At 8 ½ her Binet IQ was 92. On this occasion a different psychologist noted: "Yetta does not seem bright and in some tests she gave somewhat strange stupid answers." (3) At 16 ½ her IQ score on the WAIS was 98.

At school Yetta's attainment tended to be below average. At 6, she was not moved up with her classmates. At 8, her teachers thought her dreamy and withdrawn, but doing reasonably well except in arithmetic. At 11, she did not pass the selective examination to grammar school. When she came into analysis she had difficulties in several subjects. In the course of analysis her learning improved so much that she was transferred to a grammar school, where she obtained several "0" levels.

Her analyst, an experienced psychologist, thought that Yetta's real IQ was closer to 115–120. Yetta's intellectual underfunctioning showed itself more during the intelligence testing than at school. In this respect she differed from Jane; but, like Jane, she impressed several trained observers as being dull. To quote from one observation: "Yetta gives the impression of being very dull intellectually and of having just picked up phrases from her mother."

Yetta was the child of an unmarried mother; her father deserted the mother as soon as he knew that she was pregnant. Yetta was brought up by her mother with the help of lodgers, a childless couple who "doted" on the little girl.

Yetta was born prematurely at 6 months, weighing about 4 lbs., and was kept in the hospital for the first 6 weeks. She was breast-fed for 4 months and was weaned gradually to a bottle, which she had till she was 12 months. She did not suck her fingers or a dummy.

In a letter to the Clinic, headed "Complaint," the mother wrote: "Only one thing troubled me—her insatiable thirst. She screamed when we stopped feeding her, so sometimes I had to give her double amount. At that time navel trouble developed so that I was frightened to let her cry too much. In spite of a danger of strangulation the doctor refused to operate on her . . . after a week the navel became alright after all." The "insatiable thirst" may well have denoted the mother's lack of experience, but it also points to her ambivalent feelings toward her baby. The reference to strangulation seems to confirm this.

Toilet training started at 9 months and was carried out "according to the book," i.e., Yetta was held out every two hours. She appeared never to have achieved bladder control at night and enuresis was a major referral symptom. At about 12 months she started to play with her feces, smearing herself, her bed, and the walls. She was not prevented from these activities because her mother did not believe in "interfering with her pleasures." She apparently stopped of her own accord at the age of 2.

Yetta walked at 17 months and started to talk at 2 years. She suffered from sleep disturbance, and at the age of 3 began to refuse to sleep in her own bed. At the same age, she was said to have had "an enormous appetite." She stole food from the larder and from stalls. At that time, her mother began to work, and Yetta was looked after by a neighbor. Subsequently, she was placed in a large nursery.

She was reported to be "very attached" and very clinging to her mother, whom Yetta cuddled and stroked when mother was upset.

At 5, Yetta had a long period of separation from mother and home. She contracted pneumonia and spent two months in a hospital and convalescent home. When she returned home, she again went at night to her mother's or the male lodger's bed. This man was highly disturbed. He was said to have been amused by Yetta's overtures to him and permitted her to handle his penis.

Yetta did not know about the circumstances of her birth, which for years remained a "secret." She was merely told that her father was working overseas. Only during Yetta's analysis, at the instigation of her analyst, did the mother tell Yetta the truth.

The mother's attitude toward Yetta's intellectual functioning was highly ambivalent. She reported that she was glad that Yetta was not "an infant prodigy," because her very clever nephew had shot himself at the age of 12 following his parents' divorce and his father's suicide.

Several observers noted that Yetta identified with her mother in her speech mannerisms and use of "wrong words." The mother, too, impressed all the workers who were in touch with her as being dull, yet her dullness also turned out to be a "pseudo" rather than a true dullness. We learned that when she was a child her father had lovingly called her "dumme Liese." As a child the mother had been unable to learn and had been sent to a school for retarded children until it became obvious that she did not belong there. She had almost no education.

There were indications that she needed to have Yetta repeat some of her own experiences. The mother revealed that she herself had been exposed in her childhood to excessive sexual stimulation and had been seduced; and like Yetta, she had been a bed-wetter until she was 10 years old.

The mother claimed that she had very much wanted Yetta. She thought the child was very beautiful and described her as "that wonderful thing that came out of my belly." Later she had fantasies that Yetta would become a "ravishing film star." The child was often photographed, and the mother even managed to attract the attention of journalists to the child. These fantasies appear to reflect the positive side of her ambivalence toward the child. Feelings reflecting the negative side were inherent in many of the mother's worries during Yetta's childhood, for example, that Yetta might suffer from a road accident; in her conflicting wishes about the girl's achievements and future; and others mentioned previously.

It would seem that the underlying motive of the mother's conflicts about Yetta, and especially of the negative side of ambivalent feelings, was her unconscious need to see her daughter as an extension of the "dumme Liese" image of herself as dull, dirty, and enuretic. Apparently, Yetta unconsciously responded to this image by assuming a psuedobackward style of functioning.

Yetta's analytic material showed that her learning inhibition had several determinants. She had difficulty in history and geography, subjects affected by her preoccupation with the circumstances of her birth and the whereabouts of her father.

The therapist saw Yetta's main problem to be her self-devaluation. She reported: "Yetta feels that nothing can go right for her, and no one was more surprised than she when she won the school prize for improvement ... She celebrated the occasion by having an accident in the school playground and hurting her nose. When her improvement in language, history and geography was not matched by her math results, she felt quite sure that she could never expect that, it would be too much to hope."

Yetta brought her therapist newspaper cuttings of herself. Among them were a number of photographs of herself as a young child in fancy dress in which she had won prizes or competitions. She said that her mother had loved to dress her up. In a whisper she added, "I hated those fancy dress competitions. I wanted to be just me, not all dressed up."

The fact that Yetta had no father was seen as an important reason for her low self-esteem. She hated her name, which was her mother's maiden name. Her mother's ambivalence toward her was seen as another major factor in Yetta's devaluation of herself. The mother's conflicting ideals for her daughter—on the one hand, a fantasy ideal of a film star and, on the other, an unconscious "negative" ideal of a dumme Liese"—each affected the child. The former presented her with aspirations she felt unwilling or unable to attain (she wanted to be "ordinary"), while the latter contributed to her need to assume the role of a stupid child.

Conflicts clustering around the problem of her self image, the question of paternity, and her ambivalence toward her mother affected Yetta's thinking and learning, and these factors were more significant than the more usual developmental conflicts.

The origins of Yetta's ambivalence toward her mother must have been multiple—the early separations, the lack of a father, and her mother's dullness. The ambivalence showed itself in her conflict over being like her mother or surpassing her. Yetta's identification with her mother's speech, indeed her "backward." mode of functioning, was probably due to her attempts to find a solution for her ambivalent feelings toward her mother. These efforts would have conformed to her mother's unconscious need to have a child as "dull" as she was herself.

Case 3

Jeremy, who was referred to the Clinic at the age of 6, grew up, like Yetta, in an atmosphere of secrecy. In his case the secret concerned his older brother who was afflicted with mongolism and lived in an institution.

At the beginning of treatment Jeremy presented a picture of real retardation. He lisped, dripped mucus from his nose, could not dress himself or tie his shoelaces. From infancy he drooled continuously and extensively and required medication for lips and chin. His spasticlike hands could barely grasp small objects; his fine motor control was limited. the boy spoke so badly that at one stage his parents had been concerned that he might be "tongue tied" and need corrective surgery. At the start of his analysis his speech was slurred, there was some initial stuttering, and he was difficult to understand. The father was particularly concerned that Jeremy might be limited in intelligence. School reports were not particularly critical, yet Jeremy showed no evidence of readiness to read or write.

At the age of 6, his IQ on the Binet (Form L) was 108, but it was thought to be an underestimate by both the psychologist and the child's analyst. His parents described him as a slow developer. Jeremy started to walk with help as early as 9 months, but could not walk freely for another year. He started to talk late, but when his speech developed at the age of 3, it was fluent and precocious in form and content. Of greater significance, however, was the parents' treatment of Jeremy as a suspected defective. His play was restricted and he was prevented from mixing with other children.

He was never expected to meet any age-appropriate demands; for example, at the age of 7 he still stood passively, expecting and demanding of his mother to dress him, comb his hair, wash his hands, wipe his nose, and clean his bottom. The mother felt he was incapable of doing any of these things for himself.

Jeremy disclaimed responsibility for bowel movements, which in fact were most carefully controlled by him; he was late in achieving bladder control; he remained a soiler until the last phase of treatment, when he was 10 ½. At referral, Jeremy showed massive inhibitions in ego functioning.

The mother had told Jeremy's therapist that she had only wanted one child, preferably a girl, who could be as close to her as she herself had been to her own mother. The first child, a daughter, seemed to have been much loved. However, Mrs A. did have a second child—the mongoloid boy mentioned above. Jeremy was born shortly after the unexpected death of the maternal grandmother. Mrs A. was profoundly depressed and suffered from recurring obsessive thoughts that she had killed her mother. She felt impelled to have another child to make retribution for the mongoloid boy, and Jeremy was born two years later.

The pregnancy with Jeremy was normal, though the mother reported that she had been troubled by transient depressive moods. She claimed that she intensely wanted and eagerly awaited the birth and that she did not worry whether the baby might be abnormal. Jeremy was born three weeks prematurely; the delivery was easy. However, from the beginning the baby impressed the mother as somewhat odd or abnormal because of his poorly developed eyelashes and diminutive fingernails.

Mrs A. had suffered from tuberculosis and was unable to breast-feed any of her children. Jeremy took to the bottle well. Semisolids were introduced at 4 to 6 months and the bottle was given up at age 2, reportedly without difficulty.

Jeremy was always cared for by nannies and au-pair girls, but the mother could not allow any other woman to become close to him. In fact, she selected girls who were soon bound to leave. Jeremy was not supposed to mind the loss of au-pairs or the absence of his parents. The parents themselves denied the importance of separations. For example, when Jeremy was 18 months old, he was sent to the country with a nanny. Mrs A. instructed this nanny to start

Jeremy's toilet training during their absence from home. He began urinating in the pot at age 2 and was dry at night when he was 3, but continued to soil. The mother herself tried to train him, alternating between angry demands and permissiveness. Later she abandoned the attempts to force him because he became furiously upset and she hoped that he would "eventually assume responsibility" when he was ready. Between the age of 5 and 6 he began to be constipated. During treatment the extent of the mother's unconscious collusion with Jeremy's soiling became apparent.

Jeremy's father always thought of his son as a stranger who was better left to his wife's care. He was rather obsessional in personal cleanliness and during Jeremy's treatment it became apparent that he bitterly resented his son's drooling, wetting, and soiling—so much so that he involuntarily shuddered if Jeremy approached him. In fact, the father had very limited emotional contact with his son. He was away from the family frequently.

From Jeremy's birth onward the parents continually looked for evidence of damage. On the father's side of the family, there was a history of mental illness. The birth of the mongoloid son reinforced fears of hereditary defect for which the father felt responsible. He looked at Jeremy's odd development with anxious trepidation, and found his worst fears confirmed by Jeremy's behavior. The mother, intensely guilty about her "abandoned" mongoloid son, had a distorted view of Jeremy, and thereby encouraged his passivity. Her fear of being "unkind" to Jeremy was so great that she failed to appreciate his pleasure in mastering tasks, achieving control, and becoming independent. She could hardly believe, for example, that he might want to walk to school on his own, or wash and dress himself. At the time of referral Jeremy seemed to have developed in ways that realized his parents' worst fears; he seemed hopelessly effeminate, infantile, and intellectually defective.

Jeremy's therapist had the impression that the mother could not tolerate a masculine child and that her permissiveness with regard to the boy's anality masked her aversion to phallic sexuality. In his infancy she dressed Jeremy as a girl; she still bought him petticoats at the age of 3; she provided him with a dollhouse he did not want. She was terrified by Jeremy's temper tantrums and tried to avoid them by giving in to his wishes at almost any cost. Signs of aggression in Jeremy aroused her fears that he might become a criminal. Yet, at the age of 7, Jeremy's aggression was anything but age-adequate in expres-sion, quality, or quantity. He had outbreaks of rage when frustrated at home, but otherwise he was pathetically passive and restricted.

Jeremy was not supposed to know about his mongoloid brother, who was never mentioned by the parents. However, during treatment there was ample evidence of fantasies about this brother and of Jeremy's identification with him. He frequently presented himself as a stupid, defective, clumsy, neglected child who, in fantasy, was ultimately sent away and killed.

Secrets and mysteries were recurrent themes in his treatment. The connection between his soiling and the secret surrounding his brother became clear. More and more often, a reference by the therapist to Jeremy's soiling or to his fear of rejection, would be followed first by resistance, then by material about mysteries and secrets. Sexual curiosity was perceived as dangerous by Jeremy, who clearly showed his fear of looking at, or knowing about, forbidden things.

At the start of treatment, Jeremy's self-esteem was depressingly low. He considered his body as bad (smelly) and not functioning properly (it could not retain feces). He felt he could neither do nor learn anything. This view of himself accurately reflected his parents' view—that he was a child who needed to be constantly looked after and handled physically, yet who remained distressingly distasteful.

During treatment Jeremy's fear of failure and its consequences began to emerge in his accounts of John, his other self, a boy who was afraid to try, because if he failed, he would be punished by being sent away and destroyed. This explained why Jeremy did not allow himself to try anything until he was certain of a high degree of competence.

In addition to seeing himself as a passive, dependent, soiling child, Jeremy perceived himself as tyrannical, violently aggressive, and omnipotent. He felt isolated and ignored by his parents and peers. He retreated into self-isolated fantasies or regressive anal gratifications via toilet and body care. During analysis he revealed that he both feared and wished to be his parents' defective child.

His work improved considerably in the course of analysis. At the end of treatment Jeremy showed an ability to undertake hobbies, to master games requiring concentration and competition, and to learn new skills. All this confirmed that his tested IQ had, indeed, been an underestimate.

The parents' intense guilt over the conception and subsequent abandonment of the mongoloid son heavily impinged on Jeremy's development from the start. The ongoing fears that he, too, would become abnormal had a later counterpart in Jeremy's fear of failing and being sent away or destroyed. However, there were other factors which also affected the mother's feelings about this son. Originally, she had not wanted another child, and particularly not a boy. Jeremy was conceived to help her cope with her guilt feelings about the death of her own mother and about the birth and abandonment of the mongoloid child.

The mother's negative attitude to Jeremy's masculinity, coupled with her preoccupation with the question of his normality, entered into her tolerance for his soiling and his general incompetence. Jeremy complied with her unconscious demand that he remain a passive baby. Her handling of him conveyed to him her image of an inadequate child. The father's ambivalent attitude to Jeremy reinforced rather than counteracted this image. Apart from these impingements, the mother's physical illness and depressed states during Jeremy's infancy interfered with the early mother-child relationship. To a large extent she was an emotionally unavailable object. In addition, the departure of his first nanny (who left suddenly two months after returning with him from the country) interrupted an intense relationship with a mother substitute. The subsequent coming and going of au-pair girls repeatedly undermined any stability of relationships he may have experienced.

Case 4

Clement's referral to the Hampstead Clinic, when he was 10 years old, was instigated by his headmaster. Clement worried excessively about his work; although he seemed to be trying his best, his scholastic achievements were rather poor. His parents alternated between the view that Clement was mentally retarded and the view that he was "morally retarded" and did not apply himself sufficiently to his work.

The father had had a previous marriage which was dissolved after only a few months: The parents wanted to avoid repeating such a mistake and waited several years before they married. Clement was a planned and much wanted baby, but there were problems from the beginning.

Both parents were emotionally unprepared for the care of their first baby. They were totally unsupported by relatives, since Clement was born abroad in an American hospital. Already at birth he did not fit in with his parents' prearranged plans. Mrs C. showed signs of preeclamptic toxemia toward the end of pregnancy and birth was induced. Breast feeding, too, presented difficulties and had to be supplemented. Clement had colic during the first three months, cried a lot, and both parents resented the disturbed nights. The mother felt tired and depressed and found it difficult to cope with the baby, especially when the family had to move six weeks after Clement's birth. Although a proper sleeping pattern was soon established, Clement continued to be a poor feeder. The mother expressed guilt about having forced him to eat; she had always worried he was not getting enough. Now she regretted that she "had not done what one does with animals; let them eat and leave what they want."

While the mother-child interaction during the first year established a significant pattern for later development and was characterized by the mother's disappointment in her "inadequate" baby and the baby's apparent noncompliance with his mother's expectations, the major pathogenic influences in Clement's life occurred in his second and early in his third year.

Except for a brief separation from mother at 6 months, when the parents went on a holiday, and at 16 months when the mother went to the hospital for her second confinement, the mother always looked after Clement herself.

Clement's toilet training was described as "a great struggle." Although it was started in Clement's first year, he did not become toilet trained until he was 3 ½ years old. In fact, he gained bladder control at more or less the same time as his younger brother, but continued to wet his bed intermittently until 9. Irrespective of the accuracy of the developmental history, there is ample evidence in the analytic material relating to the effects of the tremendous battle with mother over toilet training.

The problem of gaining bladder control was undoubtedly increased by the fact that Clement developed phimosis. The mother had constant difficulty in retracting the foreskin, a circumstance which must have caused considerable discomfort to Clement and involved extensive examinations and manipulations of his penis. Eventually he was circumcised at the insistence of the family doctor, but afterward the mother wondered whether the operation had been necessary. Although she stayed with him in the hospital, Clement is said to have reacted with great distress to the treatment.

These experiences, colored by unresolved anal conflicts, may even have led tQ a premature entry into the phallic phase, and certainly contributed to the intensity of his castration anxiety. The combination of sexual stimulation, pain, and attack on the penis shaped the form of the subsequent phallic and Oedipal conflicts.

Following the operation Clement experienced his mother as even more omnipotent, rejecting, and now also as castrating; and the mother, too, probably now saw her "inadequate" son as even "more damaged." There is ample confirmation from the analytic material that the experiences surrounding the circumcision constituted a major sexual trauma for Clement. The excessive handling of his penis, both exciting and painful, mobilized a massive aggressive response at a time when he already felt rejected by his mother because of the arrival of the new baby. The operation, and especially the anesthetic, was experienced as an assault by his mother on him and his body.

At first, Clement's revengeful hostility found expression in messy and destructive bevahior, but this was met by his parents with severe reprimands and physical punishment, which carried the threat of total abandonment and loss of love for Clement. The rigid standards held up by his parents eventually became internalized and acquired enormous reinforcements from aggressive and sadistic instinctual sources. This punitive, harsh, and sadistic superego largely contributed to Clement's unhappiness and his inhibited and restricted functioning.

When Clement was 16 months his brother was born. He was in the care of his grandparents for 12 days and, although on this occasion he showed signs of distress over the separation, according to the parents there were no signs of jealousy afterward. Much stress was laid on the good relationship between the brothers and by parents and teachers, but the analytic material certainly did not bear this out. Clement's deep-seated hate and envy of his brother was an ever-recurring theme in the analysis and was only thinly disguised at the beginning. In part this was a displacement of his hostility and anger toward his mother for having produced this child and for ostensibly favoring the baby.

The parents described the younger brother as an altogether more satisfactory, bigger, and easier baby; and comparisons must have been made from the earliest time. Physically, the boys were soon of the same size and, as the baby was always developmentally advanced while Clement's development began to lag during his second year, the parents commented that they often thought of their two sons as twins. Clement walked only when he was about 2 years old, while his brother did so when he was just over 1; and in this way the developmental gap gradually narrowed. Clement's speech development was so retarded that his younger brother was said to have talked first. This delayed speech development may well have been linked with the enormous aggression he was trying to contain. Speech certainly became in due course an "aggressivized" activity. In analysis some of his most guilt-ridden material was "unspeakable" and had to be brought in writing. His speech was always difficult to understand, it was slurred, and it was often inaudible.

The younger brother quickly became more successful in almost every area, and especially in his scholastic achievements. While Clement attacked other children as rivals, or provoked their attacks on himself, his brother made friends wherever he went—thus confirming Clement's idea that his brother was better loved by everyone. The unfavorable comparisons with the brother became an integral part of Clement's life. They not only increased, and kept alive, his hostility and murderous wishes; they had a devastating effect on his self-esteem. He felt that his brother was not only better loved but also superior in every respect.

Clement started school when he was 5 and had four changes of school in the next four years. From the beginning he was unhappy and unsettled and his progress was slow. This was usually attributed to his difficulty in adjusting to the many changes. However, his scholastic achievements remained poor. At the time of referral he was in a form below that of his younger brother. Yet, tested on the WISC, he had a verbal IQ of 131 and a performance IQ of 91.

Both parents were irritated by Clement's lack of interests and disparagingly referred to him as "bored and boring." Although the mother was well aware of her disappointment in him, she felt guilty about her irritation, boredom, and impatience with him. There is some evidence to suggest that these attitudes in the mother stemmed from her own unconscious conflicts around penis envy.

Clement clearly experienced his mother as a seducer and attacker, both aspects being reflected in many of their interactions. His highly ambivalent relationship to her not only was based on his need to repeat the early sexual trauma, but also was a way of contacting her, getting close to her, and trying to get her undivided attention. Symbolically, he appeared to relinquish possession of his penis to her; unconsciously, the mother appeared to demand and respond to this. Throughout Clement's development, even during the analysis, the mother appeared to seize every opportunity "to handle" his body. As she was a trained nurse before her marriage, she could readily rationalize these interactions.

In spite of an open preference for the brother, the father, at times, showed sympathy with Clement on the basis of an identification with him as a solitary, withdrawn, and depressed person. As the more compliant partner in the marriage, he at first left the care and upbringing of the children to his wife. He was unable to give her adequate support and help. In later years he began to play the role of martinet; in accordance with his wife's wishes, he became the strict and punitive father who put all the emphasis on discipline. Thus, for Clement, father reinforced mother's rejecting and denigrating attitudes, and failed to provide a satisfactory object for masculine identification.

At the beginning of treatment Clement was a severely inhibited and very depressed boy. His frail appearance, his awkward movements, his inability to communicate, and his initial anxious overcompliance all added to the picture of severe impairment of functioning. The diagnostic assessment raised the question whether he was organically damaged. In spite of his good intellectual potential, indicated by the result of the intelligence test, Clement presented a picture of slow and delayed development from earliest childhood.

It is likely that the mother's disappointment in her baby, based in part on unrealistic expectations about birth and the mothering role, affected her handling of her firstborn. These early experiences probably interfered with the baby's feeling of omnipotence. Furthermore, the experiences surrounding the birth of his brother and the traumatic circumcision caused such severe narcissistic depletion that development henceforth was interfered with by his lowered self-esteem and highly ambivalent object relationships. Clement's aggression, which may at first have been largely reactive, became intolerable and conflictual in the face of his later experiences of retaliation and threatened abandonment by his mother. This forced him into a role of passive submission toward the mother on the basis of a sadomasochistic interaction with her and was at the root of his deep-seated conviction of being unloved, inferior, stupid, damaged, evil, and unlovable. The complete lack of understanding of his difficulties and dilemmas of that time led his parents to react to manifestations of disturbance and stress, which emanated from feelings of rejection and low valuation, in a manner which reinforced them. In the end he completely identified with his parents' disparaging picture of him.

Clement's learning problem was intimately linked with this devalued self image and his inability to compete with his brother; but he also had a problem with concentration. The latter was linked more directly with his sexual problems, his fight against masturbation, and the intrusiveness of his sadomasochistic fantasies. These conflicts were in turn condemned by the superego and thus secondarily contributed further to his devalued and denigrated self image.

Discussion

It is apparent that none of these four children grew up in an environment conducive to healthy development. Their social backgrounds differed, but there were some common and striking features in their emotional backgrounds, most notably their mothers' attitude toward them. This attitude, whether overtly or covertly conveyed, was highly ambivalent on the part of all four (indeed, all seven mothers and it contained a striking need to denigrate the child. Moreover, this attitude appeared to be prevalent from birth onward and, as far as could be ascertained, in some cases was already present during the pregnancy. It may also be significant that three of the children were firstborn babies (six out of seven in the original sample); one, Jeremy, followed the birth of a mongoloid brother.

One can infer that these mothers' fantasies about and expectations of their babies affected their mothering role from the very beginning.

Several of the mothers had a fantasy that they would produce a damaged child. Yetta's parents were not married, and the father deserted the mother during the pregnancy. Jeremy was born three weeks prematurely, and his mother thought that his faint eyelashes and thin fingernails were evidence of mental abnormality. Clement's mother had definite, inflexible expectations of her baby and found him wanting right from the start when he arrived a few days too early and there were slight complications at delivery.

These mothers perceived their children from earliest infancy as damaged or inadequate. With the exception of Jeremy (who was not breast-fed), there were difficulties in feeding. None of the three mothers enjoyed breast feeding and none felt that her baby enjoyed it. All three mothers felt that their crying and dissatisfied babies rejected them and made too many demands on them.

Almost from the beginning the mothers' concern about the physical growth of their babies was matched by their fears about their children's limited intelligence. Although there was no real cause for such anxieties insofar as the early development of the children did not appear significantly deviant, these mothers seized on any unusual aspect in their children in a derogatory and damaging manner. The degree to which maternal attitudes influence the actual developmental processes is, of course, open to speculation. In all our cases the early development was somewhat slow. One may question how far this reinforced the mother's idea that her child was backward, and how far these developmental lags were responses to maternal attitudes and expectations. It is likely that there was a mutual interplay between the two factors in that lack of pleasure and pride in their babies and inadequate maternal stimulation and encouragement may have exacerbated whatever initial difficulties the babies may have had.

It is important to note that the denigrating maternal attitudes centered on only one child and did not extend to the other siblings. In every case in which there were siblings the mothers compared the "denigrated" child unfavorably with them and often showed overt preference for the siblings. This was more prominent in the original sample of seven cases, where Yetta was the only child without siblings. Although we have relatively little information about the fathers' attitudes to these children, the fathers tended to share and reinforce the mother& negative attitudes rather than to counteract them. Yetta, of course, never met her father; Jeremy's and Jane's fathers were frequently away from home because of their professions. In fact, none of the fathers seemed to have actively participated in the care and early upbringing of their children.

Some insight into the origin of such ambivalent and denigrating maternal attitudes could be gained from the analyses of two of these mothers. Their pathology centered around a severely devalued self image and the conviction that they were incapable of achieving or producing anything good. It is likely that the attainment of motherhood mobilized conflicts and intensified their anxieties.

In our small sample of cases we can discern a pattern: the mother assigns a specific role to her child, who is perceived as a not-quite-good-enough baby, an inadequate and damaged product. While three of the mothers almost constantly looked for evidence to confirm signs of damage in the children, Yetta's mother strenuously tried to defend against this by denial and reaction formation. There was little evidence of overt guilt in these mothers about having damaged their children. Rather, they used the children as a vehicle to rid themselves of unwanted aspects of their self images. The role assigned to the child might be viewed as an externalization of those aspects of the mother's denigrated self that she wanted, defensively, to disown. Another important factor may have been the mother's need to perpetuate, in the relationship to that one child, the denigration she herself had experienced from her own mother.

The children we studied appeared to have been unusually compliant in accepting the role allotted to them by their mothers. We assume that this compliance was motivated by a wish to preserve a sense of safety and retain the mother's involvement on whatever basis of mutual interaction existed. In the absence of positive emotional involvement by the fathers, this probably was the only way out for these children.

The analyses of these four children revealed that their main pathology centered around a severely devalued self image and depleted self-esteem. The other presenting symptoms can be viewed as attempts to adapt to this basic problem. Jeremy was encopretic; Yetta and Jane were enuretic; and Clement remained enuretic well into latency. All four children were described as solitary, sad, and unhappy. Their tendency to cling to early body pleasures (soiling, wetting, masturbating) can in part be understood as an attempt to find some pleasure and satisfaction, but this inevitably perpetuated their low self-esteem.

While the functioning of all the children substantially improved with treatment, considerable vulnerability in the area of self-confidence and self-esteem remained. This was least in evidence in Jane, the youngest child in our sample. This suggests that the analysis of the sources and influences of a devalued self image may have greater success in changing the self representation if the denigrated role has not yet been fully taken over by the superego. One could also assume that all four children benefited from some by-product of analysis, such as experiencing the therapist as a new object valuing the child and offering alternative and more beneficial identificatory ideals. Moreover, in their contacts with the Clinic, the mothers' attitudes were sufficiently modified so that they could allow their children to progress. They did not appear, however, to have been profoundly changed, and this seemed to have been true even of the two mothers who were analyzed.

In her study of mothers of children with intellectual inhibitions, Heliman (1954) stated that "the mothers' capacity to understand their children was confined to certain areas only, areas in which the child played the role unconsciously assigned to him . . . To keep the child passive and stupid was a necessity for these mothers" (p. 266). It was linked up, as Hellman illustrates, with the mothers' need to deny the impact of their secrets on their children.

Two of our children grew up with the burden of family secrets. Yetta had to cope with the secret of her paternity as well as with her own secret, sexual experiences with the lodger. But even her secrets were not the only, or even main, cause of her distorted personality development. Nor was the secret in Jeremy's family (the existence of a mongoloid brother) the only reason for his "backwardness." The secrets played, of course, a part in Yetta's and Jeremy's inhibitions of curiosity and therefore in their inability to learn, but they formed only one aspect of the generally pathological attitudes shown toward these children. And there were, to our knowledge, no special secrets in any of the other cases.

Our findings are in agreement with those of Hellman insofar as the mothers in our study also needed to keep their children passive and stupid. However, we found that this need arose from deeper seated motives than a need to preserve a secret. The fact that they saw in their children undesirable aspects of their own selves seemed to us to be crucial. For some of the mothers, their "damaged" children represented their "castratedness" or stupidity; for others, their entire despised self images.

That such impositions of parts of their own self representations upon their children can be carried out by fathers as well as mothers is illustrated by Sprince's case, a boy whose pseudostupidity "was based on a conviction that his father viewed him as part of himself" (p. 106). Underlying this conviction there was a history of sexual play between the father and the child.

In her study of 17 cases of intellectual retardation, Nancy Stayer hypothesizes that in each case the mother had some unconscious need for the child not to learn. She found that some of the mothers themselves had intellectual inhibitions and appeared to encourage their children, whom they identified as parts of themselves, to develop such inhibitions. In at least one of our cases (Yetta), intellectual inhibition was both the mother's and the child's way of adapting to reality.

In researches based on simultaneous psychotherapies of mothers and their children, Johnson and Szurek (1952) described the impact of unconscious parental expectations on the pathology of their children. They observed a specific superego defect in the child which was "a duplication of a similar distortion in the organization of a parent's own personality" (p. 342).

Berta Bornstein (1930) and use Hellman discuss the link between difficulties experienced in the oral phase and intellectual inhibitions. The equation of oral intake and the intake of knowledge was recognized as far back as the writings of Abraham (1927), Fenichel (1937), Glover (1925), and Strachey (1930). Subsequently many analysts stressed the role of oral fixation in reading difficulties and the link between conflicts over oral aggression and such difficulties (M. Klein, 19313); (Blanchard, 1946); (E. Klein, 1949); (Pearson, 1952).

The tendency of these and other contemporary authors is to stress multiple causation of learning difficulties rather than to connect them only with oral conflicts. Among the children of our study, three (Jane, Yetta, Clement) had early feeding problems of one kind or another. Of the three, only Yetta had difficulty in learning to read (Jane's analysis may have forestalled the emergence of such a difficulty). Even in Yetta's case, however, it was the generally disturbed mother-child relationship which had repercussions on the child's development and learning rather than just the feeding aspect of the relationship.

Summary

In the four cases we have described, as well as in the remaining three that were studied, the inhibitions of ego functions were far-reaching. We have defined their pseudobackwardness descriptively, taking as a point of departure the parents' or educators' view of the child. We found, however, that the child's presenting himself in this way was due to his unconscious compliance with the image imposed on him by his mother. To be sure, all the children had neurotic conflicts, but it was not the magnitude of their conflicts which accounted for their generally "backward" way of functioning. We assume that quite early in their development these children adapted to their mothers' perception of them, in order to ensure their mothers' cathexis and to preserve feelings of safety. In that sense these children may be said to have developed as distorted personalities rather than as neurotically disturbed children.

Note

* In collaboration with Don Campbell, Sara Lundberg, and Randi Markowitz. This paper forms part of a Research Project entitled: "Childhood Psychopathology: Pathogenic Processes and Overt Symptomatology." The paper also forms part of the work carried out by the Index Research Group, Chairman, Dr Joseph Sandler. We are grateful to the therapists, staff of the Well-Baby Clinic and the Nursery School for making their data available to the Index.

References

Abraham, K. (1927). The influence of oral erotism on character-formation. In *Selected Papers* (pp. 393–406). London: Hogarth Press, 1949.

Blanchard, P. (1946). Psychoanalytic contributions to the problems of reading disabilities. *Psychoanalytic Study of the Child*, *2*: 163–87.

Bornstein, B. (1930). Zur psychogenese der pseudodebilität int. *Z. Psychoanal.*, *16*: 378–99.

Buxbaum, E. (1964). The parents' role in the etiology of learning disabilities. *Psychoanalytic Study of the Child, 19*: 421–47.

Fenichel, 0. (1937). The scopophilic instinct and Identification. *International Journal of Psychoanalysis, 18*: 6–34.

Glover, E. (1925). Notes on oral character formation. *International Journal of Psychoanalysis, 12*: 131–54.

Hellman, I. (1954). Some observations on mothers of children with intellectual inhibitions. *Psychoanalytic Study of the Child, 9*: 259–73.

Johnson, A. M., & Szurek, S. A. (1952). The genesis of antisocial acting out in children and adults. *Psychoanalytic Quarterly, 21*: 323–43.

Jones, E. (1910). Simulated foolishness in hysteria. In *Papers on Psycho-Analysis* (pp. 141–53). London: Ballière, Tindall & Cox, 1913.

Klein, B. (1949). Psychoanalytic aspects of school problems. *Psychoanalytic Study of the Child, 3/4*: 369–90.

Klein, M. (1931). A contribution to the theory of intellectual inhibition. *International Journal of Psychoanalysis, 12*: 206–18.

Landauer, K. (1929). Zur psychosexuellen genese der dummheit. Z. *Sexualwiss, 16*: 12–22, 87–96.

Mahler, M. S. (1942). Pseudo-imbecility. *Psychoanalytic Quarterly, 11*: 149–64.

Oberndorf, C. P. (1939). The feeling of stupidity. *International Journal of Psychoanalysis, 20*: 443–51.

Pearson, G. H. J. (1952). A survey of learning difficulties in children. *Psychoanalytic Study of the Child, 7*: 322–86.

Sprince, M. P. (1967). The psychoanalytic handling of pseudo stupidity and grossly abnormal behavior in a highly intelligent boy. In: E.R. Geleerd (Ed.), *The Child Analyst at Work* (pp. 85–114). New York: Int. Univ. Press.

Siaver, N. (1953). The child's learning difficulty as related to the emotional problems of the mother. *American Journal of Orthopsychiatry, 23*: 131–41.

Strachey, J. (1930). Some unconscious factors in reading. *International Journal of Psychoanalysis, 11*: 322–31.

CHAPTER SEVEN

Some Reflections on Infantile Neurosis*

Rose Edgcumbe, Hansi Kennedy, Joseph Sandler and Clifford Yorke 1978

Anna Freud has, among much else, stressed a number of important discrepancies between infantile and adult neuroses and has underlined our recognition that a particular type of neurotic disturbance in childhood is not necessarily the forerunner of a similar type of adult disturbance. She has reminded us of the existence of pre-oedipal compromise solutions in addition to those which arise when the superego is more fully structured, and has emphasised the influence of early personality development on subsequent pathology.

In this paper we shall not concern ourselves with the wide variety of childhood disturbances which cannot legitimately be considered neurotic in the traditional sense. We shall confine ourselves to three clinical vignettes of children, analysed at the Hampstead Clinic, who present clinical pictures which appear to arise, at least in part, from internalised conflict. In each case, we shall approach the child's disturbance from the standpoint that it represents the best possible adaptation at his disposal to the inner and outer forces which operate upon him.

Internalised conflict, and its solution by compromise, describes one particular process by which the interaction of these inner and outer forces may be dealt with. It varies in degree, stability, and kind. While all three cases will illustrate the process of internalisation, the role of external factors is different in each one. In the first and simplest of our examples external factors play no more than a precipitating role, and the case shows a classical, regressive retreat from the oedipal stage to a pre-existing fixation point. But as the work of such investigators as Anna Freud and Winnicott has amply shown, there are other children where external reality, however coloured it may otherwise be by externalisations and projections, continues not only to take part in, but to foster and maintain an apparently internalised conflict. This will be illustrated by our second example. And there are yet other children where the external contribution to the internalisation includes the impact of past parental pathology where this has been externalised by the parents on to the child during the course of the child's development, and has now become an integral part of his personality structure. These points will be amplified in the material which follows.

It is convenient to begin with the case of *Clare*. When Clare was seven-and-a-half, her persistent wish to be a boy was so intense that her parents referred her for treatment. Her refusal to wear dresses was absolute and had existed for at least four years. Widely regarded as graceful, beautiful and intelligent, her popularity and social accomplishments did little to offset her unhappiness; and her dissatisfaction was typified when she said to her mother: "There is something spoiling my life because I want to be a Daddy when I grow up."

Clare was the third child of warm and affectionate parents. Her two brothers were two and four years older than herself. Father was able to spend much time at home, both parents shared in the handling and care of the children and Clam was reported to be close to her father even at ten months. When she was two-and-a-half a baby sister was born. By the age of three Clare's fondness for her father bordered on the excessive. It led, on his part, to some irritation and mild withdrawal. During this period the family moved to a new town. Father found a new job which took more of his interest and time, and matters were hardly helped by the six weeks which father spent away from the family while making the necessary arrangements.

There is little doubt, from the diagnostic material alone, that Clare had a close and pleasurable relationship to her mother during her early infancy. This was confirmed in treatment, where she tried to recreate an early, blissful state where mouth-play, bodily pleasure and non-verbal communications prevailed, and where she had not yet encountered any narcissistic blows. The first of these came at the time of her mother's pregnancy. Clare responded by making a premature step towards an even closer relationship with her father, thus fostering an unusually strong and early oedipal tie. Frightened perhaps by this incestuous bond, father appeared to withdraw, and Clare's feelings of sexual rejection reinforced her conviction of maternal disaffection in favour of the sister. The changing family circumstances occasioned by the move may have served to strengthen Clare's view of these experiences. Her response was to abandon her feminine role, and there followed an enormous intensification of her penis envy.

Clare's case shows the classical sequence described by Anna Freud. The child enters an oedipal phase coloured by what has gone before. Oedipal conflict fosters regression, old anxieties are re-aroused, conflict at an earlier phase—namely, the phallic one—is revived, and a compromise solution is found at that earlier level. The wish to be a boy now finds ego expression in that she abandons her femininity and with it, ostensibly, the wish to possess the father. But although she displaces her father and in fantasy regains the mother, she maintains her tie to him through identification. The pattern is therefore one of neurotic compromise, but the solution lacks both the structure and the symbolic quality of an adult symptom. As Anna Freud's work reminds us, the child's solution remains much closer to the conflict it tries to resolve.

Such a classical picture will serve as a point of departure for our next example— the case of *Robert*. While the picture is ostensibly a neurotic one, it is less straightforward than Clare's. We hope to show how the child's disturbance includes an attempt to adapt to a frightening reality.

Robert was in treatment with one of our colleagues from the age of four-and-a-half to six. He had attended our nursery school from the age of three-and-a-half, and his very disturbed behaviour there led to his referral. He was restless, distractible impulsive and unpredictable. He was unable to make friends with any other children or to share in activities with them. On the contrary, he frightened them by his threats and hostility, and the staff needed to protect them from physical danger. His own anxiety was intense, and often issued in screams and panic. His size and sturdiness added to these problems, and reinforced the anxieties of both himself and others. His neat appearance and precocious verbal development appeared oddly adult in contrast with his behaviour, but did little to mitigate matters. Robert therefore presented a behavioural disorder in which lack of impulse control appeared a leading feature. It was not at all clear from the presenting picture what this disturbance signified. We shall now try to indicate how some of these problems were clarified, beginning with some preliminary points which emerged from interviews with the mother.

Robert's mother was a small but explosive woman, whose speech was loud, harsh, rapid and excited. When she spoke of Robert her face was frequently twisted with rage. She attributed her anger with him to his disobedient and provocative behaviour. However it soon became clear that she used him as a vehicle for all kinds of externalisations, and that her contradictory handling provoked a good deal of his confused and anxiety-driven behaviour. For example, she was sexually overstimulating towards him and, although she allowed him to share her bed with much kissing and cuddling, she became instantly punitive whenever his excitement got out of control. Her seductiveness was matched by her distaste and embarrassment in talking of sexual matters. At home, she required instant obedience and could make no allowance for Robert's own wishes and needs. Whenever he complied with all her wishes he was praised as "a good boy"; whenever he failed to do so, or followed his own inclination, he was "bad". Outside the home, however, this mother made endless excuses for Robert whenever he got into trouble. She angrily blamed other children and adults, roundly asserting that Robert was a good child unless provoked. Yet, at the same time, she reproached him endlessly for being "bad" and constantly enquired of teachers and others whether Robert "had been a good boy today?" She was visibly embarrassed and shamed by his public behaviour.

It is not clear when these difficulties between mother and child began. The marriage, of which Robert was the only child, lasted only two-and-a-half years. The mother, who at first found her husband a "charmer", said that she quickly came to see him as selfish, work-shy and unreliable. She suspected him of affairs with prostitutes, of dishonesty, and of criminality. But there is no way of knowing the extent to which this picture was influenced by her own projections. When the parents separated, Robert was only six months old; and he never again saw his father. There followed a period of some depression, and she and her son were confined to a one-room flat until the boy was three. She then seems to have pulled herself together, and began taking him to the park for exercise.

It is difficult to trace the early history with accuracy. The mother described him as a "good baby", and it seems possible that battles between the two began when Robert made the transition from being a passive baby to the relative independence and self-will of a toddler. By the time he entered nursery school at three-and-a-half, the mother complained both of his clinging and of his running away from her. She was acutely embarrassed by his tantrums when she was out with him, and felt compelled to enforce obedience lest he develop the supposedly criminal characteristics of his father. Her loud and furious tirades about his naughtiness, as well as damaging physical attacks on him, bore no relationship to the seriousness or triviality of the occasion.

We turn now to Robert's treatment and to certain theoretical implications. At the very beginning, Robert made violent and uncontrolled physical attacks on his therapist, as well as presenting her with an abundance of destructive and sadistic fantasies. These terrifying fantasies not only indicated his fear of external attack but also his fear of destroying everyone with whom he came into contact. While much of this material was phallic in content and was associated with much castration anxiety, the existence and influence of pre-existing conflict over his sadism and destructiveness, derived from earlier development levels, was readily apparent. Robert's terror, and with it his physical attacks on the therapist, began to diminish in the analysis when certain important aspects of his behaviour were established and recognised. Among these was a major defence of identification with the aggressor which, however, had hitherto only served to increase his anxieties of injuring, and thereby losing, his objects. The sadness, loneliness, and fear of rejection began to come to the surface.

In attempting to analyse and work through the material, a central problem which faced the therapist can only be understood if the terrifying and confusing reality presented by the mother is taken into account. It became necessary to distinguish between those aspects of Robert's self-representation which derived from his own impulses and wishes and those which derived from his introjects and identifications; and also between contributions made to his object-representations by the reality of those objects, as well as by the externalisation on to them of his own instinctual derivatives. His defensive identification with the aggressor included identification with a real aggressor and with an aggressive introject.

The point we wish to emphasise, and the reason we have chosen this example, is that external reality played a great part in determining the clinical picture. Much of Robert's disturbance can be seen as an adaptive response to disturbed reality as it became internalised in him. He was constantly faced with the reality of a mother whose behaviour alternated from sexual seductiveness to hostile reproach and rejection. She gave him a view of himself as dangerously bad and unacceptable and behaved towards him in a way which wholly failed to take into account his wishes and needs. She could neither understand, nor help him deal with his feelings and experiences in a constructive or helpful way.

We can summarise some of the points emerging from this vignette. Robert's therapist felt that, at the time of entering into treatment, he had internalised frightening aspects of his mother, but that these were based on an alarming reality as well as on his projections of his own aggression. He subsequently dealt with this fear of aggression by identifying with the internalised mother. Although this frightening reality and its internalisation preceded structuralised superego formation, it also continued through the oedipal phase and contributed to the subsequent viciousness of the child's superego.

In emphasising these points, we stress the role and the power of projection and externalisation and assert that an introject may be more frightening than a real parent. But we do want to draw attention to the possible effects of the internalisation of a really terrifying parent upon the child. Robert's identification with his frightening mother, while unquestionably defensive, was never fully integrated into his self-representation. He never wholly accepted his mother's view of him in spite of an attempt to integrate this with his own experiences of anger and aggression. While, therefore, his basic self-representation contained the elements of an angry and destructive person, it also contained the picture of a sad and lonely boy who longed for understanding and acceptance from his objects. His aggressive and destructive impulses were therefore all the more conflictual and frightening to him, since he never abandoned the idea of becoming a loving, protective, and constructive person. But the achievement of such an ideal required not only the resolution of his own internal conflicts over aggression, but also the capacity to differentiate between those aspects of himself which were contributed by his mother and those which were contributed by his own processes of externalisation and internalisation.

Our third and last clinical illustration refers to the case of *Sally*, who came into treatment shortly after her sixth birthday. The presenting problems were an extensive learning inhibition, a long-standing disturbed relationship with her mother and asthma. The clinical picture therefore contained a disturbance of ego functioning, a behaviour disturbance the diagnostic status of which had yet to be determined and a condition which might or might not prove to be psychosomatic. In this instance both mother and child were taken into analysis, one with a senior analyst, the other with a therapist at the Clinic. We were thereby afforded an unusual opportunity to see how strongly Sally's early history had been influenced by that of her mother. Indeed, the mother's painful recognition that Sally was, in many ways, recapitulating the experiences and miseries of her own childhood had led her to bring Sally for treatment. She had already managed to see that she reacted to the child as her own mother had done to her. Indeed, it is of some interest that the symptoms of both Sally and her mother were almost identical.

The mother's psychoanalysis suggested that her own parents had been very disappointed that their only child was not a boy. This disappointment was evidently intensified when the child appeared not only dull, but fat and unprepossessing because of overeating. Her learning inhibition was so severe that she could neither read nor write until, in her early teens, she was sent to boarding school. Once there, she thrived both academically and socially, and eventually attained a professional qualification. She married in her late twenties and was upset by an unplanned pregnancy. When her baby turned out to be a girl, her disappointment was intense and lasting.

The mother's early experiences had raised grave doubts about her own capacity for motherhood. Such doubts were at once enhanced by Sally's early feeding difficulties. An attempt to breast-feed the child was soon abandoned as unsuccessful. Sally cried, seemed "colicky" and showed no appreciable gain in weight until she was three-and-a-half months old. She remained a finicky eater until the age of six, when a ravenous appetite soon led to severe obesity. Yet, apart from the feeding difficulties, and two short spells of disturbed sleep at the ages of eight and eighteen months, Sally was described as a sweet and placid baby.

When Sally was four months old the mother returned to her professional work, though not without conflict. Sally was cared for by a trained nurse until she was seven months, and subsequently by a maid until she was two years old. This maid was much beloved and may well have afforded the child her happiest experiences. Sally began to thrive in a gentle and loving relationship. Unhappily, this situation did not last. Not only did the maid leave when Sally was two but, at the same time, the mother gave birth to a boy. The mother quickly returned to work, leaving the children in the hands of a new maid who openly preferred the baby boy. Among other things, this maid would try to force Sally into passing motions and would punish her when she did not comply. By the age of three Sally was becoming so unhappy that the maid was dismissed by the mother. At roughly the same time, Sally was admitted to hospital with a severe attack of measles. When Sally returned home, she began to suffer from attacks of asthma. She already had a tendency to develop a wheeze whenever the pollen count was high, and this had been understood entirely in terms of somatic allergic sensitivity. Mother, too, was similarly allergic to pollen. But now, and henceforth, the attacks increased in both frequency and intensity, and occurred in response to respiratory infections, at moments of excitement, after physical exertion, as well as on occasions when no external stimulus was obvious, though it may be significant that, on such occasions, the mother was always about. Sally would now often wake at night with distressing attacks which would frighten and anger her mother, who anxiously and uncertainly administered medication.

One possible explanation of the increasing attacks is that any form of excitation beyond a certain threshold, whether psychical or not, discharged itself through an available somatic pathway. Further speculation will, however, be postponed for the moment. Whatever the facts of the matter, Sally's disturbance was not confined to the asthma. On leaving hospital, her relationship to her mother became truly and progressively miserable. She became exceptionally demanding, controlling, and abusive. She flew into rages and tantrums, insisting nevertheless that she loved her mother and begging for similar assurance in return. Her clinging to mother increased, but the latter's ambivalence was far too intense to permit consistent action. Her attempts to meet Sally's demands were as helpless as they were hopeless, so that, in the end, she could only react by resorting to rage herself. She found the child "unbearable" and spoke of Sally making "a misery of our family life". Through all this her clear preference for the boy was manifest.

Before turning to the treatment itself, it seems worth remarking that a child who feels of little value to an ambivalent mother internalises a comparable self-image the strength of which is reinforced by the child's own ambivalence. Under such circumstances experience of object loss further reinforce such a poor self-valuation and heightens the conflicts arising from the anal-sadistic phase. The latter found expression in her need to denigrate her objects and control them omnipotently.

The treatment material indicated the nature, origin, and consequences of Sally's profoundly damaging attitude to herself which was keenly experienced, actively defended against, yet constantly acted upon at all phases of her analysis. This was evident from the very beginning of treatment though it was initially centred around her remarkably undefended penis envy. She would say, for example, "I'm a girl, not a boy. Wish I could be king. But I'll be ruler of the land."

Violent swings between love and hate were always evident in the transference relationship. This ambivalence was invariably intensified by holiday breaks and weekends, and represented her response to past experiences and present threats of object loss. She would sometimes deal with this by storming prematurely from the room, shouting at the top of her voice that the therapist was "no good", "horrible" and "stupid". At times her provocativeness and sadism made it almost impossible to get beyond her verbal denunciations, distortions of affect and her imperious and peremptory demands. Nevertheless, her "nastiness" was not simply a response to a failure to meet her needs, but also masked her underlying feelings of extreme anxiety and helplessness,

Sally's great longing to have a uniquely close and binding relationship to her mother appeared to be linked with her early need for a satisfying caring and pain-relieving object; and later interference with need-satisfaction with the subsequent loss of the maid reinforced a premature object tie. It is partly in this light that the early colic and the later asthma have to be viewed. The entire vicissitudes of this child's early development influence the nature, quality and extent of her later difficulties, so that it was by no means simply orality or its residues which coloured her later phases. Nevertheless, oral elements were prominent. Even material which, on the surface, seemed plainly oedipal, nevertheless had a pronounced oral colouring. Some of her doll play illustrated this clearly. For example, the baby girl wants to go to bed with her Daddy. Once there she asks for a drink. The Daddy rejects her with the remark, "you are old enough to do it yourself", whereupon the child cries out "but I am only two".

Treatment now centered around the battle for control. She would threaten to kill the therapist unless the latter read to her. Sally would demand that the therapist choose pleasing stories while she herself would not have to say a word. Reading in the analytic hour came to be understood as a feeding situation in which she obtained exclusive and undivided attention. Yet confrontation with her oral longings aroused tremendous guilt, partly through the re-experience of concomitant and powerful primitive oral aggression. This oral fixation, related to her enormous need to be loved and valued, coloured all subsequent stages of her drive development.

While her wish to be a cared-for and comforted baby was unattainable, so was a conflicting wish to grow up. The mother's lack of pleasure in Sally's achievements meant that forward growth could not be valued and might even invite further rejection. These fears were not without some validity, since Sally was constantly experienced as an extension and revival of the mother's own derogated self. This conflict over growing up played an especially important part in Sally's learning inhibition. Disturbance in her ego achievements had been present from early times. Even as a toddler she often preferred "just to sit and look". Although she initially adapted well to nursery school, she failed to settle down after her hospital admission and became diffident, dependent and dull. Although her IQ. was "high average", and on the test for abstract reasoning even very superior, her intellectual functioning remained far behind her potentialities. Her fear of failure and its association with her self-devaluation seemed important in this respect.

It remains to say something of Sally's asthma and its vicissitudes as these were reflected in the treatment. From Sally's point of view it was her "curse" and, as such, evidence of her damage and castration. There is little doubt, too, that its existence allowed it to be exploited in the interest of regressive phenomena, in that it controlled the mother and kept her tied to Sally, fulfilling need-satisfactions through special bodily care. In this respect the ego development, object relations and libidinal ties, formed in a particular fashion by the realities of this child's early colic as well as by the role of the maid as a comforter, allowed a pre-existing pattern of psychological response to be carried forward into a later phase, where it provided a behavioural matrix in which the asthma was embedded. In addition to all this, the asthma subserved a sado-masochistic relationship, as well as keeping the parents separated at night. In the treatment, one of the most fascinating features of the asthma was the way in which it would disappear soon after the analytic hour began, only to return when Sally again saw her mother at the end of the session. There is, however, no justification for saying that any of these factors were in themselves causal and it is of interest that, as the child's sadness and depressive affect were worked through in the treatment, the asthma also appeared during the analytic hour. One day when the child appeared for her session she was wheezing and ill. The therapist wondered whether Sally should perhaps have stayed in bed. Sally retorted angrily: "You're like my mummy. You don't like the wheeze either." For days she remained cross and distant.

It has been suggested that the asthma, which originated as an allergic response to pollen, may have offered a pre-existing somatic pathway whereby states of excitation, whether psychical or not, were sometimes able to find discharge. We would like to elaborate this suggestion by putting forward the view that, under certain circumstances, the asthma afforded an avenue of discharge for affective states which would otherwise have been intolerably painful. This view is partly supported by the relationship of asthmatic attacks to the working through of depression and sadness in the sessions.

Furthermore, it was striking to observe how, following a rage reaction—in itself an attempt to ward off depression and sadness—she would first become wheezy and then much calmer. It was as if the asthma removed the psychic pressure for the time being. It therefore seems possible that, if the asthma had not existed, depressive affect would have been far more pronounced in the clinical picture.

Some Concluding Remarks

We began our clinical illustrations with the case of Clare. To recapitulate: an internalised conflict arose when a premature move to the oedipal phase, fostered, at least in part, by disappointment in the mother, was followed by feelings of rejection and further disappointment. There was a subsequent regressive reinforcement of phallic wishes and strivings. Nevertheless, reality factors were not wholly unimportant and the profound regressive shift in the treatment situation indicated how significant the earlier phases were in their influence on later development. For Clare, her early positive experiences appear to have fostered an excellent ego development and to have played an important part in restricting and localising her disturbance within the framework of an otherwise intact personality. This may serve to exemplify one of the ways in which past experience contributes to the limitation of later pathology and continues to foster progressive trends.

In Robert's case we also saw the importance of internalised conflict in the clinical picture, but, in addition, we saw how some of his anxieties were appropriate to the situation in which he found himself. Furthermore, in Robert's case, it would not be true to say that we *only* see a revival of fixation points at pregenital levels due to regression from oedipal anxieties. Although there are many elements of neurotic conflict associated with earlier phases, we also observe an overall deviant development occasioned by the fact that the child had to deal with a deviant reality. In particular, we were able to understand the way in which that deviant reality impinged upon him. In Robert's case, his internalised conflict was also maintained and kept in being by the reality. This latter point raises the question of whether, under such circumstances, analysis can do more than achieve limited gains.

Although Sally's case is different from Robert's and is complicated by widespread disturbance in ego-functioning as well as by psychosomatic illness, she illustrates some similar points. While her case again clearly indicates the presence of internalised conflict, it equally demonstrates how profoundly her internalisations are affected by *past* external reality relationships, as well as by present ones. And while, for Sally, the disturbing current reality is more consistent than Robert's, the origins of her internalisations are by now so remote and firmly established that they can be said to have acquired a degree of independence. But more than this. The parental contribution to those internalisations derives, to an appreciable extent, from the *mother's* externalisation of her own past. And while Sally's self-devaluation derives from the mother's projection of her own lack of childhood self-esteem, this again has by now acquired a certain autonomy. Nevertheless, the fact that both mother and child are in analysis affords therapeutic possibilities not present in Robert's case.

It should be emphasised that, in both these children, we are not dealing with any confusion between inner and outer in the sense that this may be experienced by borderline children. Neither Robert nor Sally have any ego defect, though their egos have been strongly affected developmentally by their previous experiences and by the adaptations they have had to make both to internal and external reality.

In our opening comments we referred to infantile neurosis in terms of internalised conflict and drive regression to the fixation points of earlier phases. But this is not the only way in which the past shows its influence on the present in the kinds of disturbance under discussion. In Sally's case it was not difficult to see that later conflict included and reflected the influence of pre-existing conflict which had remained unresolved from earlier phases, and the influence of fixation points is very clear. But in considering, for example, the way in which problems of an oedipal kind are influenced by pre-oedipal development, we must also bear in mind other possibilities. We have to differentiate the continuation of the anxieties of the pre-oedipal phases into the oedipal one from the *regressive* revival of such conflicts and anxieties. The child will try to integrate his new experiences with the old. Some of the old may be revived, but a situation may develop which is essentially different from the reactivation of silent fixation points under the influence of regression.

The beginnings of early character traits in pre-oedipal development may influence the way in which later conflicts are dealt with, though it is a matter of some surprise how wildly at odds symptom-formation and character-formation may be in many children. It is of great interest to study this problem from the standpoint of object relations and to see how modes of relating, which have begun to develop in earlier times, are carried forward into the oedipal period. In some instances, these ways of making relationships develop a certain autonomy. Thus it may be a technical error to regard, for example, some derivative of anality as if the child's wish to defecate on the mother was on the verge of accessibility. This reminds us that the *developmental* viewpoint is not the same as the genetic, let alone the dynamic one; and that questions of economics and structure are also concerned in the problem of adaptation to both internal and external reality. This may mean no more than that, when we speak of the importance of pre-oedipal factors in infantile neurosis, we need to bear in mind our metapsychology. This is not a very novel conclusion, but it may be worth restating.

All of this may give us food for thought about what actually occurs when we make our reconstructions in adult analysis. For we are, perhaps, too readily tempted to take for granted the notion that what unfolds in the treatment of the adult accurately reflects past developments in the internal life of the child.

Note

* The clinical material on which this paper is based is derived from cases analysed at the Hampstead Clinic.

CHAPTER EIGHT

Childhood Neurosis vs Developmental Deviations: Two Clinical Case Histories

Hansi Kennedy and Clifford Yorke 1980

This paper concerns certain important aspects of psychoanalytic therapy with children and presents material from the intensive treatment of two very different cases. One of these concerns a childhood neurosis; the other a disorder of much greater complexity.

It is a unique feature of the Hampstead Clinic that we have some forty to fifty cases in five-times-a-week treatment. Such intensive therapy is at the heart of our program because our work at the Clinic has a threefold function. Two of these arise from the fortunate circumstances that, in psychoanalysis, the method of treatment and the method of clinical research are closely linked. The third arises from the historical circumstance that our organization was founded to meet the need of professional workers who wished to undertake training in the psychoanalytic psychotherapy of children. The advantages which such an intensive approach offers to the trainee are fairly dear. While, in non-intensive work, with its inevitable discontinuity, the operation of the unconscious and its influence on the child's difficulties is often a matter of inference, daily therapeutic contact permits the gradual unfolding of material and allows the student to listen to the voice of the unconscious and to discover for himself its ineluctable effects on the psychic life of the child in a way which cannot escape conviction. For this reason, a training of this kind is not only a valuable preparation for the practitioner of child analysis, but also provides a sound basis for the wide range of clinical approaches which the therapist may later be called upon to practice.

But what, otherwise, are the advantages of five-times weekly treatment when it is such an expensive and time consuming method and when it often imposes further burdens on the child and his family? In truth, five hours a week is little enough in the whole of the child's life, and barely permits the intimate and detailed contact needed for him to share, confide, and expose his thoughts and feelings; and it is little enough time for the therapist to gain insight into the child's inner life, to help him to form a treatment alliance with her which will sustain him through the difficulties of the analytic work. It is scarcely time enough for the detailed unfolding of the analytic material which permits the exposure of past and present phantasies and their ramifications which have contributed to his present conflicts and dilemmas; and which affords adequate opportunities, not only to frame interpretations in the light of analytic understanding, but to work through the manifold aspects of the child's conflicts to facilitate his growth of self-awareness and insight.

These considerations apply with special force to neurotic disturbances where *psychoanalysis* is the treatment of choice. But of course a child's appearance in the consulting room on five occasions each week does not in itself constitute psychoanalysis. There are many children who are unwilling to participate in treatment or who will need an extended period of preparatory work before analysis proper can be undertaken. There are others whose ego-immaturity or impaired capacity for relationships precludes interpretative work of this kind: e.g. children with developmental defects or deviations may need a modification of technique. But the intensity of contact may still be needed to lay the foundations for work with the child, and the therapeutic interventions deployed will remain firmly grounded on a psychoanalytic knowledge of child development.

Last but not least, five-times weekly work with children can be justified in the light of the fact that only intensive study of them by the psychoanalytically informed observer can throw light on the many aberrant forms of development, complex psychological difficulties, and the considerable gaps in our knowledge of which every worker in the field is painfully aware. Psychoanalysis is a method of treatment, to be sure; and restricted in its scope. Applied psychoanalysis extends therapeutic work to a wider field. But psychoanalysis as science is inseparable from all our work and it is the extension of our knowledge which will, in the end, benefit all those therapies, brief or otherwise, which rest securely on the bedrock of a sound psychology.

Harvey: The Case of a Neurotic Boy

We begin the clinical part of our presentation with a brief account of the treatment—as yet incomplete—of a boy who was referred to us at the age of nine years and whom we have called Harvey. We have chosen him because we believe he illustrated the formation and operation of a neurosis of a comparatively straightforward kind.

Harvey's early history was uneventful. His only sibling, Bernadette, was born when he was two and three-quarters; and on this account he was separated from his mother for ten days. On the mother's return from hospital with the baby, neither parent noticed any reaction. He was, however, a quiet child at this period, and his subsequent fights with Bernadette, together with a sense of unfairness and oversensitivity, point to the jealousy he must have experienced. It is not known whether it was around this time that he became indifferent to food; but the indifference persisted up to the time of referral, and food was refused whenever he was upset.

Harvey was about three when he began to attend Nursery School where, after some initial difficulty in separating from the mother, he settled happily. At five he moved to a small school where again he was happy and where he made one or two good friends. Academically he was an able child who learned easily and showed good concentration. Soon after his eighth birthday he moved to his present school, and it was shortly after this that the parents became concerned about him. He became a loner and a worrier. He was increasingly reluctant to go to school. In the mornings be was miserable, listless, and pallid. He complained of headaches and stomach upsets, though he improved as a rule during the day. He was unable to look forward to any event with pleasure. His school performance rapidly deteriorated, and he did badly in nearly all his subjects in spite of a full-scale I.Q. of 150. He became increasingly afraid of fights with, and bullying by, older boys. He disliked team sports or any games in which there was a chance of being hurt. At home, his only close friend was a girl with whom he spent time listening to records. Otherwise he spent hours alone, drawing and painting—creatively, it should be added.

At the interview with Dr Yorke, Harvey made a good impression. He was bright, articulate, and communicative, and readily conceded his anxieties. It was thought that he would make a good treatment relationship; and this expectation was borne out when he started analysis. From the he first he showed an enthusiasm for his visits, and an interest in the various play materials available, but, to begin with, preferred to play games. He wanted to play chess, at which he was supposed to be very good, but made the most elementary blunders in ways which invited crushing defeat. It was not difficult to make links between his invitations of overwhelming defeat and his provocations of bullying by bigger boys at school.

If his fears of attack included a fear of being overwhelmed by the older boys, the provocations of such attacks were very real. As Harvey himself put it: "sometimes, when you do little things to bigger boys, they do bigger things back to you." Climbing over other boys' desks, for example, and flicking pellets at them from rubber bands must, in the context of Harvey's anxieties, have provoked the very things he feared. These fears of, and wishes for, retaliation, had already been indicated at the time of psychological testing. In one of his drawings, a man with a big sword tackled a big tree which promptly fell on top of him. In another, a man lit a log fire to burn down a tree, and a new population of trees grew so quickly that they entangled the man.

At this earlier stage of treatment, however, these matters were rather less readily expressed since the anxiety about going to school was still in the picture. He told of his fears of being bullied or attacked on the way to school, and spoke of a phantasy in which he was kidnapped and tied up. It was not, as yet, possible to get in touch with the exciting elements in such phantasies. But when he said that, recently, his relationship with Bernadette had improved, it was suggested that, currently, it might feel safer to be with girls rather than with boys. Harvey agreed that this might be so, and referred to his friendship with the girl next door.

Dr Yorke already had in mind, in this exchange, a very unusual response to one of the T.A.T. cards shown to Harvey during assessment. The card concerned depicts a *boy* leaning on a violin with his head on his arm. Harvey told a story about a *girl* called Jean, sitting in her room in a girl's boarding school, making a drawing to send home to her mother; and in his account of this he emphasised the girl's loneliness. He had also drawn a girl who appeared remarkably similar to a boy previously outlined, observing as he did so that: "if it were not for her hair she would look just like a boy."

We return to this matter later. We shall also need to say, in a similar connection, something about his castration complex which had also figured prominently in referral material. But, in the initial stages of the analysis, this showed itself only in the enjoyable and quasi—sublimated form of conjuring. Harvey delighted in mystifying the therapist, in repeatedly making things appear and re-appear from nowhere, using his magic wand with gusto and enthusiasm.

But, although he asked the therapist to show him tricks in return, he could not bear not to know just how the trick was done. He was free of anxiety only when he kept control over the penis substitute which he could ensure was present or absent at will. Interpretations at this point were, however, fairly generalised, as it was felt important to cement a treatment alliance as a first objective.

As such an alliance became established Harvey showed a particular liking for plasticene and for modeling with it. He worked quickly and well, with great imagination. Human beings disappeared altogether from his communications as he reproduced, through his modeling, a phantasy life currently dominated by monsters. Harvey would talk as he worked, weaving imaginative stories about his productions, and soon giving important indications of the kind of preoccupations underlying them. He would fashion enormous and voracious fish, with huge teeth and prominent eyes. Big fish ate little fish; occasionally, little fish ate big fish. It was evident that he was so interested and preoccupied with the activities of his fish that phantasies about them preoccupied him and precluded an interest in anything else—including work at school. Furthermore, all these aggressive and competitive phantasies had an unmistakable pleasurable tinge and betrayed their instinctual origins. In addition, he fished actively on every available opportunity.

His sexual phantasies soon began to express themselves with a similar piscatorial relish. In one of these phantasies the big fish laid eggs. Were they Daddy-fish or Mummy-fish?, asked the therapist. They were neither, said Harvey: all big fish were the same sex and were neither male nor female. The eggs they laid sank to the bottom of an extremely dark ocean where the little fish were hatched. Were these little fish also of only one sex? asked the therapist, or were there boy-fish and girl-fish? "Oh yes," said Harvey: "there are boy-fish and girl-fish," observed the therapist: "So it's the children who have all the fun!"

From material of this kind it was not too difficult to move a little closer to primal scene anxieties. In all his work with plasticene, and in all his drawings, the children-fish had enormous eyes. Why? To see in the dark, in the depths of the ocean, said Harvey. Perhaps there were things going on in the dark that the Harvey-fish needed to see, that were upsetting perhaps, or even too exciting. Harvey didn't always respond to comments of this kind very directly, but sometimes he took them in. And, if he answered with a "perhaps", his reply could generally be regarded as confirmatory. But, at this stage, he found it particularly difficult to respond to comments about "Mummy-fish" and "Daddy-fish" and to accept their sexual differences, and to look at his phantasies about their activities in the dark. Nevertheless, when he was asked if his penis became stiff when, in the dark, he thought about his parents, he was prepared to acknowledge that it did become stiff when he watched a particular T.V. program which concerned itself with monsters. So, little by little, we were able to get closer to some of these major concerns. And soon there was an interesting development in the material.

The fish quickly became monsters which not only possessed enormous eyes but enormous teeth as well. He modeled them in plasticene and put them in a prominent position over the fireplace in readiness for the next day's session. On one occasion the therapist said to him: "I don't think I'd like to sleep here overnight, Harvey. Not with that great big monster keeping such an eye on me and baring its teeth as if it couldn't wait to eat me up!" Harvey laughed. "Don't worry," he said: "It's only a model!" Nevertheless it was not very long before we were able to get at Harvey's excitement at the thought of eating people or being eaten, though he was still somewhat resistive to the idea that he might want to eat the therapist:

after all, he still needed him around. But it was interesting that the idea of being eaten was even more exciting, suggesting an oral basis for the later wish, however conflictual, to be aggressively and sexually overwhelmed by the big-boy/father.

As these links were established in treatment, it was possible to re-explore Harvey's night time phantasies and his difficulties in getting off to sleep because of sexual excitement. Again he was able to speak of his fears of burglars, of people breaking in; and soon of his wish that they should. Now, however, he described, with greater directness, how a burglar might attack his mother and how he would save her—inferentially, by taking her place. His wish to be attacked was portrayed repeatedly in his drawings; and he was enabled to acknowledge the excitement aroused by these phantasies. He still showed some resistance to transference interpretations, but he retained them, and sometimes acknowledged them later. Let us give an example. When there was a shift from passive to active in his phantasy life, and an aggressive masculinity was beginning to reassert itself, Harvey drew, in the most convincingly graphic and dynamic manner, a classroom revolt against a teacher who, for reason unknown, be had called "Mr Buffy". The therapist took up with him his feeling of excitement and revolt against the teacher-therapist, and the expected retaliation. Harvey said nothing. But, at the end of the session, as he was leaving, Harvey turned to the therapist and said, "See you tomorrow, Mr Buffy!"

These fragments from an analysis will allow us to reconstruct, however imperfectly, a picture of the pathology in developmental terms with, perhaps, one reservation. We need a working hypothesis to account for the fluidity with which the material moved from the devoured to the castrated and the intrusively penetrated in a way which suggested significant links between them. This is not a simple matter of an equation between breast, penis and whole body. Such an equation can be expected to the general significance; but we must look for more *specific* factors in Harvey case. We know that he fed at the breast for seven months with pleasurable industry; and continued to enjoy his food, especially milk, for some time thereafter. Yet at some point he became indifferent to these gratifications. Was his reaction to a suckling Bernadette observed by him at the age of two-and-three quarters a matter for jealously, matched only by envy, and which became a focus for defensive indifference? And did it lead to a conviction that, in order to be loved, one had to be a girl? Were his later fights with Bernadette not simply an expression of hostility to his rival but also an expression of his envy of her femininity? And did his observation of female genitals at an age when his phallic anxieties might be expected to be developing, help to forge the link between oral and phallic phantasies?

However this may have been, both parents and child are agreed that a decisive precipitant in Harvey's disturbance was a change of school. Harvey moved from a co-educational establishment to an all-male one. The impact of this wholly masculine world, with its games, its compulsory showers, and its fighting, appears to have mobilised Harvey's anxieties and set a regressive experience in train. Oedipal trends would be reactivated and further regression occur, since the various feminine identifications, and their roots in ambivalence to the mother, would foster a retreat to the negative oedipal phase, that is a phase in which the boy imagines himself a girl loved by the father. It was precisely around this pre-established fixation point that symptom formation occurred. The resulting compromise consisted in the co-existence of the fears of aggressively masculine attack side by side with its provocation; but the compromise retained a certain fluidity, in contrast with the more structured kind of symptom-formation one would encounter in an adult.

The identification with the mother as the victim of aggressive sexual attack by the father was based on primal scene phantasies, in their negative-oedipal form; and these in turn were intimately linked with intense sexual curiosity. The *content* of the curiosity was dealt with by the initial compromise formation, including the various displacements involving the boys at school. The curiosity itself was not. This was dealt with by simple inhibition: but by an inhibition which progressively spread to greater and greater areas of learning *as the process of taking in information from others became increasingly sexualised and therefore linked with the forbidden wish to observe the parents at night*. In modeling and drawing, on the other hand, the phantasies depicted were "self-created", and for this reason were in no way subject to the inhibiting process. Hence, before treatment, school failure existed side by side with these creative and absorbing activities.

It is characteristic of neurosis and inhibition that solutions of this kind cannot always be maintained in the face of increasing instinctual pressure. Life becomes joyless as pleasures of all kinds are drawn into the domain of forbidden sexuality. In some children the resulting restrictions are so crippling that developmental arrests supervene which are not only refractory to external influence but step outside the boundaries of childhood neuroses.

This kind of arrest did not happen to Harvey. His psychic resources and flexibility were such that the failure of the initial attempts at conflict-solution by compromise and inhibition could yet be replaced by a more effective, if still maladaptive illness. The preoccupation with fish replaced the presenting symptom-formation with a new one which, while concerned identical conflicts, had the advantage, to say the least, of considerably greater economy. The disavowal of sexual curiosity in the form of a learning inhibition *gave way* to a preoccupation with sexual phantasy which replaced every other interest. The initial displacement from *people* to *fish* was the ingenious if unconscious point of departure. From then on, the symptom formation was subject to a powerful process of condensation of dreams, added to the vividness and compelling quality of the mental imagery involved. The fish combined phantastically, both in its body and its activities, the instinctual body and instinctual activities of Harvey himself. It was a phallic body, to be sure; but it also expressed its anality as it deposited its eggs, the products of its cloaca, into the dark sea bed of the water-closet; and the orality which it presented so vividly needs no further elaboration. His exhibitionistic and voyeuristic wishes likewise reached ready expression. As for the defensive aspects of the ego and the operation of the superego, these too contributed to the symptom-formation. The fish was repeatedly *caught* in action (catching real fish) as well as in phantasy. And Harvey himself *suffered*, for all his excitement, by the circumstances that his preoccupation with sexuality effectively interfered with his learning and achievements at school.

Lastly, there is one other important presenting symptom, which we have not yet discussed: namely, Harvey's sickness and headaches in the mornings. These can be accounted for by the fact of Harvey's identification with his mother who suffered from migraine and sickness. But the identification with the sufferer, with the victim, is only one of many meanings: it may also represent a wish to take over the mother's illness and protect her from phantasied sexual attacks.

Peter: A Case of Developmental Arrest

Harvey's disturbance, then, is dearly a neurosis of a classical kind. This cannot be said for Peter, a narcissistically vulnerable adolescent whose developmental deviations were strikingly displayed in his severely disturbed object relations, and who was in five-times a week treatment with Mrs Kennedy from the age of 13–19 years.

In spite of a long, and in many ways successful, analysis, Peter has remained unable to relinquish entirely his sado-masochistic tie to his mother. He remains rather depressed and dominated by pervasive feelings of inadequacy and resentment from which he tries to escape by sexual activities. He has masturbated compulsively from early childhood; but in late adolescence he bean a practice which enhanced his orgasmic pleasure. He ties a plastic bag over his head, so that his masturbatory phantasies, in which a female partner castrates and suffocates him, are given an added dimension of reality. He longs for a girl friend who will love him and with whom he can strike up a sexual relationship; but on the few occasions when he has managed to get into bed with a girl he became so terrified during foreplay that he simply had to take flight.

Peter comes from a military background. The family have no permanent home, often live abroad, and have never stayed more than two years in any one place. Peter had to change school several times until, at the age of 9, he was sent to boarding school in England where he stayed for four years.

Peter was a planned and wanted baby and the pregnancy was easy and straightforward, but both parents were emotionally unprepared for the care of their first baby. Even at birth Peter did not fit in with the parents' pre-arranged plans. He arrived 12 days too early and there were complications necessitating forceps delivery. Breast feeding too presented difficulties and had to be supplemented. Peter was unsettled, cried a lot and during the first 3months his parents resented the disturbed nights. Mother felt tired and depressed and found it difficult to cope with the baby, especially as the family had to move yet again to another country when Peter was only six weeks old. Though a regular sleeping pattern was soon established Peter continued to be a poor feeder. The mother expressed guilt about having forced him to eat; she always worried he was not getting enough. When he was 8 months, the mother again became pregnant.

The difficulties in the mother-child interaction during the first year of life established significant patterns for later development, in particular forcing things upon him, worrying about his health and bodily growth and her being disappointed with him. However, the major pathogenic influences which affected Peter's development occurred during the second and early third year and culminated in a circumcision operation at 2 years 8 months—the "traumatic" event around which his later conflicts became organised.

Peter's toilet training was described as "a great battle." Though it began before Peter was one, was not accomplished until he was 3 or 3½ years old. In fact, he gained bladder control at more or less the same time as his younger brother. Difficulty in gaining bladder control was undoubtedly increased by the fact that Peter developed phimosis. This must have caused considerable discomfort and pain when urinating and involved extensive examinations and manipulations of his penis. It was this which eventually led to the circumcision operation. Mother stayed with him in hospital and Peter is said to have reacted very badly to the anesthetic.

These experiences, coloured by unresolved anal conflicts, may even have led to a premature entry into the phallic phase; they certainly determined the intensity of his castration anxiety. The combination of sexual stimulation, pain and attack on the penis shaped the way in which phallic and oedipal conflicts were later experienced.

In analysis Peter maintained to have a memory of mother driving him to the hospital for the operation, though this memory lacked any affective colouring. There also appeared to be some somatic memories of the panic experienced when given the anesthetic. In retrospect it is clear that these were quickly brought into treatment. Periodically, he would freeze into a motionless stare and sit with fixed staring eyes and a mask like facial expression, for several minutes, in almost every session. He would emerge from this trance-like state, either spontaneously or in response to the therapist's intervention, only after a violent jerking movement of his head, which was suggestive of a deliberate effort to rid himself of something terrifying and gripping. At the time, various hypotheses were suggested to account for this puzzling behaviour. Was it indicative of "petit mal" and due to organic impairment? Did it suggest a kind of hysterical twilight state or even hallucinatory experiences? Or was it an attempt to immobilize his body in order to control sexual excitement and terrifying phantasies? As soon as Peter's fear of treatment lessened and he could begin to permit himself to communicate his phantasies, these "trance-like" states completely disappeared and the possible contribution of organic factors could be dismissed. But his defensive use of "withdrawal into phantasy" in the face of any kind of internal or external impingement which mobilised painful feeling states, remained. This suggested that his disturbance could be understood as a result of psychological conflict, probably superimposed on earlier personality distortions, in the development of which his early life experiences had played a substantial part.

When Peter was 17 months his brother was born. He was in the care of his grandparents for 12 days and showed signs of distress over the separation; but the parents failed to notice any signs of jealousy of the baby. Indeed, they emphasised the good relationship between the brothers, but the analytic material certainly did not bear this out. Peter's deep seated hate and envy of his brother was an ever recurring theme in the analysis and was only thinly disguised at the beginning. In part this is a displacement of hostility and anger towards his mother fur producing the brother and for favouring him.

The parents described the younger brother as more satisfactory in every way and comparisons must have been made from the earliest time. Physically the boys were soon of similar size and, developmentally, the baby was always advanced; and Peter's own development began to lag during his second year. The parents often thought of their two sons as twins. Peter only walked when he was 2 years, his brother when he was just over one; and gradually the developmental gap narrowed. Peter's speech development was so retarded that his younger brother is said to have talked first. This delayed speech development may well have been linked with the enormous aggression which Peter was trying to contain. In analysis some of his most guilt-ridden material was "unspeakable" and had to be brought in writing. His speech was always difficult to understand: it was slurred and often inaudible.

The unfavourable comparisons with the brother became an integral part of Peter's life. They not only increased and kept alive his hostility and murderous wishes, but had a devastating effect on his self-esteem. He felt that his brother was not only better loved but also superior in every respect.

At the time of referral to the Clinic Peter gave the impression of being a very depressed boy. His frail appearance, his awkward movements, his inability to communicate, and his anxious over-compliance all added to the picture of misery and severe inhibition. Peter referred to his learning problem as backwardness and complained of excessive fatigue, thus drawing attention to his devalued self—a boy damaged in mind and body.

Though initially Peter was ostensibly brought for advice about his future schooling, the parents noted his general unhappiness and excessive worrying but linked this with his learning difficulties. They were baffled by his poor scholastic achievements, as his good intelligence (Verbal I.Q. 131; Performance I.Q. 91; Full Scale 114) was generally recognized.

It was clear even at the diagnostic stage that severe conflicts around aggression had led to inhibitions and ego restrictions. Early in treatment, Peter scribbled on sheets of paper, thoughts which at first looked bizarre and out of context. For example: "God save our gracious Queen"—"Jack Chariton is the greatest footballer in the world"—"Mrs Kennedy is mad". These were later understood as phantasied destructive attacks on his mother, brother and himself and led to an understanding of Peter's intense preoccupation with thoughts of killing and torture. It emerged that Peter's affective life was completely caught up in his masturbation phantasies. Nothing in his life gave him interest or enjoyment, save sexually arousing activities. If he read the newspaper it was only to scan the pages for reports of atrocities, sexual murder, rape and persecutions.

Masturbatory activity aroused severe guilt and it is significant that he referred to them as "his sins". In fact, the intensity of the masturbatory conflict suggested the existence of a punitive, harsh and sadistic superego. It would seem that the rigid standards held up by his parents were internalised and were enormously reinforced from aggressive and sadistic instinctual sources.

Long before there was any verbal communication Peter enacted the battle against masturbation in the analytic sessions. He played a highly exciting game with a ruler. He repeatedly threw it into the air and caught it. He tapped it against his legs or the chair; and the masturbatory quality of these activities was betrayed by the concomitant erections. Whereas, in the waiting room, he would sit calmly doing his homework, he could hardly wait to get to the treatment room, where he would bring out his ruler and often spend the whole session tossing it.

In this context the inner struggle against masturbation was externalised in the treatment situation. He reproached himself for wasting treatment time and his parents' money by playing with his ruler. Periodically he would throw the ruler across the room, declare that he wanted to get on with analysis, but a few minutes later be would retrieve the ruler and start tossing it all over again. Eventually, he would begin to reproach himself for not trying harder to talk about his problems, for not making any progress, and for not being a good patient.

The activity with the ruler was a key to his phantasy life and opened up many aspects of the analytic work. The significance of the ruler itself emerged later. It represented the mother's penis, and replaced a long shoehorn, also originally his mother's, which he used at home. It therefore had fetishistic qualities in as far as it enhanced his sexual excitement; but it also had the qualities of a magic wand which transposed him into a phantasy world where he was an omnipotent ruler of thousands of slaves who depended on his mercy for their survival. These presented the most conscious layers of his masturbation phantasies.

It is difficult to know with certainty whether Peter's compulsive need to masturbate followed, or preceded, the circumcision. Masturbation problems have certainly existed for a long time although they were either not observed or not remembered by his parents. For Peter, masturbation conflicts became inevitably linked with his feelings about his damaged penis and his devalued self.

An important feature of his *masturbation practices* was the need to create simultaneous, or quickly alternating, experiences of sexual excitement, pain and anxiety. This suggests a link with the traumatic experiences surrounding his circumcision.

The content of his sado—masochistic *masturbation phantasies* are particularly relevant in establishing links with the early traumatisation. Their gradual unfolding during analysis can be roughly grouped into phases. In the first phase Peter was absorbed in phantasies about being beaten, being castrated and being murdered which had a masochistic flavour. In the second phase he was turning passive into active and sadistically, in phantasy, first raping and then killing "attractive females" to cover his crimes. Eventually his phantasies had both active and passive versions and centered around themes of painful assaults on the genitals. For example, he wanted to get his young female teacher sexually excited by tickling her and then pulling at her clitoris very hard so that it would stick out. Similarly he phantasied that she would pull at or pull off his penis. This material confirmed that he had experienced the past assaults on his penis as exciting and seductive; but the resulting painful erections had also evoked retaliatory wishes in him. These phantasies also reflected Peter's persistent need to cling to the notion of the phallic mother, in order to defend against castration anxiety.

The technical problems in analysis with this type of patient are well known The transference and the treatment process itself can be used fur vicarious gratification For example Peter suggested that, instead of just waiting for him to talk, which was so difficult, the therapist should ask him questions This was the prelude to a longing for a Gestapo kind of interrogation where he would be tied down and forced to confess his crimes under torture.

Peter's need to cast the therapist in the role of enemy, or at least of hostile opponent, has been a persistent feature throughout treatment. His initial anxiety about what was going to happen in treatment could be related to his notion that all women were potentially dangerous and powerful castrators. He was disturbed by the therapist's foreign accent and origin and thought that Austrian females were worse than any others. In the first week of treatment he talked about a skiing holiday in Austria where the food was so terrible that he fell ill; and the local doctor misdiagnosed his stomach upset as suspected appendicitis. Of course, he could not let this doctor come near him again otherwise "his appendix would be whipped away".

Whatever the therapist said or did in the early stages of analysis was experienced as an attack, and Peter defended against such dangers by becoming the attacker. He hurled pillows and abuse at the therapist, always threatening more violent action if she would not submit to his attempts to silence and control her. He omnipotently asserted that he had superior strength as the therapist was only a female bag. Whereas this may have temporarily reduced the anxiety engendered by the initial treatment situation, it also heightened his conflict around aggression. Attacking was as dangerous as being attacked, and equally aroused guilt and anxiety. He now began to worry about people looking in or listening to what was going on in the session, or that the therapist would complain to some higher authority about his aggressive behaviour. While holding menacingly a chair above the therapist's head, he reassured himself that the therapist would enlist "outside help" from male members of staff or the police, in case he really attacked her. The oedipal content of these sexualised attacks was not interpreted at that point. The analytic work was focused on his defensive attempt to reduce the intensity of inner conflict by externalising the criticising and threatening superego introjects.

The analysis of these various defensive maneuvers helped to curb his need to repeat these physical attacks and led instead to complex transference developments organised around his anti-Semitism.

His interest in current affairs shifted. He now became preoccupied with the Arab-Israeli conflict and with the Jews in general. He condemned Israel's aggression, scorned her military successes and advocated the destruction of the Jewish race. He became an avid reader of reference books in order to learn which public figures were famous and Jewish. He read all he could on Jewish persecutions, exterminations and migrations. He could readily quote statistics on the present world distribution of the Jews. In a very short time he built up an impressive fund of knowledge, all the more striking in view of his learning difficulties elsewhere.

The sessions were now filled with anti-Jewish ranting which Peter referred to as "Mrs Kennedy baiting". He questioned why the therapist permitted his attacks and abuses just retaliation. This was a clear *attempt* to establish a sado-masochistic relationship, but it became obvious that it was also unconsciously designed to avoid depressive feeling stares by providing himself with sexual excitement. He began to talk about "Jew baiting" as a disguise which served no useful purpose in the session if it failed to make the therapist feel bad. He suggested that the therapist might even be proud of being Jewish. Later he said with real sadness that he knew why the therapist did not retaliate. She thought that he "was only a poor psychiatric patient" and she "a clever Jewish psychologist". He even began to question whether the Jews were really a chosen people, and not an inferior race.

He was often preoccupied with the therapist's status, position and wealth and had sometimes expressed envy of her cleverness and success. On rare occasions he had even shown signs of admiring her, for example when he responded to a meaningful interpretation with "How *do* you know all that?" Any fleeting acknowledgement of her omniscience was invariably followed by a scathing attack on her uselessness and stupidity: "Anyone could sit there getting paid for doing nothing."

As we explored the links between his feelings of inferiority and his need to make others feel inferior, we came to understand that his hate of the Jews also reflected self hate. Peter began to talk about feeling "a bit Jewish himself". He felt inferior, discriminated against, and he began to bring material about his circumcision. He expressed disgust with the Jews who were smelly and had terribly ugly noses which made them conspicuous and repellent. In describing a Jewish boy with whom he felt a sudden affinity, he said: "It's difficult to describe him—perhaps I should say he is a bit trimmed."

The dual notion of the Jews as a chosen and inferior race, endowed with superior qualities but as damaged and castrated, made them particularly suitable for expressing his problems. He was forever trying to decide whether he admired or hated Jews; and in this way expressed the confusion occasioned by his highly ambivalent transference feelings. From his exclusive experience of hate towards the therapist, he began to make his declarations of hatred sound like declarations of love. He questioned the therapist saying, for example: "Tell me, do I love you or do I hate you? I really do not know." Other remarks included: "Look at her sweet face—but look at her awful Jewish nose" and later in treatment he said seductively: "Sweety—I want to kill you." These acute ambivalent conflicts contributed to his experience of himself as split and divided, so that he never knew what his "real self" was. This intensified his fear of madness.

All these elements emerged more clearly when his complex identification with Hitler became the focus of the analysis. His admiration for Hitler as omnipotent ruler of a master race and as sadistic persecutor of the Jews was matched by his contempt for the beaten ex-enemy and his view of Hitler as a castrated, evil and mad person.

The first references to Hitler came long before his anti-Jewish transference phase. He alluded to Hitler as a denigrated and castrated object. The "Leitmotiv" for bringing *castration anxiety* at that time was a schoolboy's ditty, "Hitler only has one ball, the other is on the Albert Hall"; and this featured very prominently in the material. Almost a year later Peter added a significant second verse: "his mother took it when he was only small".

The significance of balls related to all phases of psycho-sexual development. They had an anal significance when he bombarded the therapist with ping-pong balls; and be later accused her of stealing his precious balls. Much of this aggressive investment in feces as weapons for attack applied equally to the phallus. Moreover, there was an equation of balls and breasts linked with the phantasy of the phallic mother which Peter was unable to relinquish and which contained his most primitive anxieties over loss. The oral aggressive and phallic-aggressive components in his varied rape phantasies were especially clearly illustrated when he wanted to make love to the therapist by sticking pins in her breasts. Much of the phallic castration anxiety was experienced and enacted as attacks on the testicles. This he said was how bullocks got castrated and how males in India get sterilised. At boarding school, in a favourite punishment by boys in his dormitory, the naked victim was forced to stand facing the rest of the boys who aimed pellets at his genitals.

Though guilt was the inevitable consequence of masturbation, it seemed to have no effect on curbing it. Peter was at the mercy of his unchanneled, uncontrollable sexuality. One reason for this, suggested by the content of the masturbation phantasies, was related to the need to repeat the early traumatic childhood experience. However, *analytic insight into this did not bring about any significant changes in his sexual problems.* The recognition that Peter worked hard to get himself into a state of sexual excitement, for example by "Mrs Kennedy baiting", suggests that *sexual excitement served to avoid depressive feelings states and therefore bad to be understood in terms of his narcissistic vulnerability.*

His reiteration that "Jews must die" soon became personalised. If anything emerged that remotely suggested positive feelings towards the therapist, he at once followed it up with "but you are a Jew and Jews must die". His death wishes appeared to stem mainly from retaliatory revenge. Oedipal rivalry was now brought into the transference, with phantasies about the therapist's family, her sexual activities and his intrusion on them. He accused her of putting others before him and of not having time for him. Hitherto he had hardly mentioned his parents but he now spoke of intense resentment he experienced as soon as father entered the house. He was irritated by everything father did, the way be sat, the way he ate, and even the way he breathed. These outbursts resembled primitive rage responses and were followed by a longing to be loved. He sadly spoke of a mutual hate relationship with father, in which he felt hated by the father as much as he hated in return. Though he also expressed envy of the good and loving relationship between the brother and the father, both were ultimately experienced as rivals for mother's love. Perhaps it would be more correct to speak of Peter's hate of the object who, he felt, "possessed" mother. More resistance was encountered when a mother transference dominated the material. By using his young English teacher as an extension for his transference feelings, he attempted to split his ambivalence. The therapist was hated and attacked as a depriving, rejecting object who did not provide nice drinks but only lousy water, and who did not relieve his physical discomforts—he was suffering from hay fever and a blocked up nose at the time. The English teacher became the object of intense sexual longings and featured prominently in his erotic phantasies. In many ways she was an idealised and also a loving object; but she was also experienced as a dangerous sexual seducer. Peter was afraid of being alone with her, afraid of sitting next to her when they met on the train; but in his phantasies he embellished what he experienced as her sexual advances and planned to put on a disguise, visit her at night, and sexually assault her.

The reconstruction of early childhood experiences when the mother was experienced as the sexual seducer and castrator led to material which revealed continuing sexual seductions by the mother, experienced partly as attacks. At one time he had wondered what the therapist would do if be stripped in the session. Would she like it and get excited? Would she admire or find fault with his penis? He now spoke of the parents' display of their nudity at home and their expectation that the boys do likewise. Whenever he complained of pains his mother massaged his neck and back; and she even tried to convince the doctor that it was more convenient if she gave Peter the prescribed course of prophylactic injections against hay fever. Thus it appears that Peter was unable to prevent his mother's manipulations and her ownership of his body. It is as if they were fighting over possession of his penis, which he is prepared to relinquish in order to retain mother's love and interest in him.

In the next phase of the transference Peter fell in love with his English teacher and began to invest her with power to control him and thereby his wellbeing. She had the power to give or take, to love him or leave him, to make him feel good, or to make him suffer. The realisation of this made Peter wish he could forget her altogether. He said he "hated loving her" and wanted to "destroy his love for her". He became very depressed and said he felt hated by everyone and in return hated everyone else. The therapist too would soon throw him out or his parents would terminate treatment. He spoke of feeling hopeless, beyond therapeutic help, and said he wanted to kill himself Such suicidal thoughts always contained the wish to attack and punish his parents. Indeed, as treatment progressed he became more openly critical and hostile towards them. The sado-masochistic battles reached a peak when, one rainy evening, the parents told him to leave home and never come back. Peter considered throwing himself in front of a passing car but instead decided to denounce his parents to the police. He felt triumphant when the police drove him home by car after speaking to the parents on the telephone. Later, when he told his mother that he had considered throwing himself in front of a car she reproached him for being inconsiderate of the driver. Following this incident the parents decided that treatment made Peter too difficult to live with and that he could only continue if he lived away from home. Peter now responded with despair and feelings of total rejection. It revived all the unhappiness and feelings of abandonment he had experienced when he was sent to boarding school at the age of 8. Fortunately, leaving home at 17 turned out to be an altogether different experience for Peter, giving him a change to gain distance and some independence from his family.

The attainment of self-esteem for Peter is tied to the acquisition of power and status. Peter worries excessively about his future and longs for a job with power and status—a solicitor, perhaps, or even a judge. Such longings for a position of power and status are invariably followed by thoughts that he is not good or clever enough to achieve this. While in this respect he is more realistic in his appraisal of himself and shows a reduction in defensive externalisations, it is also exploited in the interests of masochistic self-derision.

Space precludes further discussion of Peter's case and the many questions it poses. But, in conclusion, we want to revert to the distinction between neurotic pathology and pathology resulting from developmental disharmonies. For all the *temporary* dislocation in Harvey's life, the battlegrounds of childhood have simply been re-visited, and the resolution of the conflicts enacted there affords once more the chance to leave them behind. In Peter's case, some of the battles which started so early in his life have decisively affected the developmental process. Lack of adequate narcissistic investment by the mother, constant criticism and derogation, have failed, at every step, to meet his ordinary developmental needs. The experiences of pain and excessive sexual excitation were inextricably bound up with his earliest object relationship. The resulting distortion of personality has meant that his self-structure and potential for normal object relationships have been distorted. Love, while longed for, cannot be met with love: but only with demandingness, accusation, envy, and attack.

CHAPTER NINE

Different Types of Sado-Masochistic Behaviour in Children*

Marion Burgner and Hansi Kennedy 1980

Introduction

Work with sado-masochistic patients has occupied analysts over several decades, both because of the complex structure of their pathology and the technical difficulties they present in treatment. In this paper we shall examine the meanings of the term "sado-masochistic" mainly by drawing on child analytic material from the Hampstead Clinic. We hope that such material will introduce a developmental viewpoint that will aid theoretical conceptualization and clinical understanding. Our presentation is a reflection of work in progress rather than a comprehensive or new formulation. We shall examine our cases principally from the viewpoint of their object relationships, since instinctual drive pressures and the contributions of the ego come together most clearly in this area of functioning.

The term "sado-masochism" is frequently used so descriptively as to lose all psychological meaning. It is employed to describe normal, aggressive behaviour; clinging, dependent behaviour which is experienced by the object as excessively demanding; domination and obsession of the object to assert separateness and independence and to gain control; hurting and tormenting the object or eliciting attack from the object; as well as perverse sexual activity. Sometimes we find that behaviour labeled sado-masochistic has in fact more the stamp of the anal-sadistic level of development. At other times we are puzzled how sadomasochistic manifestations in children can be compared with adult perversions. We can put it no better than Freud who, in 1905, wrote in the Three Essays: "In ordinary speech the connotation of sadism oscillates between, on the one hand, cases merely characterised by an active or violent attitude to the sexual object, and, on the other hand, cases in which satisfaction is entirely conditional on the humiliation and maltreatment of the object. Strictly speaking, it is only this last extreme instance which deserves to be described as a perversion. Similarly, the term masochism comprises any passive attitude towards sexual life and the sexual object, the extreme instance of which appears to be that in which satisfaction is conditional upon suffering physical or mental pain at the hands of the sexual object."

It is also relevant for us to note that children are the passive recipients of their parents' ministrations and feelings. They are loved and hated by their parents; they are controlled, frustrated and even punished, long before ego structualisation is mature enough to organise and express their own feelings. Thus, the child inevitably takes up a passive posture in relation to his parents in his early years though he will continually attempt to assert himself and reverse this position. This assertion starts in the first year of life and reaches a peak in the second year, as the child makes the change from a predominantly passive position to a more active one, a change which is facilitated by motor, cognitive and affective development.

It is in the second year of life that the toddler becomes behaviourally aggressive and since his battles with his mother are sometimes responded to by her as if they were an attack, confusion may arise in the observer as to the content of the relationship and the type of gratification sought. Making the anal-sadistic phase our starting point, we shall examine how the difficulties encountered within this phase affect later stages of development and, eventually, may result in a personality structure that is sado-masochistic.

Object Relationships of the Anal-Sadistic Phase

This phase is defined by Laplanche and Pontalis as follows: "Freud's second stage of libidinal development, occurring approximately between the ages of two and four. The stage is characterised by an organisation of the libido under the primacy of the anal erotogenic zone. The object-relationship at this time is invested with meanings having to do with the function of defecation (expulsion/retention) and with the symbolic value of feces." This definition incidentally, makes no reference to the role of aggression in this phase.

Abraham (1924) has suggested "two different pleasurable tendencies in the anal-sadistic phase: a more primitive one of expelling the object (evacuation) and destroying it, and a late: one of retaining and controlling it". Both these stages are seen by Abraham to involve "partial-love" rather than "object-love" and to be characterised by feelings of ambivalence.

Margaret Mahler and her co-workers (1975) have made an extensive contribution to our understanding of development during this period in terms of ego processes and self-object differentiation. The latter three sub-phases of the separation-individuation phase fall within the anal phase: the sub-phases of practicing, rapprochement, and the consolidation of individuality with the beginning of emotional object-constancy. Their demonstration of the varied behavioural phenomena which gradually contribute to the child's internal structuralisations and to the establishment of separate self-object representations has brought into focus the complexity of the issues involved in becoming a psychologically separate individual.

We should now like to examine more specifically what makes for a normal anal phase or development which each individual child has to negotiate and, in some measure, adaptive leave behind for the dominance of the phallic phase. The terms themselves *anal* and *sadistic* describe various phenomena in all areas of functioning: an anxiety about disappearance an loss of highly valued bodily products and a consequent wish on the toddler's part to retain his feces; a pride in the explosive production of large, well-formed feces and, if time and place are right, a mutually pleasurable interaction between toddler and mother. Characteristic behaviour of the phase— to keep for oneself, to control and to destroy— patterns itself on anal drive derivatives; but these wishes also quickly translate themselves into behavioural manifestations in the self and object world. The pleasure in messing and messy activities is paramount.

Typically, the toddler also derives inordinate pleasure from his increasing motility and activity (Mahler's practising sub-phase, the child's "love affair with the world"); he is self willed, obstinate, by turns clinging or demanding, given to battling and temper tantrums. All of this behaviour has, optimally, the pleasurable stamp of self-assertion, an increasing awareness of the power of the self. But this glorious sense of omnipotence is subject to frequent disillusion and demolition from all sides: from the ego's immature capacity to contain anxiety and other affects; from the mother who is experienced as arbitrarily loving and punishing, coming and going; and also from the internal world where emotional object ties have not achieved constancy. Thus, neither omnipotent feelings nor a positive narcissistic investment can be maintained for very long and the child returns time and time again to the battling behaviour of this phase, with its undercurrent of anxiety over separation from, and loss of, the object and over the multiple onslaught on an omnipotent self. All of this is normal behaviour in the toddler. Similarly, he does not have that degree of ego structuralisation which requires control and containment of ambivalence; seemingly contradictory feelings of love and hate are freely expressed toward the same object in quick succession. Emotional object constancy, with its pressure to tolerate and contain the ambivalence, has not yet been achieved, it is only toward the end of this phase that ego structuralisation leads to conflicts over ambivalence, to splitting and to problems over death wishes and consequent talion fears. When such ambivalence is nor at least partially resolved in the phallic phase, we may expect a harsh and punitive superego structure in which aspects of a more sophisticated anal-sadistic drive expression may be lodged. But—and this is very important to note—the toddler in this phase only *appears* sadistic, since the intentionality to hurt is lacking and the emphasis is not on obtaining pleasure from the causing or suffering of pain. As Freud noted (1915): "a sadistic child takes no account of whether or not he inflicts pain, nor does he intend to do so".

As therapists, we only consider intervention when such a mode of relating persists into, and beyond, the phallic phase of development in a relatively unmodified form or when there is evidence of regression at the phallic-oedipal stage back to the anal phase.

Derek aged 4 years illustrates a developmental problem in this area. He is a child in our Nursery School whose parents, though separated, maintain a continuing sado-.masochistic relationship expressed in verbal and physical abuse. Both parents are seemingly devoted to their son. It has been noted by the teaching staff that the mother also rakes a masochistic stance toward Derek, a stance which is subtly dominating and controlling and which gives him no room for individual expression. Toward his mother, then, Derek is at present overtly compliant and placatory, retaliating only by an extensive sleep disturbance and an occasional sulky, negative response. He is markedly ambivalent to both parents, subtly and omnipotently playing off one against the other in contrast, his behaviour in the Nursery School toward the other children is physically attacking and certainly affords him some gratification—he smiles as he hits; when questioned by the teacher, he will invariably maintain that such attacks are "accidents". Chronologically, Derek is moving into the phallic-oedipal stage of development, a move which is likely to be distorted by his anxieties over object loss, the disturbed parental relationship, the confusions generated by the father's unplanned appearances and disappearances, and the inadequacies of the father as a satisfactory masculine model for identification. In these circumstances, adequate negotiation of the phallic-oedipal phase is gravely endangered and it seems likely that he will partially remain in or regress to the anal-sadistic phase; a further danger for his future development lies in his adopting the parental sado-masochistic style of relating, so that his own relationships could eventually become similarly organised and his sado-masochism become superimposed on the regressed anal mode of object relations.

At this point, a brief vignette from an adult case may assist our argument in differentiating between anality and sadomasochism. Mr A., in his early twenties, asked for analysis because of his difficulties in relating to women; he also had problems over his creative work as a sculptor and over his gender identity; and fantasy and reality were not always clearly differentiated. When he entered analysis, Mr A. worked mainly with clay and, quite without inhibition, he talked of the clay as "shit", saying how much he loved handling and fashioning it. He went on to describe a part of his work which gave him much pleasure: it was to have in front of him an enormous block of wet clay to press the whole of the posterior part of his naked body into the clay so as to leave an imprint; he would then embellish the imprint, giving it carefully fashioned limbs. In this patient we see very clearly a direct derivative from the pleasures in anal messing; in fact, he involved his entire body in the gratificatory activity. But Mr A. was certainly not sado-masochistic his sexual orientation or in his relationships and he did not specifically wish to harm his objects or himself.

Before leaving our discussion of the anal-aggressive phase, we would emphasise the pleasure derived from anality and self-assertion; further, that the battling with and the controlling of the object are normal manifestations of this phase. The so-called sadism within the phase is not truly sadism since the intention to inflict pain and to derive pleasure from such action is absent. The normal child who, in the anal phase, is angry with the object will nor hesitate to show his anger by hitting out at the person involved. Indeed the manifestations of this phase should more aptly be referred to as *anal aggressive* rather than anal-sadistic. It is worth remembering that, when Freud coined the description of the anal-sadistic phase, he based this on analytic material, often taken from severely disturbed adult patients.

Sado-Masochistic Object Relationships

When does behaviour merit the hallmark of *sadism*? We suggest that together with the regressive move back to the anal-aggressive phase, there are other elements retroactively superimposed to give sadism its specific hallmark. There is the more sophisticated drive expression of the phallic-oedipal phase; there is the increasing complexity of the ego and its functions; there is the maturation and strengthening of the physical apparatus; there is the proliferation of a vivid imaginative and fantasy life; and there is the involvement of the object in a collusive and mutually pleasurable interaction.

We know that the sexualised pleasure in causing pain is one element in sadism. We also know that sadism usually has a complementary masochistic stance and that the roles become interchangeable within a partnership. In describing an adult sado-masochistic relation, we assume that sado-masochistic interchanges often substitute for, or are a prelude to, sexual intercourse and that sexualised excitement will either be apparent or thinly disguised.

An adult analytic patient said in her initial interview that for some years there had not been a sexual relationship between her and her husband. However, she went on to describe a recurring pattern of inflammatory verbal quarrels between them which culminated in her triumphantly biting her husband so that she Left him marked; he would then plead with her to have intercourse with him; she would refuse him and he would threaten suicide. It seemed that for this patient the specific sexual gratification lay in her fantasies about murdering him. It was not too difficult, as the analysis got under way, to understand that for this woman the interchangeable roles of sadist and masochist served to ensure the object's involvement with her. Undoubtedly, sexual excitement was experienced in the rows, but the attainment of such an excited state was not the sole aim; what seemed important as well for both husband and wife was the need to retain the object within that specific relationship. Later in the analysis it was understood how this sado-masochistic mode of relating generalised onto other relationships and how it had originated in the patient's childhood relationship with her mother. When, at one point, her pleasurable need to be the victim in each and every interaction was interpreted, the patient's reply was: "You see, I *know* it there, it's like being at home".

Thus we have to account for other aims apart from the wish to obtain direct sexual gratification, namely the more distanced aim of securing and underpinning the object relationship and of protecting the self from object loss. And if we have to do this for adults, it is even more necessary in the case of children where the level of genital sexuality has not been reached and where the relationship to the primary object, mother, continues for so long to be of utmost importance. In our clinical practice we have all met with disturbed children and adolescents where the mode of relating could certainly be described as sado-masochistic. In such a pattern of relating, the gratification of narcissistic and ego needs is often as important or even more important than drive satisfaction. Such gratification is sought via the omnipotent controlling, dominating and denigration of the object. Though such object-related behaviour is often understood in an analysis as an attempt to safeguard the integrity of the self, the self representation is in fact frequently subjected to the same devaluation and attack as to object representations. Perverse sexual activity as such is not always discernible though a measure

J drive gratification is, of course, involved within the relationship. The collusion of the object within this sado-masochistic type of relationship becomes indispensable, a collusion which permits an interchangeability of role between victim and persecutor and an externalization of unwanted aspects of the self.

The clinical vignettes we now present are selected to illustrate the continuum along which anal drive derivatives are taken up into modes of sado-masochistic functioning and relating; these modes are seen to culminate in behaviour which is certainly akin to adult perverse activity with its accompanying sexualised excitement.

Case 1

Benedict, aged 6:0 years when analysis began, straddled two worlds: his continuing enuresis and encopresis belonged initially to the anal phase of drive development and regressively provided anal gratification, though his incontinence also became firmly embedded in his relationship with his mother; the parents also complained of his antisocial and manipulative behaviour, aggression directed particularly against his younger brother, fears of dying and of falling asleep and dreaming about monsters that would kill his brother. Benedict was said to have had some of these symptoms from an early age. Just after the brothers birth when Benedict was 1 year 8 months old, he began withholding his feces for several days at a time; he experienced intense pain and eventually suffered an anal prolapse. This became the pattern of the defaecatory process and mother was taught by the doctor how to replace the prolapse. When Benedict was 4 years old, his father went abroad for several months and retention and diurnal enuresis recurred. It appeared that Benedict's demanding, clinging, manipulative behaviour, as well as his soiling and enuresis, were directed in the main to his mother who was emotionally unavailable; he would try and make contact with her by provoking her to anger. Benedict sado-masochistic relationship to his father was best seen in repeated play during treatment, play which bore a painful resemblance to Benedict's reality. A baby waited for his father at the airport; as the plane arrived the baby became excited and eager to see father; the plane would either land briefly or not at all and the baby was left disappointed and often in tears. Through his play Benedict gave a vivid picture of his internal world: it was a place in which one either inflicted hurt or was hurt.

Benedict was destructive, messy and aggressive in his treatment, often soiling and wetting during sessions with sexualised excitement and defiance. He would plead with his therapist to control him, that is physically to restrain him, and he became very clinging at the end of each session. He tried to provoke his real objects and the therapist in the transference into controlling him and caring for him, into nor leaving him. The seeming contemptuous and denigratory feelings Benedict expressed toward his objects were understood as an externalisation of his devalued self. The baby who frequently appeared in his play in treatment was described by him thus: "the little boy is not one year old, he is nothing".

The parents were more than adequate models for Benedict for a sado-masochistic pattern relating. They were both self-absorbed artists who, by their own admission, were unable to make contact with their children. They fought together, denigrated each other, had affair the father was away for months at a time and the mother too was often absent. But we have also to take account of the experiences of acute physical pain in the latter half of Benedict's second year and of the intimate involvement of the mother both in his pain and its alleviation. It seems possible that his relationships became organised round these experience of pain and that, later in his development, Benedict needed to recreate pain, with inadequate differentiation between physical and psychic pain, in order to bind his objects to him. Thus his attempts to control everyone and everything could be understood as an omnipotent response to experiencing his parents as rejecting, punishing and abandoning objects. He viewed himself as a dangerous, murderous boy who was repeatedly left, physically an emotionally, by his parents because he was destructive and dirty. The analytic outcome was disappointing one—there was a symptomatic improvement in soiling and wetting but no marked improvement in his relationships. This is hardly surprising in that he remained ensconced in the unhealthy, sado-masochistic family environment.

Case 2

Let us now, by contrast, look at a young boy whose actual behaviour was extraordinarily sadistic. Alan was referred to the Clinic when he was 4½ years old for aggressive and violent behaviour resulting in expulsion from one Nursery School and in the present Nursery School teacher recommending referral for treatment. His attacks on animals were even more vicious than on other children. He had killed a kitten by biting and squeezing it to death. His parents were even more shocked by the cold-blooded and provocative way he had recounted the incident afterwards, saying boastfully "I am a cat killer". Soon after treatment began, he was reported by mother to have killed a pigeon and then to have pulled out its feathers. In the Clinic, he would capture insects and torture them to death by pulling out their wings and legs; at these times his excitement and fascination were intense.

Although Alan's violent and murderous attacks on animals and other children and the way h became excitedly engrossed in such attacks, suggested direct sadistic drive expression, treatment also revealed other contributory elements. Alan had been a victim and a witness of violent and sadistic attacks by his father from babyhood onwards. Thus, his aggressive and violent behaviour was also a defensive identification with the aggressor. The father had a serious drinking problem and, in the face of any criticism or opposition from his wife an others, became abusive and physically violent.

Alan was born in the first year of the marriage, a strong and healthy baby who soon became physically very active, self-willed and determined. He sat up at 3 months, walked at 9 month and, according to mother, "ruled" her. There were battles over feeding, sometimes lasting, more than an hour and, by the time he was one year old, Alan had many temper tantrums and was said by the mother to be aggressive toward her. The father alternated between pride in his "strong" and powerful son and experiencing him as a rival. The mother often had to protect. Alan from the father's rages; even when he was an infant, the father would stand over him furiously shouting "he is defying me"; at other times he would unpredictably cake the baby side and blame the mother for thwarting him.

Alan's second year of life was full of potentially traumatic experiences. When he was one year old he began to attend a play-group every morning while mother went to work to pay off sort of the family's debts. A few months later the mother's parents were killed in a car crash and she became very depressed for several months needing medication and some psychiatric intervention. The father took over some of Alan's care and in particular his toilet training. According to the mother, this was carried out with brutal violence. Often, when Alan wet his pants, father bear him with a hairbrush until his buttocks bled. Alan became dry and clean early and never lost sphincter control. A series of accidents and admissions to hospital followed. When Alan was 1:9 years he walked into an unattended room at the play-group and fell some 50 feet off a balcony. He was shocked, broke his arm and was hospitalised for one week. He was unhappy in hospital and the mother visited daily. Soon after his discharge the mother had herself to go into hospital for two weeks; there was yet another separation and hospitalisation when Alan was 2 years old and contracted pneumonia.

At this stage mother began seriously to worry about Alan's unhappiness and her inability to control and contain him. He seemed hostile and rejected her affection and he appeared to provoke punishment from his father. The mother decided that he needed more affection from her and this took the form of sexual seductiveness. Alan was encouraged to come to mother's bed, in keeping with her way of controlling and pacifying her husband. The parents decided to start another pregnancy "for Alan's sake". When he was 3:9 years his brother was born and he at once became the mother's favourite, a happy, contented and loving baby. Although there was no overt aggression towards his nine months old brother at the time of referral, Alan's anger and jealousy were only thinly disguised and we felt real concern that he might murder him, indeed, on one occasion when the mother left him in charge of the brother, he dragged the screaming baby to the mother's sickbed saying that he had rescued him from trying to hang himself on the curtain cord; the baby had red marks round his neck.

Alan was destructive, provocative and difficult to contain in every situation. He was afraid of his father but told his mother that he wanted to kill father and pull his teeth out. The father reported that Alan was oblivious to physical pain, that only he was strong enough to hurt him, and that his wile could neither control nor punish him. The inflicting and experiencing of pain had obviously become sexualised for Alan, and the continuous exposure to violence acted as a stimulus to his own aggressive and destructive wishes. In treatment Alan once referred to his therapist as a lion tamer; he described himself as facing a lion outside and a lion inside. He tended to meet the dangers lodged in the external world by becoming aggressive, but the exploding of his "inner lion" mobilised massive anxiety. When stripped of his defensive bravado, he often presented as an anxious and fearful boy.

The future development of this boy is endangered even with therapeutic help; however, the final pathology will remain uncertain until he has negotiated latency and adolescence. The sado-masochistic mode of relating and the sexualisation of pain may lead to perversion. Moreover, his parents' sado-masochistic relationship is very pronounced; when the mother was once warned during treatment that the loaded gun her husband kept by his bedside endangered her and her children's lives, she responded that her husband could also kill her with his bare hands. In the course of their marriage, she left him, with or without the children, on many occasions but always returned when he pleaded that he needed her. The sado-masochistic interplay between Alan and his mother also became clear. For example, he once terrified his mother by pretending to step off the platform in front of an oncoming train and then saying quite calmly and gleefully: "that scared you". In fact, during treatment Alan began to curb the expression of extreme aggression toward the external world and increasingly caused hurt and injury to himself. It was almost as if the developing superego condemned hurting others and recommended hurting the self instead. This process may expose him to the danger of a suicidal attempt, possibly one that indirectly attacks the internalised object.

Case 3

With the entry into puberty and psychological adolescence, the sado-masochistic personality structure begins to resemble the adult model more closely. Katie illustrated a pervasive form of sado-masochistic relating when she began analytic treatment at the age of 17 years. Referral complaints were listed as a constant involvement in verbal and physical fights with everyone. She was described as cruel, obstinate, retentive, controlling, and with no regard for objects. She was extremely self-critical and despised both herself and objects for being weak and cringing. Treatment was seen by Katie as a punishment ordained by her mother; to accept analysis implied for Katie the acceptance of mother's view of her as mad and intolerable, like her paranoid grandmother. Katie told her analyst that her mother has said to her: "I want to vomit when I look at you, not you physically; you are very pretty; but you; yes, I want to throw up every time I see you." Katie's reply to mother was: "You don't like me; you never have. Nothing gives me greater pleasure in life than making you suffer, I am sick and I enjoy giving you pain." The pervasive sado-masochistic relationship was immediately transferred to the therapist and treatment was inevitably experienced as a form of torture.

Katie's fantasies involved a wish to be beaten, forced into surrender, a search for libidinal gratification on the functional genital level. She was also compelled to repeat her childhood experience of being the victim of her nanny's and her parents' beatings. Day-dreams—in which "poor Katie" suffered and was pitied—indicated a wish to use her suffering as an attack on the object.

In terms of aetiology, there was an anal fixation originating in severe battles over toilet training. There were pronounced anal character traits; cruelty, obstinacy, doubting and indecision. Relationships were seen by Katie, in terms of controlling or being controlled, of treating or of being treated "like dirt". Her expressions of aggression remained explosive, destructive outpourings of abuse or physical attacks. The parents' sado-masochistic relationship and the mother's overt hostility to her daughter was viewed as important. Her need to denigrate and control objects seemed to originate in a childhood passive-into-active defence against feelings of helplessness toward the parents; her feelings of omnipotence seemed to have been shattered too soon and she constantly tried to reinstate them.

Analysis was terminated after two years at the analyst's suggestion. Katie could not use treatment constructively, could nor establish a viable treatment alliance and evinced a negative therapeutic reaction throughout; she constantly came very late for her sessions and fought against every interpretation. The difficulties were such as to make the analyst feel despairing at times, yet hopeful at other times when Katie did seem able to use treatment; and this would appear to be a characteristic of the sado-masochistic patient.

In a followup interview over a year later, Katie explained her resistance to analysis on the basis of mother having placed her in treatment. The analyst considered that Katie's marked improvement in her work capacity was only definitely established after the termination of analysis and after she had left home. Until then, Katie was too embroiled in the sadomasochistic interaction with her analyst and her mother to make full use of her ego capacities. She then became able to relate more adequately to professional colleagues and her capacity for friendship improved somewhat, though her sexual relationships still carried a sadomasochistic hallmark.

Case 4

Our last case demonstrates the developmental path which led to perverse sexual activity in a young adult whose analysis extended throughout his adolescence. As Peter's story has been reported elsewhere, it will be only briefly summarised here.

He was a depressed and narcissistically vulnerable young man whose life was dominated by a pervasive feeling of inadequacy and resentment from which he could only escape through sexual excitation. He masturbated compulsively from early childhood and, in late adolescence, he enhanced orgasmic pleasure by tying a plastic bag over his head—a practice which was accompanied by fantasies of a female partner castrating and suffocating him. He longed for girl friends but on the few occasions he managed to get into bed with a girl, he became so terrified during foreplay that he took flight.

While the mother-child interaction during Peter's first years was characterised by the mother's disappointment in her "inadequate" baby and the baby's apparent non-compliance with his mother's expectations, the major pathogenic influences occurred in the second and early third years. Toilet training started in his first year, was a "great battle". Bladder and bowel control were only achieved at 3:6 years, and intermittent nocturnal enuresis continued until he has 9 years. The problems over gaining bladder control were undoubtedly increased by his developing phimosis; this led to many examinations and painful manipulations of his penis and eventually necessitated circumcision at the age of 2:8 years. There was ample confirmation from the analytic material that the experiences surrounding this operation, including the anaesthetic to which he had responded with terror, constituted a major sexual trauma for Peter. The excessive handling of his penis, both exciting and painful, mobilised a passive aggressive response at a time when he already felt rejected by his mother. The birth of his brother when Peter was 1:4 years caused a major narcissistic hurt. This brother, always favourably compared with Peter, quickly became more successful in every area with further devastating effects on Peter's self-esteem. He always perceived his brother not only as favoured by both parents but also as superior in every respect, in body and mind.

Peter's aggressive and negativistic behaviour, stemming from the anal-phase and reinforced by the reactions to his life experiences, should have been recognised as signs of disturbance and internal stress; but instead they were met by severe parental punishments and further rejection. He was frequently beaten, humiliated and threatened with abandonment, responses which only reinforced his difficulties and dilemmas. He was forced into a role of passive submission toward his mother on the basis of a sado-masochistic interaction with her. In order to get close to her and gain her attention, he relinquished possession of his penis to her, and unconsciously the mother seemed to demand and respond to this. In later years she seized every opportunity to handle his body, giving him physiotherapy and injections which he consciously hated. Thus, Peter continued to experience his mother both as seducer and attacker, based on his masochistic need to repeat the early sexual trauma and to attain and maintain a close sado-masochistic tie to her. Despite his long, and in many ways successful, analysis, Peter was unable entirely to relinquish this tie to the mother and this particular way of obtaining drive gratification.

Discussion

To conclude, we should like to summarise some salient points arising from our discussion of these descriptively sado-masochistic patients. Central to the formation of a sado-masochistic personality structure seems to be an experience of pain in early life, and particularly in the second and third years when the child is negotiating the tasks involved in separation and individuation, in sell and object differentiation. Such pain originates in the unpleasure of a stressful mother-child relationship and is further accentuated by the actual experience of physical pain. All our cases had certainly experienced inadequate mothering in the first two years of life, due either to the mother's depression or emotional unavailability, or to the mother's marked ambivalence because this particular infant represented unwanted aspects of the mother's own self, her parents, or siblings.

This usually contributed to acute feeding or toilet training problems in which both mother and child were involved. In some cases the birth of a sibling who was more positively invested by the mother enhanced these difficulties.

In his paper on Masochism (1957) Loewenstein describes the mechanism of "seduction of the aggressor", behaviour which seeks "to change an unloving attitude to a loving attitude in a parent", and he suggests that it would be more appropriate to term such behaviour "protomasochistic" or "premasochistic" in that "involvement of the genital apparatus is absent". This behaviour ensures "the existence of parental love, at a time when parental love is as necessary for the development of sexuality as it is for survival". This formulation can be aptly applied to the sado-masochistic children we have described. By the time they entered treatment our patients showed that such mutual tormenting and recriminatory relationships were, for them, tantamount to love relationships and that only these had come within the gamut of their experience and were available to them. Just as a defence mechanism takes on the fit of the wearer and the individual becomes habituated to it, feels safer and more in control when he uses it, so too did these patients use their sado-masochistic mode of relating to ensure the constancy of the relationship, but with a masochistic and sadistic rather than positive stamp. The repetition of this mode of relating both in action and in fantasy not only perpetuates the relationship with the object but may also create the illusion of never having to separate from the object, in that a fit becomes established between the internal and external object relationship.

What also seemed crucial in our patients was the inadequacy of the self-investment. Their grandiosity, egocentricity and self-inflation were paralleled by an underlying, hidden self-denigration which was based on the internalised parental denigration and had its counterpart in their treatment of others. Such narcissistic investment served to defend against the pain inherent in the rejection anticipated from the object as well as against the patient's feelings of being unloved and unlovable, hopeless and depressed. In some patients such defensive grandiosity interfered with the learning process since, in their view, the object was incapable of imparting knowledge to their omniscient selves; and a similar interference was, of course, manifest within the analytic situation. In other cases, the interplay between the superego introjects and the self perpetuated feelings of worthlessness, guilt and masochistic suffering.

In those cases we have, described where actual experiences of physical pain were woven into the fabric of the disturbed mother-child relationship, sexualisation of pain resulted. This was particularly striking in two of the cases we discussed in which the mother's intrusive manipulation of the anus, and the penis involved pain as well as excitation. Similarly, the excessive beatings described in two of the other cases resulted in a sexualisation of pain. The child then repetitively seeks such excitingly painful contact with the object and paves the way for possible sado-masochistic perverse activity in adolescence and adulthood.

The attachment to painful feelings so evident in our patients is well documented in the literature, as is the link with the negative therapeutic reaction. Valenstein (1973) proposes that "the core of the negative therapeutic reaction . . . comes from the patient's attachment to pain"; these painful experiences sometimes occur before self-object differentiation or signify an "original attachment to painfully perceived objects and inconstant objects at that. It appears that in the development of such individuals, instead of the early pleasurable object experiences being consolidated into love and a sense of trust, the opposite occurs. Early affects are predominantly painful and as such recur consistently, crystallizing in the direction of attachment to pain and distrust of objects. The painful affects are then held to, both as a defence and as an instinctually charged concomitant of object experience."

With regard to treatment, it seems important to differentiate at the diagnostic stage between the child whose predominant mode to relating is anal-aggressive as opposed to the child whose pervasive mode is sado-masochistic. Such a differentiation helps to evaluate the collusive role of the object in the patient's problems, as well as to predict more accurately the nature and content of the transference relationship. This is also of technical relevance for the analyst if he wishes to avoid an interminable engagement with the patient in an endless re-enactment of the sado-masochistic mode of relating in the transference; instead the patient has to be confronted with his destructive wishes to self, object and analysis and, by analysing this defensive stance, reach the all-important underlying depression and self-denigration. Further, the constant monitoring of the analyst's counter responses to such patients is important, in that the analyst has to be scrupulous in examining whether the patient's relentless accusations may not eventually trigger off responses which partially fit the sado-masochistic pattern which the patient seeks to impose on the analytic situation.

Conclusion

In summary we have attempted in this paper to approach so-called sado-masochistic behaviour in children from a developmental point of view. Features of the anal-aggressive phase were common in all the cases we discussed. We have also suggested that, from a phenomenological as well as from a dynamic standpoint, we may discern a line of development starring in the disturbed mother-child relationship and affecting the normal processes of separation and individuation. The specific drive organisation of the anal-aggressive phase emphasises the battle between mother and child and subsequently colours the more sophisticated and later sado-masochistic manifestations. In such a schema, behaviour and relationships of the anal-aggressive phase can be viewed as precursors of sado-masochistic functioning. But we suggest that we should only speak of sado-masochistic relationships or sado-masochistic perverse activity if we can demonstrate that such functioning has been superimposed retroactively on the original anal-aggressive mode.

Note

* We are grateful to the contributions made by members of the Research Group on Sado-Masochism, Debbi Bandler, Marion Burgner (Chair), Pauling Cohen, Rose Edgcumbe, DorothyLuciani, Karen Marschke, Katherine Wangh, Marie Zaphiriou, and to the staff and students at the Hampstead Clinic whose cases we have used in this presentation.

References

Abraham, K. (1924). A short study of the development of the libido viewed in the light of mental disorders. In *Selected Papers on Psycho-Analysis* (pp. 418–501). London: Hogarth Press, 1949.

Freud, S. (1905). Three essays on the Theory of Sexuality. *Standard Edition, 7.*

Freud, S. (1915). Instincts and their Vicissitudes. *Standard Edition, 14.*

Laplanche, J. & Pontalis, J. B. (1973). *The Language of Psycho-Analysis.* London: Hogarth Press.

Loewenstein, F. A. (1957). Contribution to the psychoanalytic theory of masochism. *Journal of the American Psychoanalytic Association, 2*: 197–234.

Mahler, M., Pine, F., & Bergman, A. (1975). *The Psychological Birth of the Human Infant.* New York: Basic Books.

Valenstein, A. (1973). On attachment to painful feelings and the negative therapeutic reaction. *Psychoanalytic Study of the Child, 28*: 365–92.

CHAPTER TEN

Steps from Outer to Inner Conflict Viewed as Superego Precursors*

Hansi Kennedy and Clifford Yorke 1982

The existence of a vast literature on the superego bears witness to the many difficulties encountered by those who attempt to conceptualize its formation and its functioning. Our paper, however, is simply an attempt to clarify, within the framework of existing knowledge, the principal steps in the progression from outer to inner conflict, insofar as these can be viewed as superego precursors. We try to do this, wherever possible, in the light of inferences drawn from child observation and clinical practice.

It is true that the analyst of adults usually can trace the beginnings of internal conflicts, based upon interference with drive satisfaction, back to the external conflicts which preceded them; indeed, this constitutes a substantial part of reconstructive work with patients. For example, important checks and prohibitions with which internal impulses are met can generally be seen to derive, through careful historical scrutiny, from certain external controls and interdictions.

The child analyst, on the other hand, and the psychoanalytically informed observer of children, can follow directly the means and the pathways by which external prohibitions become internalized; but in doing so, he will be aware that by no means all such prohibitions can be regarded as superego precursors. We shall therefore try to trace, in this brief opening statement, the pathways by which the child meets the earliest restrictions and prohibitions; how and why they become internalized; what role they play in internal conflict; and the basis on which some of them proceed to play a significant part in the formation of the superego.

At the beginning of life the infant's needs and wishes are met by the mother's facilitation or restraint. Within this interaction some affective mutuality is established, which opens up new areas of gratification and well-being for the child and marks a departure from purely biological to psychological needs. In due course this interaction will modify the peremptory quality and urgency of the infant's demands, to that extent marking the beginning of a capacity to tolerate frustration. The manner in which the mother exercises her functions as a guardian and auxiliary ego; the way she recognizes her baby's needs; how she provides satisfactions or substitute satisfactions; and the means by which she makes frustrations more bearable—all these have an important part to play in the building up of the child's inner representations. Those experiences which enable the infant to tolerate delay in the face of mounting excitation, and which themselves become increasingly pleasurable in terms of the child's well-being, enable him to lay the foundations for inner controls, though it is axiomatic that sooner or later these measures will yield to the imperative demands of drive expression. In all these matters the influence of innate givens, maturational factors, and of course the *experiential* contributants will together determine the individual variations in the ways in which these structures are built up in each child.

With the child's growing awareness of the differentiation of self and object, with his expanding cognitive and motor development, his wishes and pursuits are increasingly interfered with by the external world. The toddler is repeatedly frustrated by limitations imposed by external reality, by an incomprehensible series of maternal interventions designed (unknown to him) to protect him from danger, by the need to gratify contradictory wishes at one and the same time, and by otherwise unattainable drive demands.

Before he can begin to adapt to these early demands and restraints, certain steps in ego development will have to be taken. The child will have to move from an understanding of the immediate wishes and prohibitions to the capacity to remember these experiences in terms of their connotations of approval or disapproval. He will have to learn to generalize his experiences from the particular to a whole new set of similar situations. These cognitive skills will facilitate a growing capacity to *monitor* and to classify, in however rudimentary a fashion, his various wishes and activities in terms of the mother's approval and disapproval. The child thus becomes able to designate; but this new capacity does no more than reflect his mother's view of these different situations. He simply apprehends the models of "goodness" or "badness" which his mother holds up to him.

These models do not as a rule reflect his own wishes. Indeed, they create formidable struggles which persist for a considerable time. For example, a 3-year-old who particularly wanted to get her mother's approval repeatedly asked, "Am I good?" As soon as she was reassured of this, however, she would add, with a certain immediacy, "But I don't like doing what I am told." Another little girl, aged 4 at the time, clashed with her mother whenever she failed to get her own way. In these circumstances, the child would say, "You don't love me, or you would not say 'no.' I don't love you." Elements of these primitive barter systems can, of course, also be detected much later in life. It is one thing to understand a prohibition and quite another to accept it. And without acceptance there is no possibility of making adaptations and modifying behavior on the strength of internal resources alone.

Let us look more closely at the line which leads from dependence on the mother as controller, through physical restraints, verbal restraints, interdiction or forbidding glance, to internal impulse control. External prohibitions originally operate against a multitude of childhood wishes, not all of which are libidinal or aggressive, but some of which nevertheless endanger the child or, for that matter, the security of the brother, the cat, or things in the home.

To begin with the child is unable to differentiate between these different prohibitions. But as ego functions mature, some of these external restraints acquire meaning through increased reality appraisal, through a growing capacity for logical reasoning, through advances in motor control and growing independence, through an increase in the child's capacity to bear frustration, and through the diminishing urgency of certain drive demands as the child moves into a further stage in instinctual development, and so forth.

While all these developmental achievements contribute to the child's capacity for inner control and self-regulation, the wishes which remain closest to drive derivatives are still the hardest to give up, and it is these wishes which continue to mobilize anger with the restraining adult. Toilet training often provides the most striking examples. Tony, who at the age of 3% was excessively messy in his water-play and required repeated physical restraint, became very angry with his therapist whenever she interfered with his wishes. On such occasions he called her a "bloody cow" and defied her in fantasy by pretending to be a fireman and douse her with hoses, though he was careful to emphasize that this was for her own protection. Another young patient invariably called his therapist "naughty" whenever his own aggression was aroused and he anticipated her disapproval and "talion punishment."

Externalization, projection, rationalization, and a number of other defenses are frequently employed to deal with these inner struggles, with which the child has to come to terms before he can establish what Ferenczi (1925) has so appropriately called "sphincter-morality." Nursery observations have furnished us with lots of examples of how children begin to internalize prohibitions. A first step is to direct the adult's prohibitions against others. A common example is provided by children who have not yet attained bladder control but who point with indignation at puddles on the floor put there by other children.

Until the child is able to identify with the ideal held up to him, and thereby turn against his own impulses, full toilet training cannot be achieved; and true, if rudimentary, internal conflict cannot be said to exist. In this respect, one of our War Nursery children, Brigit, who had difficulty in acquiring bladder control, reached a turning point when she was able to announce, with a great deal of affect, "No more wee-wee on the floor: Mummy doesn't like it; Nurse doesn't like it; Brigit doesn't like it."

The crucial point that Brigit makes is that *she* doesn't like it; *she* doesn't like wee-wee on the floor. She takes an *affective* attitude toward unrestricted wetting; her ego begins to find repugnant, if not to hate, an unrestrained instinctual activity or impulse. Her early defensive structures therefore contain an important affective component which lays the ground for reaction formations, and there will be similar affectively toned defenses against aggression, narcissistic wishes, and the like which, as Edith Jacobson (1964) has pointed out, together constitute important superego precursors. Structural refinement and affective differentiation continue to go hand in hand and will ultimately be augmented by the enduring countercathexes of repression proper in the postoedipal period.

What we have tried to describe so far is a move from the use of an external policeman to the use of an internal one; but it does not follow that both constables exercise identical functions, even though they recognizably belong to the same force. At first we see, internally, an incomplete representation of the external policeman, a mere cadet, who is able to discharge only limited functions, and who repeatedly needs reinforcements, orders, and support from outside. It may well be that, for obsessional children, in whom the superego precursors develop particularly early, the need for external reinforcement is unusually urgent. Such children seem constantly to seek external reassurance that they are "good" in order to deal with the sense of "badness" which accompanies any failure to live up to their own severe and premature internal strictures.

To return to our metaphor of the police cadet, compelled to rely for effective action upon external support. It is at this stage that, harassed though he may be, he can draw strength from an unexpected quarter and can turn to the id itself, in the form of aggressive derivatives, to reinforce internal prohibitions. This can be observed in certain changes in the fantasy play of children. Whereas in the beginning such play may tend to repeat, through imitation, the child's day-to-day experience in, for example, turning passive into active, it now begins to reflect a stand against the impulse. For example, one small boy who had always used dolls to represent either himself or other children and repeated with them the various activities of his daily life around mealtimes and bedtimes began to scold his dolls for their "naughtiness" and "dirtiness," for doing "wee-wees" and "poos," and for being smelly or stinking. The dolls were dealt with harshly: they were often smacked or even thrown about. It would seem that the anger and humiliation aroused in the child by external restraints and threats of punishment mobilize his aggression and the anxieties associated with it, so that they are defensively directed against the self. Paradoxically, part of the id rages against itself.

It is not possible to understand these moves, and the motivations behind them, without taking the ego's fear of the Id into account, and thereby giving due weight to anxiety as a powerful motivating force in human development. Indeed, it could be said that it is precisely the fear of loss of love which threatens the child with overwhelming anxiety and which only appropriate internal measures can effectively keep at bay. Thus, on the one hand the pleasure principle makes it difficult for the child to accept external prohibitions, while on the other hand these selfsame prohibitions become an indispensable ally in the fight against the id. We know, for example, how so-called progressive education repeatedly brings adverse consequences, much to the surprise of its protagonists, by its insistence on the absence of external controls for the child. Since the child's instinctual wishes are not sufficiently restrained, and indeed are often overstimulated, the child may have to resort to unusually severe internal controls fostered by the ministrations of a superego which borders on the malign. This is not, of course, the only possible outcome. The absence of restraints may itself become, for the child, a powerful parental ideal with many different consequences for subsequent development.

This touches on the important question of early ideal formation. The fact that this is based on the child's idealization of his parents and on his wish to be like them is obvious enough; but it is only one of the ingredients of those ideals which are so important in providing the child with the aims, guidelines, and models in the conduct of his everyday life. To these may be added: the way in which the child perceives the parental behavior in its sexual and aggressive manifestations and the degree to which, in this respect, he will identify with the *real* parents; the manner in which the parents convey their concept of the ideal child, that is, the child they would like him to be; and whether father and mother convey *different* ideals and whether there are discrepancies between what they consciously or unconsciously convey. All these elements will be compounded in the foundation of the child's *own* self-ideal, which in addition will include the attainment of his pleasure-seeking and narcissistic wishes before these have become modified by later developments in the postoedipal and subsequent phases.

We have addressed ourselves primarily to the question of how external prohibitions become internal interdictions and, in particular, of how these contribute to impulse control. We have not addressed ourselves in any detail to the contributions to these processes made by concomitant affects such as shame, anxiety, and, ultimately, guilt as the child moves from fear of the (external) loss of the mother's love to fear of the (internal) loss of the love of the superego. But these more extensive considerations would take us beyond the perimeter of our purpose. We do not, after all, set out to describe the formation of a structured superego as this takes shape during the resolution of the oedipal conflict. But the fact remains that until the child has achieved the manifold developmental advances we have outlined, no basis exists for further progressions by which part of the ego becomes stabilized as an effective internal agency with more or less enduring independence and authority and which can then serve to guide the rest of the ego in the exercise of its executive and adaptive functions.

Although our scrutiny is limited to certain aspects of the child's protohistory, we hope it contributes to a wider, and more embracing, developmental perspective against which the subsequent structuralization of the superego can be viewed. It may, furthermore, indicate how early developmental tasks, and the success or failure with which they are tackled, can foster, delay, or distort the ultimate formation of the superego proper. None of this gainsays the fact that, in certain respects, many of these early steps contribute to the formation of the ego itself, and not exclusively, or even necessarily, to its presiding overseer. A developmental perspective is, after all, an observational viewpoint for the serial study of facilitation and interference with the progress of interrelationships within the unfolding personality, as well as between that personality and the outside world.

Note

* The paper is based on discussions by a Study Group on the Superego. The other members of this group were: Anna Freud, M. Berger, M. Burgner, C. Elliott, A. Gavshon, J. Hodges, A. Holder, G. Moran, and I. Wineman.

References

Ferenczi, S. (1925). Psycho-analysis of sexual habits. In *Further Contributions to the Theory and Technique of Psycho*-Analysis (pp. 259–97). London: Hogarth Press, 1950.

Jacobson, E. (1964). *The Self and the Object World*. New York: Int. Univ. Press.

CHAPTER ELEVEN

The Developmental Roots of Self-Injury and Response to Pain in a 4-Year-Old Boy*

Hansi Kennedy and George S. Moran 1984

Anna Freud (1977) considered the principal task facing child analysts to be the extension of psychoanalytic child psychology through the more detailed study of developmental processes, anomalies, and disturbances. She firmly believed that child analysts were in a unique position to undertake this task and that, through both treatment and psychoanalytically informed observation of children, they could significantly clarify and extend our knowledge of early development. She took the view that child development could only be understood if due weight were given to the relative contributions of constitutional, environmental, and maturational factors and their mutual interactions, in all their variations; and she saw how the outcome was further affected by factors of timing, intensity, and the extent to which the contributants were suitably matched. Such complexities would determine how far development proceeded in harmony or disharmony, and would lay the early foundations for normative adaptation or for neurotic or nonneurotic disorder.

Anna Freud (1965) viewed personality formation in terms of a continuum of different lines of development from immaturity to maturity. Such lines trace, sequentially, developmental pathways with various intermediate steps. The line from suckling to rational eating, for example, sets out the developmental tasks which have to be accomplished before a child can regulate his food intake rationally, on the basis of his own needs, irrespective of his relationship to the provider of food and without interference from fantasies. Each step along the line presents not only an outward sign of developmental progress, but also an important indication of the child's internal situation. Advance along this line also depends on other developmental achievements, and these can be charted along other relevant lines. Thus, attainments on the line to rational eating, and on the line from wetting and soiling to bladder and bowel control, will affect progress on the line from irresponsibility to responsibility in body management (as our case presentation will exemplify). A conceptual model emerges of a multitude of lines of development which interact and mutually influence each other. These ideas were developed gradually in Anna Freud's writings and gained increasing momentum in her papers of the 1970s and 1980s. In this paper we apply and illustrate these aspects of her thinking.

A study group at the Hampstead Clinic was recently set up to clarify the concept of "developmental disturbance" and the technique of "developmental help." Initially we studied a number of treatment cases whose early development was followed through infant observation, attendance at our well-baby clinic, mother-toddler group, and/or nursery school, before their referral for assessment at the Clinic. By relating data observed in statu nascendi to the subsequent diagnostic assessment and the later psychoanalytic treatment material, we endeavored to examine where and why development began to deviate from the expectable norm and to what extent progress was delayed or obstructed. Such unique clinical data permit the scrutiny of early developmental processes and their interactions, and thereby lead to the detection of the roots of pathological development. In one such case, we trace the developmental roots of self-injury and response to pain in a boy, Tom, who was referred to treatment at the age of 4.[1]

At the time of the referral to the Clinic, Tom showed age-adequate advances in ego functioning, including orientation in the external world, an understanding of cause and effect, and some appraisal of external danger, but was unable to exploit these achievements in the service of control of dangerous and self-damaging behavior. We could trace various interferences with his capacity to protect himself from injury from the time he became mobile and accident-prone to the time, just prior to the referral, when he deliberately threw a cricket ball into the air and watched it fall onto his eye. The study of this case soon forced us to examine the subjective and objective meaning of "pain" and to formulate a working definition which we could apply to the clinical and observational material of Tom.

Psychoanalytic conception of pain

It is not easy to distinguish conceptually between the psychic experience of physical pain and "psychological pain" as we generally understand it. This difficulty has occupied many psychoanalytic writers beginning with Freud (1920), who described the "specific unpleasure of physical pain" with reference to a breach in the "protective shield" (p. 30). In 1926, Freud likened the phenomenon of mental pain to physical pain.

In the psychoanalytic literature there are two major conceptual approaches to a definition of physical pain. One is to define pain as a more or less localized sensation, and the other is to conceptualize pain as an affect, because, in addition to being a sensation, the experience of pain connotes emotional and ideational components. Szasz (1957) goes so far as to attribute to pain a signal function, analogous to the signal function of anxiety. Pain signals to the ego injury or damage to the body, just as anxiety signals to the ego anticipated danger of loss. But Szasz's conceptualization proceeds from the perspective of the mature adult ego, and leaves us with many problems in assessing pain from a developmental viewpoint. In her paper "The Role of Bodily Illness in the Mental Life of Children" (1952), Anna Freud states:

> Where the direct observation of infants in the first year of life is concerned, the relative proportion of physiological and psychological elements in the experience of pain is an open question. At this stage, any tension, need or frustration is probably felt as "pain," no real distinction being made yet between the diffuse experience of discomfort and the sharper and more circumscribed one of real pain arising from specific

sources . . . From what age onward the bodily event is supposed to carry psychic meaning for the infant will depend altogether on the analytic observer's theoretical assumptions concerning the date when unconscious fantasies begin to exist [p. 76f.].

It is widely assumed that the infant's sense of his body and its boundaries evolves on the basis of initial differentiation of pleasure and pain. This is based on Freud's (1930) original idea that pleasure tends to be linked with the self and unpleasure with the outside-the-self.

Hoffer (1950) suggested that in addition to this mode of differentiation, the infant has "another differentiating system in the [his] body, that between 'pain' and 'not pain'" (p. 159). Building on Freud's early formulation of a pain barrier, Hoffer postulated that this barrier, operative from birth onward, was a potent safeguard against the turning of the aggressive instinct against the infant's own body. Gradually this barrier against self-destructiveness is reinforced by a progressive libidinization of the body and self.

Spitz (1965) concluded that the development of the drives, both libidinal and aggressive, is closely linked to the infant's relationship to his caretaking object. Due to the functioning of the developing ego the child learns to distinguish between the "bad" object (preobject) who refuses to gratify his needs and against whom his aggression is directed, and the "good" object (preobject) who gratifies needs and toward whom his libido is directed. Around 6 months of life memory traces of innumerably repeated experiences and interchanges between the infant and his mother begin to be integrated. This results, Spitz said, in a fusion of the drives and a fusion of the two preobjects, good and bad, into one.

The influences of the early mother-infant interaction on stimulating or taming the infant's aggressive strivings have been a focus of many studies. Greenacre (1941), for example, observed that ambivalent and aggressive mothers increase the child's anxiety proneness and aggression. Examining the role of the mother in bringing about a harmonious initial fit with her baby, Weil (1981) noted: "A relaxed warm libidinally infusing and gently limiting mother may tone down even markedly aggressive tendencies and, in consequence, soften the potential aggressive tinge of ego and superego, thus diminishing the later potential superego anxiety" (p. 141).

Joffe and Sandler (1965) expressed the ideas that "From the point of view of the drives, the normal response to pain is aggression, directed at whatever is considered to be the source of pain" (p. 421). "If a state of pain is experienced in the self, then the actual self may become an object of the child's anger or even hate. It is an unsatisfactory self, and will be invested with aggressive cathexis" (p. 413).

Fraiberg (1982) described toddlers from the age of 13 months whom she observed to tolerate high levels of pain without discernible reactions; she argued that in these cases, the tolerance could not be attributed to a biological fault in the pain threshold. She considered the aberrant development in object relationships, which was found to be present in each case, to be closely related to the deviant course of the aggressive drive which became manifest when the children became mobile at the beginning of the second year of life. "When our therapeutic work is successful, . . . when the parents become the protectors against danger, these children begin to look like normal children. Aggression is discharged along normal pathways, it is modified in the service of love of parents, it is no longer turned upon the self, and pain is experienced in a measure that is appropriate to circumstance" (p. 631).

In reviewing some of the relevant literature we are left with the problem of defining and conceptually differentiating the experience of pain, anxiety, painful affect, and unpleasure. As early as 1958, Ramzy and Wallerstein posed this question in their thoughtful paper on "Pain, Fear, and Anxiety." Valenstein (1973) revisited the problem and concluded:

> For all its omnipresence as the watchdog alarm guarding life, pain is nonetheless extraordinarily difficult to define succinctly . . . The term encompasses pain and affects associated with it, whether the pain is initiated physiologically and has psychic concomitants, or whether the pain is predominantly psychic in origin in consequence of interpersonal or intrapsychic unconscious conflict and has physiological concomitants. The connotation will be a specific affect (Schmerz) or related affect within the psychoanalytic concept of unpleasure (Unlust) [p. 366f].

It may be helpful to keep some of these contributions in mind in considering what follows.

Case Presentation

Developmental Assessment

Those at the Clinic who were in contact with the T. family had been concerned about Tom's development and his difficult relationship with his mother before his referral for assessment at age 4. By then he showed more obvious signs of disturbance. He was extremely negativistic toward his mother and was struggling with his aggression toward his 2-year-old sister. He was often frightened, restless, anxious, and uncommonly prone to injury. At the time of the referral, he still wet his bed at night. There was a history of feeding difficulties.

The developmental lines in the Diagnostic Profile displayed the unevenness and aberrant features of his development, On the line from suckling to rational eating, we trace his development as follows: Tom's mother was desperately unhappy and breast-feeding was fraught with anxiety for her. She gave it up after only a few weeks and put Tom on the bottle. He soon settled down and fed well. But this served only to convince Mrs T. that she had starved him during the first few weeks of life. When he was weaned from the bottle at 12 months, feeding once more became a problem. He restricted his intake and enjoyed only milk and juice. His lack of interest in food caused Mrs T. to feel anxious and guilty, and this continued until the age of 3½ years when the feeding pattern changed. He ate well for a short time, but then passed into a phase in which he stuffed food and vomited. In the intervening period, he developed whooping cough, which may well have laid a foundation for the vomiting. Tom was a messy eater and had not accepted the use of fork or spoon. Feeding involved battles, and he had not outgrown the equation of food and mother.

The line from wetting and soiling to bowel and bladder control provides another example of Tom's difficulty in moving forward. Toilet training was started at the age of 2 and intensified before the sister's birth and his entry into a play group. His mother felt bad about this afterward. Although Tom became clean and dry by day, his bladder control at night was still unreliable up to and beyond the time of diagnostic assessment. In various respects his reaction formations were tenuous. On occasions, he wet the parents' bed in the morning. The entire house was strewn with his toys which he habitually refused to clear up, and on his visits to the well-baby clinic he likewise left the room in disarray.

Since it is directly relevant to the focus of this study, we shall examine in detail Tom's severely impeded progress on the developmental line from irresponsibility to responsibility in body management. Apparently, he had never fully accomplished the first step along the line in which aggression is turned away from the body. From the time he became mobile he had a long series of injuries; and these continued throughout his second year. Several were sufficiently serious to call for treatment in the emergency department of the local hospital. During the period of observation made at home, he often seemed heedless of danger and was hyperactive. He was repeatedly observed to climb up the side of his cot and leap wildly on the floor; his mother's attempts to stop him were inadequate. In order to understand the origin of the disturbance on this line we shall look at the ways in which certain aspects of his environment, constitutional endowment, and developmental progress contributed to, and interacted with, his tendency to self-injury. In so doing, we shall have to retrace our steps a little.

Mrs T. was unhappy during the pregnancy and troubled by the changes in her physical appearance. She was depressed and angry after Tom's birth and felt unappreciated and unprotected, particularly by her husband. Her depression often led her to leave Tom in a state of distress, and her ministrations were inconsistent. In handling him, she was often careless and even rather rough. We concluded that, at best, the satisfaction of Tom's needs was barely adequate, and that too often painful experiences predominated in the first year of life.

Once Tom became mobile, Mrs T.'s ambivalence caused her to leave him too much to his own devices. Furthermore, her tendency to externalize her aggression led her to view Tom as hostile through successive developmental phases. His difficulties with feeding at the breast and, later, his food fads were experienced by her as rejections. She perceived Tom's pleasure in motility and his hyperactivity as intentionally and frighteningly aggressive. Since she repeatedly spoke, with a gleam in her eye, of his defiance in the company of the extended family, she may have taken vicarious pleasure in such behavior. All these matters contributed to her inability to help Tom contain instinctual impulses in the toddler phase and beyond.

Tom's hyperactivity became evident with his mobility. It contributed to his self-injurious behavior in the second year of life. In view of the relative absence of pleasure in other areas, pleasure in motility may have been particularly important for Tom. His libidinal investment in motor activity was unquestionable, and it may have contributed to the precarious quality of his libidinal investment in his objects. During treatment this was still evident in his habitual response to frustration. He would run about wildly or take dangerous leaps off furniture and relinquish his contact with the therapist.

Whatever degree of pleasure Tom derived from motility, his mother failed to provide protective limits. Hence he sustained minor injuries and the more serious accidents to which we have already referred. Tom's inability to control and protect himself increased his anxiety, which then further contributed to frenetic motor behavior. The situation was worsened by the fact that even his mother's reality appraisal of danger was inadequate.

For an infant with an imbalance in the pleasure-pain series, pain and the aggression it mobilizes may become focal organizers of experience. Tom's mother was unable to provide adequate libidinal investment in Tom and his body. His early experiences of his mother's inconsistent care and her rough handling may have laid a foundation for an aggressive taint to his relationship to self and object. Whereas normally the child's responses to frustration are mitigated by pleasurable interaction with his objects, Tom's interaction with his mother was often experienced as painful. His many accidents in the second year of life indicated that pain had become inextricably bound to his relationship to himself and his mother, and may account for the heightening of his pain threshold which remained in evidence up to and beyond his referral for treatment.

Because of his mother's earlier failure to provide safe and secure limits, Tom was prevented from sharing in the illusion that his mother could protect him from painful experiences. Lacking this shared omnipotence to help him cope with pain and anxiety, he was thrown back on his own resources. Moreover, by failing to impose necessary restrictions, Mrs T. had allowed Tom's impulse control to grow unchecked, particularly in relation to aggression. For example, when the mother tried to encourage him to urinate in the lavatory instead of on a potted plant, he became anxious and angry. He raced across the room, viciously grabbed his mother's breasts, and swiped at her necklace as she drew him on her lap. Her anxious laughter and equivocal prohibition failed either to stop him or reassure him.

Anal-phase conflicts around hurting and being hurt further reinforced the unfavorable balance between pleasurable and painful experiences in his object relationships and underscored his disappointment and anger with his mother. When toward the end of his second year, his mother's pregnancy became obtrusive, his aggressive and self-damaging behavior intensified.

In many respects Tom's ego development was quite precocious, not only in fostering motility but in promoting thought and language. His fantasy play revealed an early awareness and impressive knowledge of the world around him. He also showed a growing tendency for abstract reasoning and symbolic thought at a high level and a provocative and imaginative spirit of inquiry. His disappointment and anger with his mother led him to exploit these advanced ego capacities in the service of precocious independence, thus emphasizing the disharmony of his developmental progress. As a toddler he already had shown his reluctance to let his mother touch him, hold him, or kiss him; and his apparent inability to be loving toward his mother was later understood as a defensive stance against a fear of loss of her love.

When Tom was 2 the birth of the baby brought a fresh difficulty in his efforts to cope with his mother's and his own ambivalence. He showed expectable jealousy and frequently attacked his sister, but his mother was unable to help him control his aggression. He would hit the baby with his toy truncheon; although Mrs T. protested vigorously, she repeatedly left the truncheon within his reach. Concomitantly, her fear of Tom's capacity to hurt reached pathological proportions. She hid from him when he talked to her "like a skinhead," instead of stopping him from behaving like one. Although Mr T. at times harshly condemned Tom's attacks on his sister, he was experienced by Tom as a more consistent and therefore safer love, object than his mother.

The advent of toilet training, the birth of his sister, and his mother's insistence that he attend a play group, all of which occurred within the span of a few weeks, led to Tom's overwhelming sense of himself as aggressive and unloving; he felt worthless and cast aside like his feces. It was at this point that his development was seriously endangered, though this was not recognized by his parents. His view of himself as unsafe and unloved heightened his anxieties about object loss. By now, his association of pain with his mother was so well established that he was obliged to renew defensive measures against aggressive impulses.

As Tom felt the threats of his mother's withdrawal of love to be increasingly linked with intolerance of his aggressive attacks, especially on the baby, he began to internalize her condemnation in the form of harsh and punitive superego precursors. As a result, he felt less bad when he hurt himself than when he attacked the baby; and this feeling was secondarily reinforced by the circumstance that self-injury could elicit his mother's guilt and attract her concern and attention. In this way, hurting himself was a compromise between the wish to hurt, the desire to retain his mother's love, and the condemnation of his own aggression in the form of self-punishment. Thus, in order to defend against the painful affects associated with these conflicts, he increasingly turned to physical pain. This preference for physical pain over psychological pain had its roots in the pattern of the early mother-child interaction.

Developmental Psychopathology as Shown by the Treatment Material

When recommendations for treatment of this kind of disturbance are made, we recognize the need for daily contact with the child but question the effectiveness of a purely interpretative technique. With a clearer understanding of developmental distortions and delays, the therapeutic task must be widened to include ways and means of correcting the consequences of these disturbances. The study of such cases helps us to refine the distinction between antecedent developmental pathology and later conflictual pathology of a neurotic kind.

In Tom's case, "developmental help" in facilitating a better synthesis of developmentally acquired tendencies was intertwined with interpretation of defense and conflict. Examples of the way in which Tom's accident proneness and self-injury manifested themselves and were understood and handled by the therapist over the course of treatment will help to illustrate what we mean by this kind of therapeutic intervention.

Tom's references to, and enactments of, accidents and self-injury were numerous and served to express many affects, thoughts, and conflicts. From the outset it was clear that he blamed his mother for his hurts, and he linked the pain he experienced to his feeling uncared for by her. At home, when offended and cross, he often left the room, climbed on to high furniture, and jumped to the floor. One day, on seeing his mother arrive in the nursery school garden to collect him, Tom dropped from the slide to the ground in a dangerous manner and bruised his eye. In reporting this to his therapist, he said that he had also bruised his other eye because his mother had left a door open at home. Later in treatment Tom behaved in a similar way with his therapist: on being called for his session, he dropped dangerously from the slide. He also frequently tripped on the stairs on leaving the treatment room.

In treatment it became apparent that Tom's unconscious link between pain and his mother was associated with anxieties about aggressive wishes and concomitant fears of object loss. Describing a cut on his foot, Tom said that it did not hurt when he stepped on a stone but only when his mother put a plaster on it. In response to frustration, or when cross with the therapist, he frequently became frenetic or, at other times, pursued dangerous activities in a more deliberate way. For example, he would walk on the edge of the desk and threaten to fall and hurt himself if the therapist did not "shut up." When, after one term of analysis, a forthcoming holiday break was discussed, Tom slowly and deliberately put a little chalk dust in his eyes; although he was on the verge of tears, he denied hurt feelings about not seeing his therapist. Doing dangerous things or hurting himself when angry expressed his worries about "losing the loving feelings," and these links became the crucial verbalizations at this time in treatment.

While as a toddler Tom had appeared reckless in his motor activity, heedless of danger, and oblivious to pain, by the time he entered treatment there was evidence of intention in his self-injurious behavior. There was every indication that his tendency to hurt himself in response to feeling hurt by the object was becoming structuralized and taking shape in the defense mechanisms of turning aggression against the self and identification with the aggressor. He had to defend against the anger aroused by feeling disappointed, humiliated, and frustrated, and attacks on the object gave way to self-injury. But the earlier developmental determinants of the defense mechanisms now became increasingly obscured by the structuralization of the ego and the move into the phallic-oedipal phase.

The therapist was able to observe the way in which Tom's tendency toward overactivity and the links between pain and mother, established early in life, became absorbed in the oedipal conflict. When his uncle's death heightened the anxiety deriving from oedipal death wishes, Tom spent a session carefully and fiendishly constructing a weapon which he planned to take home to poke out "someone's eyes." In this connection Tom also recalled an occasion when his father had been away and he had jumped lustily on his mother from behind. But before leaving this session he deliberately poked his fingers in his own eyes. The following day he sneaked up behind his therapist, managed to get under the therapist's feet, and fell badly, requiring a visit to his family doctor's surgery. This incident had almost succeeded in making both the therapist and Tom feel that the therapist had brought about the fall. It led to clarification of the meaning of accidents in the second year of life, though at the time the incident signified in the transference a retaliatory punishment from father for oedipal wishes.

This incident also serves as an illustration of the way in which preverbal experiences are enacted in a child's analysis and absorbed into the context of later developmental conflicts. In subsequent treatment sessions primal scene fantasies, death wishes, oedipal disappointments, and feelings of being the rejected rival often emerged in fantasy enactments featuring frenetic activity, falling, tripping, and dropping from high places.

Verbalization and interpretation of oedipal conflicts lowered Tom's level of anxiety and overactivity. Interpretation of the manifold links between his aggressive wishes and his self-injurious behavior helped him to some extent to curb his tendency to hurt himself. But the opportunity for a one-to-one relationship with a benign and consistent adult with whom he could identify was much more significant in this respect. The therapist's capacity to accept and verbalize Tom's aggression, while at the same time endeavoring to prevent him from hurting himself by setting protective limits, gradually helped Tom to develop control over his wild activity.

Only in combination did these various technical measures allow Tom to take the steps from hurting himself to threatening to hurt himself. They helped him to redirect his aggression outward by threatening to hurt others instead of himself. He also learned to deflect his aggressive impulses toward inanimate objects. He took steps toward the sublimation of his aggression, e.g., in learning to make weapons which he used safely and with a certain skill. In the treatment situation Tom learned that his therapist would control him if necessary; in addition, the therapist attempted without negating Tom's anger to confront him with his omnipotence. These aspects of technique helped Tom to feel safe instead of destructive. In this way he learned, in relation to the therapist, that his object's anger was not as devastating as he imagined. Tom's reliance on the therapist for gaining and maintaining control and mastery of anxiety and aggression continued throughout the treatment. In addition, the value which the therapist implicitly gave to Tom's verbal facility and logical thought provided important external sources for his self-esteem. Moreover, Tom had the continuing experience that his intense interest in wild creatures and natural disasters did not promote anxiety in the therapist, as it had done with his mother.

Lastly, the therapist's genuine concern for Tom's well-being must also have contributed to a belated internalization of concern for the care of his body. There were antecedents for this care in his good relationship with his father whom Tom had preferred to care for his body in his early life. On several occasions, the therapist took active measures to protect Tom from pain and, in a gentle manner, to look after his body. On one occasion Tom became anxious and miserable about a small piece of hardened plaster which had become attached to a hair on his leg. He feared that if he pulled too hard on the plaster he would bleed. Although the therapist commented indirectly on Tom's masturbation conflict and castration anxiety, he also wet a towel and showed Tom how to get the plaster off without hurting himself. In this way Tom learned that he need not be in physical pain when anxious, but such practical help was always integrated into the context of the interpretative work.

The changes which began to accrue in the work with Tom were greatly facilitated by helping him develop psychological pathways for the experience and expression of pain and anxiety. This resulted in an alteration in his self representation and a strengthening of his capacity to choose objects he felt would like him and respond to him. The ongoing experience of the therapist's protectiveness may have augmented Tom's capacity to feel protective toward others. What was far more evident, however, was that the progressive development fostered by treatment accentuated the qualities of discernment and discrimination that underlay Tom's careful choice of persons with whom he desired a relationship. In so doing he seemed able to perceive the value and regard which others held for him, e.g., his father, his nursery school teacher, and the therapist. It was noted that in the nursery school Tom was able to make steady and intense relationships with some of the children, while he remained wary and timorous of others who he felt would not have sought him out.

The changes in his feelings about himself and others can most clearly be demonstrated in the developmental sequence of his investment in inanimate objects. For well over 2 years a large sand bucket played an important part in his life. It was put to a variety of uses. At around the age of 2 he was observed to carry it everywhere he went. His initial choice of the bucket occurred at a time when painters were in the house and appeared to represent for Tom a compromise between his wish to smear and his wish to comply with his mother's demands for cleanliness. Soon after the birth of his sister her began to wear the bucket over his head, even at night and in the bath, which suggested a desire to protect his head and his most valued attributes, i.e., his intellective functions, from injury. Sometimes the need to protect his head may have involved a displacement from his penis. His tendency to hide under the bucket also suggested an effort to contain various drive urges and fantasies. The symbolic value of the bucket as a phallic attribute was later easily discernible when he used it to pretend that he was a soldier and a policeman. The most striking feature of the bucket, regardless of the developmental processes which its use reflected, was its hardness; in contrast to the soft objects used by most children, the bucket undoubtedly was painful to go to bed with. There were, however, significant changes as treatment progressed. Once his self-injurious tendencies and aggressive wishes were linked with his worries about "losing the loving feelings," Tom developed a passionate investment in his furry mitten and lost interest in the bucket. It suggested that a modification had occurred in the balance between libidinal and aggressive cathexes of self and object representations.

After 2 years of treatment, when he was 6, Tom was well established in primary school and had stopped hurting himself for an entire year. In evaluating the beneficial factors in Tom's treatment, the work with Tom's mother was undoubtedly very important. In addition to her own psychotherapy, Mrs T. was seen regularly by Tom's therapist. These interviews were geared to the child—an approach which we consider an essential auxiliary to the treatment of young children. To some extent, this help enabled Mrs T. to free Tom from some of her externalizations and to redirect some of her anger away from him and toward other objects. She became better able to support him in curbing his impulses. The work with Mrs T. was paralleled in Tom's treatment by clarifying his experiences of his mother's inconsistency and anxiety and helping him to differentiate his worries from hers.

Whether Tom can maintain these developmental gains without the support of the therapist will depend to some extent on the permanence with which the changes in Mrs T.'s relationship to, and handling of, her son have been established. However, the fact that Tom is older, has now negotiated the oedipal phase, and is strongly identified with his father and the therapist will increase his chances of maintaining his progressive moves. In this connection, it may well have been important that Tom's therapist was a man. We cannot claim to have safeguarded Tom's future development, but we have redirected him from an aberrant path on the developmental line from irresponsibility to responsibility in the care of his body.

Conclusion

Anna Freud's (1974) systematic attempt to distinguish between developmental psychopathology and conflictual pathology of a neurotic kind led her to describe the increasing complexity of the interrelationship between the two types of pathology during the child's early years. We have tried to illustrate her view of developmental psychopathology as a fertile breeding ground for the later structuralization of defense and conflict.

Tom's experiences in early infancy led to a predominance of painful feelings which mobilized his aggression. This resulted in an imbalance between libidinal and aggressive investment in the self and his objects, so that from early on he lacked trust and was especially prone to fear of loss of love.

His mother was ambivalent and unempathic, which led to excessive frustration and inadequate need satisfaction. Normally, early pleasurable experiences consolidate and form a basis for developing love for and trust in the object and the self—factors which Khantzian and Mack (1983) also associate with the child's capacities for self-care and self-protection. In Tom's case, the opposite occurred: Unpleasure and painful affect were the organizers of early experience and crystallized in an attachment to pain and mistrust of objects. Developing against such a background, the wish to please the object was precarious. The difficulty in modifying oral and anal gratifications in the realms of feeding and toilet training, although it did not lead to battles and sadomasochistic interaction, created a situation of parental disappointment and disapproval. The difficulties in relinquishing instinctual gratification, already determined by inadequate need satisfaction in early life, were reinforced by a lack of positive feedback from the object. In this way, his parents' lack of pride in him and their failure to admire or praise him further contributed to his sense of being unlovable and unloved.

From the time he became mobile a high investment of his bodily movement may have been augmented by a constitutional tendency to hyperactivity. Pleasure in motility was a substitute for the relative absence of pleasure in other areas. It did not require the participation of his mother who all too readily left him to his own devices. His mother's inability to control and protect him from hurting himself, however, helped to consolidate both accident proneness and an attachment to pain. It was only after blatant self-injury that his mother felt guilt and on this basis provided comfort and showed concern. Pain became inseparable from his relationship to himself and to his mother. All these were all along reinforced by his experience of the mother's psychopathology, by the way she handled him, and by the father's relative unavailability.

The lack of loving reciprocity in Tom's object relationships interfered with the taming of his aggression and the building up of benign self and object representations. With the birth of the sibling and further structuralization of aggressive conflict, his self-injurious tendencies were mobilized in the service of defense and in the formation of harsh and punitive superego precursors.

Tom's developmental history thus confirms the close link between early painful experiences, i.e., unpleasure, and heightened aggression. Such an imbalance in the pleasure-pain series results in aberrant object relationships. Tom's treatment material confirms Fraiberg's (1982) observation that such distortions in object relations can lead to a modification of the threshold for physical pain. In Tom's case, we were able to take the connection between the disturbance in object relations and pain one step farther. Increasingly Tom had attained closeness to his objects in connection with the experience of physical pain.

Notes

* This work is part of a continuing study entitled "A Project to Study Variations of Normality and Pathology in Relation to Personality Development".

1. The members of the study group of Developmental Disturbances include Hansi Kennedy (Chair), Pauline Cohen, Geraldine Fitzpatrick, Audrey Gavshon, Barbara Grant, Steven Marans, George Moran, Turid Nyhamar, Sarah Rabb, Janet Szydlo. We are indebted to other group members for their many helpful comments in discussions of this case.

References

Fraiberg, S. (1982). Pathological defenses in infancy. *Psychoanalytic Quarterly, 51*: 612–35.

Freud, A. (1952). The role of bodily illness in the mental life of children. *Psychoanalytic Study of the Child, 7*: 69–81.

Freud, A. (1965). *Normality and Pathology in Childhood.* New York: Int. Univ. Press.

Freud, A. (1974). A psychoanalytic view of developmental psychopathology. In *The Writings of Anna Freud, 7* (pp. 55–74). London: Int. Univ. Press, 1981.

Freud, A. (1977). The principal task of child analysis. *Bulletin of the Hampstead Clinic, 1*: 11–16.

Freud, S. (1920). Beyond the pleasure principle. *Standard Edition, 18.*

Freud, S. (1926). Inhibitions, symptoms and anxiety. *Standard Edition, 20.*

Freud, S. (1930). Civilization and its discontents. *Standard Edition, 21.*

Greenacre, P. (1941). The predisposition to anxiety. In *Trauma, Growth, and Personality* (pp. 27–82). New York: Int. Univ. Press, 1969.

Hoffer, W. (1950). Oral aggressiveness and ego development. *International Journal of Psychoanalysis, 31*: 156–60.

Joffe, W. G. & Sandler, J. (1965). Notes on pain, depression, and individuation. *Psychoanalytic Study of the Child, 20*: 394–424.

Khantzian, E. J. & Mack, J. E. (1983). Self-preservation and the care of the self. *Psychoanalytic Study of the Child, 38*: 209–32.

Ramzy, I. & Wallerstein, R. S. (1958). Pain, fear, and anxiety. *Psychoanalytic Study of the Child, 13*: 147–89.

Spitz, R. A. (1965). *The First Year of Life.* New York: Int. Univ. Press.

Szasz, T. S. (1957). *Pain and Pleasure.* London: Tavistock.

Valenstein, A. F. (1973). On attachment to painful feelings and the negative therapeutic reaction. *Psychoanalytic Study of the Child, 28*: 365–92.

Weil, A. P. (1981). Anxiety in childhood. In: E.J. Anthony & D.C. Gilpin (Eds.), *Three Further Clinical Faces of Childhood* (pp. 135–49). New York: SP Medical and Scientific Books.

CHAPTER TWELVE

For or Against Child Placement: A Clinical Illustration*

Hansi Kennedy 1985

Introduction

In this paper I will present some case material which I hope will demonstrate the difficulties child—care professionals encounter in their work with children whose physical and/or mental health is endangered by their home environment. The task of evaluating the potential risks, physical or psychological, of growing up in such a home, against the dangers that may follow removal from the family, is formidable. The authors of *Before the Best Interests of the Child* (Goldstein et al., 1979) address themselves to these problems and suggest, as a guideline, "the least detrimental available alternative for safeguarding the child's growth and development". They argue that the least detrimental alternative is usually for the child to remain with his family and that the law should not enforce the removal of any child unless there is evidence of physical injury, physical neglect or of abandonment.

However, responsibility for taking preventive measures usually rests with the child-caring professions who carry the heavy burden of deciding what is least detrimental. In situations that pose a serious threat for a child's growth and development, the line between needing physical and needing psychological protection is often quite narrow. Even in families where the child is not the primary object of parental violence, he may at any time become so; and in any case he will be adversely affected psychologically by witnessing such scenes. Young children are physically and psychologically at risk when in the care of parents who are drunk or suicidal; and they may be neglected to the point of being physically endangered while in the care of a severely depressed or withdrawn parent. All these conditions applied in the case I am going to describe.

The Case of Peggy

Peggy was 2 years 10 months when she was referred to the Nursery School attached to the Anna Freud Centre, which provides day-care for a small group of socially and/or emotionally disadvantaged children.

The family was well known to the social services. Both parents had histories of mental breakdown and hospitalization. Mr and Mrs P had lived together for several years before Peggy was born. They had wanted a child, perhaps to compensate for their own losses and deprivations, but were unrealistic in their expectations and unable to cope with the demands that caring for a child involved. The relationship between the parents had always been difficult and turbulent, and the baby's arrival caused further strain. Peggy repeatedly witnessed arguments and physical fights between them and was often caught in the crossfire. Her name had been put on the list of "at risk" children just prior to the referral. It had followed an incident when the social worker, on a routine visit, happened to intrude on a parental fight and witnessed Mrs P hurling chairs about the room in a fit of uncontrollable rage, while Peggy cowered in a corner.

Mrs P was a very needy and vulnerable person; the slightest sign of rejection or criticism touched off violent anger and rage which was readily displaced on anyone who happened to be around at that moment. Such outbursts were usually followed by periods of severe depression, when he turned to drinking or needed medication. At times this led to accidental self—injury or suicide attempts. Mr P also suffered from depression and often used alcohol to keep going.

Peggy was a bright and demanding baby and her parents' love for her was probably the most positive aspect of their relationship. Yet caring for her had drained their limited emotional resources. Mrs P desperately wanted to be a good mother, but for her this meant never refusing her child anything. At 2 years 10 months Peggy commanded her parents' exclusive attention all day and reigned supreme in the home. Her importunity was just beginning to extend into the night with the onset of a sleep disturbance. A vicious circle had been set up in which the parents behaved like Peggy's slaves until her increasing demands drove them to hit her, which then made them feel so guilty that they again had to indulge her every wish. This had become the established pattern at home and the parents found her difficult to handle. In order to relieve some of these tensions, the social worker had suggested that Peggy join our Nursery School.

In spite of her disturbed family background Peggy presented as a well-developed little girl. She was alert, observant, articulate and her play was well organized. She related warmly to her teachers and playmates. Physically she was always well cared for, well fed and clean. She had no lack of toys and beautiful clothes, many of them made by her mother. Her good ego-functioning was sustained throughout the three years we were in close contact with her, although the strain of the deteriorating home situation showed in her sadness and depressed affect. At such times the wish to rescue her was uppermost in the minds of the staff. The question of placement was often discussed but always dismissed. Instead, we worked in the closest co-operation with the social services to set up a network of support for this family as they moved from crisis to crisis.

The first such crisis occurred even before there was a vacancy for Peggy in the Nursery School. Mr P just arrived one afternoon, carrying Peggy, who had a big bruise on her cheek and was sucking her thumb. He asked if Peggy could be admitted right away as her mother was unwell. They both looked so miserable and forlorn that the teachers agreed. Peggy separated easily from her father and settled quickly in the Nursery School. Although at first she grabbed every toy with a peremptory "I want it", she soon began to realize that the teachers were not playing the same game as her parents. She quickly learned from her own experience, and even more from scrutinizing the teachers' interactions with the other children, to accept the Nursery's social code. We soon concluded that attending Nursery School was a relief for Peggy; it was a place where she experienced safety, and consistency in regard to rules, and where she was clearly assigned the role of a child.

For the first three weeks her father brought her every morning on his way to work and collected her again in the afternoon. He shopped and cooked and took care of her at home but he could barely cope with all these responsibilities. He reported that his wife was severely depressed and had been put on medication so that she hardly talked and sat slumped over the kitchen table for most of the day As soon as Mrs P emerged from this withdrawn state and could again take over her daughter's care, Peggy's behaviour at home became more difficult and her attendance at Nursery School irregular. It became clear that the child's easy adjustment to the Nursery had an adverse effect on her mother. Mrs P complained to her social worker that she was lonely at home without Peggy, and she became quite hostile to the teachers, especially when Peggy's negativism at home took the form of telling her mother to go away and calling for the teacher's help. When Mrs P also managed to persuade her husband that Peggy was picking up "bad ways" at school, there was a real danger that the parents would withdraw her. A joint conference was held with the social services to consider what should be done, and the question of placement was raised for the first time, but was unanimously rejected as entirely inappropriate. For in spite of the parental fights and Mrs P's ambivalence and extreme mood swings to which this child was continually exposed, Peggy's physical and mental development had progressed, and her ego development was, if anything, precocious. We had all recently witnessed how Mr P was able to provide substitute care when necessary. Moreover, Mrs P's present attitude towards the teachers made it quite clear that she was not willing to relinquish her child to any other caretaker.

It was decided that the teachers should be flexible about attendance for a while and should gently encourage Mrs P to bring Peggy whenever possible. Meanwhile extra support for Mrs P would be provided by the social services. We addressed ourselves to the question of what could be clone for the mother to make her feel less envious of the child and so free Peggy of at least some of the pressures that were put on her. A grandmother figure was introduced—in the form of a peripatetic housemother—who could help the mother with special problems such as getting Peggy to sleep at night. On some evenings she would babysit so that the parents could go out together, for the first time since their daughter's birth. Eventually Mrs P was also referred for supportive psychotherapy, which she valued greatly as something that was provided especially for herself. As a result of this massive input the home situation began to improve during the next six to eight months. Some problems in the mother–child relationship continued to be enacted in the transition from home to school, but during the day Peggy seemed happy and settled. She was most co-operative with the teachers, made excellent progress and was very popular with the other children. Whereas previously it had been noted that she always scrutinized the facial expression of adults before expressing her own feelings, she now became more spontaneous. Occasionally this newly gained freedom to express her affection extended to her mother. At the time Mr P remarked appreciatively that Peggy's attendance at the Nursery School had made all the difference to their lives. This excellent progress was encouraging, though short-lived.

Following the summer holidays the mother's state began to deteriorate again and we became concerned for Peggy. Mrs P often overslept and then brought Peggy two hours late to Nursery School and she also became unreliable about fetching her at the end of the day. When the teachers objected, Mrs P became indignant, and on several occasions demanded that one of the teachers bring Peggy home. Once she even phoned to ask that Peggy be put in a taxi and sent to a pub that she and her husband frequented. Once when a neighbour had fetched her from school, they could not get into the flat as Mrs P did not answer the door-bell. The police had to be called to break a window and the mother was rushed to hospital by ambulance, having overdosed herself. When it emerged that Mr P had left home the previous day and not returned, the neighbour took Peggy in for the night. Mr P returned to bring Peggy to school but did not want to stay in the home. Mrs P discharged herself from hospital and arrived unexpectedly at the Nursery School. She was quite controlled but looked ghastly and when Peggy saw her she cried and said she wanted her daddy.

This was now a more serious family crisis, especially as Mr P had finally made up his mind to leave his wife although he wanted to go on caring for Peggy. He continued to bring and fetch Peggy from school for some weeks until Mrs P forbade this. He accepted the offer of an opportunity to discuss these problems with a member of the Centre's staff and expressed real concern about the child, but he was determined not to let his wife use Peggy to blackmail him into staying with her.

Mrs P tried hard to cope with Peggy on her own but we were doubtful that she would be able to do so in her very precarious mental state. The four-year-old was well aware of this too and responded by becoming co-operative and caring at home. Having just lost her father she knew what was at risk.

Another conference was held to discuss the changed circumstances as we were all concerned about the fact that the child now lived alone with her mother. Extra support was provided to protect Peggy and to keep a closer watch on the situation. The Nursery School agreed to provide transport to and from school, but usually when the driver called Mrs P was still asleep and did not answer the bell. The teacher then arranged to wake Mrs P by telephone every morning. Usually Peggy answered the phone and then tried to wake her mother, not always successfully. The social services made daily visits for a while and the peripatetic housemother moved in at weekends.

While these arrangements enabled Peggy not to lose her mother and her home as well as her father, and also ensured that her other needs were met by good substitute caretakers, one could not protect her from the adverse impingements of her mother's psychopathology. Mrs P was devastated by Mr P's desertion and consumed by her anger with him. Instead of helping Peggy deal with the loss of her father, Mrs P used her to unburden herself. The strain on the child was enormous and she became increasingly sad, whiny, more withdrawn and more reluctant to talk to the teachers about home. On the rare occasions she allowed herself to mention her father, it usually referred to a fantasied wish that he had visited her.

Whenever Mrs P's desperation reached a peak she began to pick fights with one of the many helpers. At such times she felt threatened and criticized by everyone and afraid the child would be taken from her. In a state of despair, about three months after Mr P left home, she requested that Peggy be temporarily fostered as she could not cope any more. But after only one week Mrs P removed her because she was critical of the way the foster parents handled Peggy and because, she said, Peggy was not happy there. However, soon after the child's return home we noticed that Mrs P was on another drinking bout. She often was unsteady on her feet and looked unkempt and neglected, although Peggy did not. The social services provided a living-in helper. A few days later an unknown social worker collected Peggy from school because her mother had been knocked down by a car and had to have stitches in her head, but again Mrs P discharged herself from hospital to look after Peggy.

Whereas it was quite obvious that Peggy was a lifeline for her mother, we worried whether the little girl's needs were being met and, how she could survive all these experiences. Another joint meeting with the social services was arranged, if only in order to assuage our doubts that this home was "the least detrimental alternative" place for Peggy to grow up in. We reaffirmed our intention of continuing to support this family, undaunted by the knowledge that the mother had interrupted her own therapy and that Peggy was due to enter school in a few months' time.

It was probably because she had always wanted for her daughter what she herself had been deprived of that Mrs P now referred Peggy for treatment. In this context Mrs P could mobilize some insight. Peggy looked sad and depressed, she had regressed in her behaviour at home, wanted to sit on her mother's lap and once even asked to suck at her breast. Mrs P said that she knew Peggy had experienced much at home that was upsetting and that she wanted her to have a happier childhood than she herself had had. Although we knew that Mrs P would not be able to sustain these insights, and that sooner or later she would become rivalrous with her daughter for the care she was receiving, Peggy was taken into psychotherapy at the Centre when she was 4½ years old.

In the diagnostic discussion which had preceded Peggy's entry into treatment it was suggested that Peggy's development had reached a danger point. Until recently she had been able to respond normally to a non-pathological environment but this was no longer the case. She had become generally depressed and withdrawn not only at home but also at Nursery School. There were signs of regression. She sucked her thumb a great deal and, at home, clung to her mother and bit her when angry. Her sleeping disturbance continued and she was now fearful of ghosts during the day too. This increasing anxiety, depression and regression to ambivalent orality were noted as indications of emerging pathology. While the strong tie with her mother was a source of good ego development, it was also the root of this pathology.

In view of Peggy's age and family situation, treatment aims were limited but it was thought that her current conflicts could be relieved. Indeed, the opportunity to explore her own feelings about her father's departure might even reduce her conflicts with her mother. Therapy might also prevent the proliferation of maladaptive defences, like regression, to which she had recently resorted.

Peggy made good use of therapy and responded well to this additional support. She began to understand that she was not responsible for either her mother's mood swings or her father's departure. She began to confide in her therapist, rather than involve her mother and thereby threaten the continuation of treatment. Eventually Mrs P even agreed that Peggy could meet Mr P on neutral ground. Nevertheless, such contacts increased the mother's anxieties and often led to arguments.

Disturbance of the mother's precarious equilibrium was caused by any changes experienced by her as loss. Peggy's move to infant school, carefully planned and well prepared on all sides, ushered in the next crisis. The mother became depressed and could not get up in the morning, and Peggy preferred to stay at home rather than arrive late. Intensive support had to be reintroduced, including wake-up calls, escorting Peggy to school, and transporting her to therapy sessions. Peggy's treatment continued for the first two terms in infant school and was terminated very gradually. When the final sessions approached, Mrs P's anxiety and rage again reached threatening proportions and her bid to placate and cling to Peggy's therapist pointed once more to her strong identification and rivalry with her daughter. Instead of bringing Peggy to her session, Mrs P demanded to be seen herself. She arrived in a state of extreme rage accompanied by her social worker as protection. She angrily insisted that Peggy needed more treatment and was "about to crack up", clearly externalizing her own precarious control. In even suggesting that Peggy should live with the therapist for a while, the mother was probably expressing concern for her child's safety. This concern was shared by the social worker who had witnessed a similar scene between mother and daughter the previous evening and felt that the child was again at risk physically. When Peggy was seen by her therapist later that day, she looked frightened and openly expressed a wish for safety and care. As Mrs P rejected the idea of temporary foster care or a joint residential placement in hospital, the social services had to provide a caretaker to live with them for the next two weeks.

Of course, further crisis situations arose but these occurred less frequently. There can be no doubt that Mrs P's psychological state gradually became more stable. The fact that the family were rehoused and that Mrs P began working part-time may have contributed to this improvement.

Peggy is now 10 years old, a rather sad and well-behaved low-keyed latency child. Her scholastic achievements are just average and she functions below her intellectual potential. She mixes with other children but has no close friends; she joins in various age-appropriate activities—a youth club, music, swimming, etc.—but pursues nothing with real zest or pleasure.

I have used this brief case story to illustrate some of the difficulties which face all who work in this field when they have to decide which of the paths open to them is "the least detrimental alternative". It is with this in mind that the work described is offered, not as a model but as a basis for discussion.

Note

* This paper was presented at the Vulnerable Child Workshop at the meeting of the International Association for Child and Adolescent Psychiatry and Allied Professions held in Dublin, Ireland, 1982.

References

Goldstein, J., Freud, A., & Solnit, A.J. (1979). *Before the Best Interests of the Child*. New York: Free Press.

CHAPTER THIRTEEN

Growing up with a Handicapped Sibling*

Hansi Kennedy 1985

It is evident to all who work with chronically ill or handicapped children that their families are often threatened by predicaments which cannot be resolved. A number of surveys point to a high incidence of marital difficulties or breakdown in such families and the adverse effects on siblings. Some studies point to the unrealistic expectations which parents have of the healthy child to compensate for their disappointment, guilt, or feelings of failure in relation to the child who is handicapped. Yet it would appear that the physically healthy children in these families are rarely referred for treatment. Their problems may seem less weighty in comparison with the difficulties facing their ill or handicapped siblings; or recognition of their problems may be precluded by the need of the parents to defend against their own conflicts in relation to their damaged child.

Describing the reactions of parents to the birth of a defective child, Solnit and Stark (1961) speak of the mother's mourning reaction. She has to relinquish the image of an expected "perfect baby," and has to adapt to the "sudden" birth of a threatening handicapped child. In our Well-Baby Clinic (Model, 1984), we have recently had the opportunity to observe how a mother's capacity to relate appropriately to her second child was impaired by her preoccupation with her firstborn. This child, who was 3 years 4 months at the time, was born totally deaf.

When, at the age of 6 weeks, the new baby was first seen, Jenny K. was failing to thrive. Her muscle tone was impoverished; she showed postural delay; she had a high-pitched cry; was miserable and had gained little weight since birth. The mother breast-fed Jenny on demand and thought that her milk supply was adequate. In a test feeding it was discovered that the baby was not getting much milk despite her good ability to suck, and Mrs K. was advised to complement her own feedings with the bottle.

Although Mrs K. was not suffering from a recognizable depressive reaction, she could neither respond to her baby's needs nor follow suggestions given with the aim of improving Jenny's well-being. Mrs K. was tense and showed a rather abstracted air: she asked many questions but hardly listened to the replies. She was evidently in the habit of reading while she gave the breast. She excused this behavior, saying, "I spend so much time feeding her, I must do something." The baby failed to gain adequate weight, and the staff learned that the mother's reluctance to introduce bottle feedings was based on her feelings of failure and inadequacy. She recalled that she had been able to feed Emily until she was 8 months. When she remarked that Jenny smiled and cooed, although "I don't talk to her very much," it was evident that she was equating Jenny with the deaf sister. When asked if she feared that Jenny too might be found to be deaf, Mrs K. denied any anxiety and stressed that Jenny was so different from Emily and that she could tell that the child could hear. She was having difficulty, however, in meeting the needs of the two children, and she expressed her wish to be available to Emily on her return from nursery school.

Emily had a profound congenital deafness, thought to be genetic in origin. Various investigations for possible mental retardation were undertaken before her condition was diagnosed at the age of 8 months. It seems likely that Mrs K. began to feel a failure as a mother when she could not experience early mutuality and responsiveness due to Emily's deafness. Mrs K.'s distress over Emily's handicap led her to dedicate herself to the task of helping her overcome the effects of her deafness; and Mrs K. had been successful in many ways. When Jenny's birth caused some withdrawal from Emily, she reacted with anger at home, with aggression at the nursery school, and with some resistance to her speech therapy program.

The revival of Mrs K.'s mourning and preoccupation with Emily ensured that she could not cathect Jenny appropriately and respond to the child's physical condition. She was unable to enjoy her normal child. When Jenny was 10 weeks old, the mother's attitude changed: she seemed to become aware of Jenny's fragile condition and to begin to follow the pediatrician's advice. She took some photographs of Jenny to send to her own parents: in some of them Jenny was naked and the mother realized just how thin she was. She looked "like an advertisement for famine relief. I was shocked, I could not send on such photos."

Jenny's needs might have remained unmet for longer without the intensive support and help provided for Mrs K. during these crucial weeks. Even today the child's future development is still at risk and further difficulties in relation to her deaf sister will arise and affect Jenny's negotiations of each and every developmental task.

In a paper written in 1979, Trevino discusses siblings of mentally retarded children. He observed that, initially, young children play with their disabled siblings on an equal basis. As they grow older, they have to redefine their role and begin to assume a superordinate position. Parental ambivalence toward the handicapped child who is often defensively overprotected and overindulged intensifies sibling rivalry. It often leads to the existence of two completely different sets of rules within the same family. Parents frequently demand that the normal child include the disabled child in peer group activities. Children close together in age often experience social discomfort when they have to deal with peer reactions and have to explain to their friends things they themselves often do not understand or cannot accept. Teasing and taunting about the handicapped child are not uncommon. While the normal child may become bitter over the extra favors and attention given to the afflicted child, the handicapped child may become intensely envious of the normality of his sibling. This affective interplay frequently results, in the siblings of the afflicted child, in feelings of guilt over their physical normality.

A number of studies consider the impact of chronic illnesses on healthy siblings (Bergmann and Wolfe, 1971); (Binger, 1973); (McKeever, 1983) and lay special stress on the resentment felt by healthy siblings vis-à-vis parental attention given to the sick child. They point to the healthy sibling's guilt which arises from having escaped the affliction— guilt further reinforced by the belief of somehow having brought it about. Bergmann and Wolfe observed and interviewed 25 siblings of their chronic patients at the orthopedic hospital in Cleveland. Just as the sick child wonders "Why did it happen to me?" the healthy sibling may wonder "Why did it *not* happen to me?" or "*When* will it happen to me?" The authors found that, as a means of coping with anxieties, defenses such as denial, repression, and reversal of affect were mobilized in the healthy children, in order to alleviate the stress of a constant awareness of the ill child's difficulties and/or deformity.

In an extensive survey of the psychoanalytic literature on siblings, Colonna and Newman (1983) draw particular attention to the dearth of in-depth studies of the reactions of healthy children to their physically ill or handicapped siblings.

At the Anna Freud Centre we have recently had a hemophilic twin and his brother in analysis. The parents first contacted us when the twins were 2 years old and expressed their concern over the healthy twin's temper tantrums. They wondered whether the necessary extra attention paid to his hemophilic brother might play some part (Lament and Wineman, 1984). The fact that these boys were twins clearly put additional strain on every member of the family, but the envy and rivalry between the children was without doubt increased by Timmy's illness. In comparing himself to his twin, Timmy felt deprived of a healthy body; while Max felt overlooked in relation to the special parental attention required for the care of his ill brother. The resultant narcissistic wounds dogged them from one developmental phase to the next, became involved with their conflicts and tasks, and greatly intensified the children's ambivalence toward their primary objects. Max's fear of injuring his afflicted twin, intensified by his death wishes, seemed to have figured largely in his passivity. For Timmy, a healthy twin was a great incentive for matching his brother's physical prowess, thereby promoting a more active role. While the healthy child's conflicts over aggression toward his twin appeared to contribute to the development of a harsh superego, Timmy's superego development was flawed by his anger, protest, and disinclination to please his parents. The twins are only just entering latency and it may be premature to make too many predictions about the future functioning of their superegos.

While there are several excellent psychoanalytic studies on children's reactions to death (especially Barnes, 1964); (R.A. Furman, 1964a), (E. Furman, 1974), these focus mainly on the child's reactions to the loss of a parent. Children's reactions to the death of a sibling have not, to my knowledge, been a focus of psychoanalytic investigation, and few accounts of brief psychotherapeutic intervention have been published (Rosenblatt, 1969). Based on a study of 58 cases seen in psychiatric interviews or brief interventions, and followed up, Cain et al. (1964) demonstrate the limitations of the notion that the impact of a sibling's death primarily produces guilt reactions in the surviving children. The children they studied suffered from a range of disturbances. In 40 percent of cases there were either immediate, prolonged, or anniversary identifications of a hysterical kind with the dead sibling's prominent symptom. Many of the children developed what they called death phobias, where talion fears and identifications with the dead sibling were particularly striking. The children were often convinced not only that they would die, but that they would die at precisely the same age or from the same cause as the dead sibling. They had a heightened awareness and fear of death, feeling that it could strike any moment at themselves, their parents, or other siblings. The authors also emphasized overprotectiveness toward the remaining children as a typical and fearful parental response which often further reinforced the children's anxiety.

In another paper "On Replacing a Child," Cain and Cain (1964) describe how the dead child often lives on in a concrete day-to-day fashion. Photographs fill every room of the house, birthdays are celebrated, and his continued presence in the family is rationalized as "We all love him and like to think of him. The surviving or replacement children always seem to know and reverberate to illness and death.

The clinical pictures may reflect a prolonged mourning process. Bowlby (1963) describes, as characteristic of childhood mourning, the unconscious urge to recover the lost object and the denial that the object is permanently lost.

Pollock (1962) found that in a random sample of adult analytic patients a significant number had suffered parent or sibling loss in their childhood. The factors which determine a child's immediate and long-term reactions to the death of a sibling ultimately depend on various preconditions. These include the age and developmental level of the surviving sibling, the preexisting relationship to the sibling and the parents, the parents' reactions to the death, and their subsequent attitude to their remaining children. The child's fantasies about the illness and the death also are important. Combinations of these variables may lead to immediate disturbance or appear only in delayed and hidden conflictual reactions in adult life.

Many of the general features described in this brief review can be illustrated in the treatment material of my patient David D. He not only grew up with a handicapped sibling, but was also in some sense a "replacement child," who experienced at the age of 8 the death of the afflicted brother. My lack of familiarity with what others had already said gave me a double satisfaction. I first discovered with David the origin of his considerable suffering in relation to the life and death of his handicapped brother; and later I found our discoveries confirmed in the work of my colleagues.

David's analysis extended over almost 3 years, but I shall confine myself to those aspects of our work which have direct bearing on the subject under discussion.

David instigated his own referral for analysis when he told his parents that he needed help because he could not stop thinking about death. The parents had been aware of his anxiety in the preceding 6 months but had attributed this to difficulties occasioned by a move into a large secondary school at that time. He complained about bullies who lay in wait for him and attacked him in the playground. He said that some of the teachers hated him. In recent weeks he had used all sorts of ploys to stay away, feigning illness or exaggerating minor injuries. His sister called him a hypochondriac. On several occasions he persuaded the school nurse that he felt ill and needed to go home, especially on days when he was expected to take part in field games or sports. He was also sleeping badly, and his anxiety was manifest in restlessness and nonstop talking. After David told his parents that he could not stop thinking about death, they noticed that he sometimes flailed his arms about, in a manner reminiscent of his dead brother. They were puzzled by this behavior. It was 3½ years since Darren had died, and David appeared to have weathered his loss much better than the rest of the family.

David was the third child of parents whose potentially warm and harmonious family life was devastated by the illness and eventual death of their firstborn son, Darren. When Darren was 3 years old, he developed symptoms stemming from a degenerative neurological disorder. The parents were told that he could not be expected to live more than a year or 2. At the time their daughter Dora was only a few months old. The parents were heartbroken, sought all kinds of professional advice, and tried to cope as best they could. They decided that Darren should remain with the family and receive the best possible care. In the event he only died at the age of 14.

After Darren's terminal illness had been diagnosed, the parents were advised to have another child, and David was born 3 years later, a planned baby conceived to replace the ill and dying child. Mrs D. had no recollection of anxiety about his birth, which was, in fact, straightforward. He was an easy and happy baby, and the mother breast-fed him for 5 months. There were no feeding or sleeping or toilet-training problems. He was described as an alert baby, advanced in his motor, speech, and social development. As a toddler, he would bang his head when he was angry; and the parents thought this linked with his need to curb his aggression on account of Darren's vulnerability. By the time David started walking, Darren was 7 years old, not particularly stunted in his growth but very unsteady in keeping his balance. He was always falling over, and the slightest push would knock him down and start him howling. On more than one occasion he broke a limb, and on many more it was feared that he had done so.

From the parents' account it seemed that the needs of each of their children had been carefully considered at every stage in their development. David was sent to nursery school at 3, but was always encouraged to have friends in to play so that he would not suffer from having a "handicapped brother." Both parents felt neither David nor Dora showed signs of stress or disturbance over Darren. They were kind and protective toward him, yet able to complain when he interfered with their activities. Although Darren was often restless and difficult to manage, he remained an integral member of the family until his death.

David was not quite 12 years old when he started analysis. He took full responsibility for his daily attendance in spite of a long and complicated journey. In periods of resistance he could develop sudden lapses of memory and go straight home after school, but he would then always telephone with profuse apologies and self-accusations, sometimes referring to himself as a "scatter-brained" boy. Most of the time the analytic work was facilitated by a genuine wish for help.

David impressed me at once as an attractive, intelligent, and articulate youngster. He was a little plump and looked more suited for intellectual pursuits than physical ones. He confirmed this impression right away when he told me sadly that some teachers and boys mockingly referred to him as "the great violin virtuoso." He felt utterly helpless vis-à-vis the bullies at school who teased him and attacked him physically. He also felt bullied by his sports master who sneered at his failures and who he felt forced him to participate even when he was feeling ill. His pleasure in learning was spoiled because he was always worrying about the next attack. In his first session he referred to his dead brother. His parents had taken him, together with his sister, to see a psychiatrist after Darren's death. He had enjoyed talking to the doctor, who had explained that it was natural to feel guilty about the death of a brother. But he did not feel guilty about Darren's death, only sorry and upset about losing him. He added, in a loving tone of voice, "Darren was such a good sport." My attempt to link this comment with his declaration that he himself was teased and humiliated for being bad at sports met with determined rejection. It alerted me straight away to the strength of his defensive repudiation of any criticism or hostility toward his dead brother.

Defenses against death wishes would seem to be an integral factor in the dynamics of the family containing a handicapped child. But with David this extended to a generalized condemnation of his own aggression which rendered him incapable of self-defense or even self-assertion. Although he expressed disapproval of the behavior of bullies, he could not express anger toward them. He even needed to mitigate his disapproval by finding excuses for his attackers. Morgan, the boy who tormented him most, "was probably so nasty because he had no one to give him affection. His mother had died a few months ago and he knew what it felt like when someone died."

David had strong reaction formations against sadism. He condemned any kind of violence, wars, revolutions, murders, and the death penalty. He was a staunch supporter of the "underdog," the victims and the weak; and his sympathy sounded quite genuine.

The dangers from the attacks David encountered in his daily life had to be rationalized and the anxiety blocked by denial or reversal. He usually arrived from school nursing some sort of injury. He sustained a bad thumb when a third-former jumped on his back, "but it was all done in fun and did not really hurt." He might, of course, have chipped a bone, but he did not really mind. Sometimes he introduced an account of his injuries by telling a joke. One of these concerned a man with false teeth which detached themselves when he ate toffees. Then he told me that a hard ball had hit his face and made his tooth bleed that day.

Long-distance running was particularly humiliating for David because he could never finish the course. His fear of straining his heart and dying made him drop down in exhaustion, hoping that an ambulance would come to his rescue. Instead he met further attacks in the form of scathing remarks by the sports master.

The analyst's office soon became a place where he gained temporary relief from these oppressing anxieties and where he could allow himself to regress. David cast me in the role of caregiver and provider and presented himself as the neglected, needy, and badly done-by child. He would arrive at the session looking a picture of misery, still dressed in sports gear, covered in mud, having "forgotten to shower and change at school and put on his coat." He would ask permission to warm himself by the radiator or wash his wounds and scratches. Sometimes he allowed himself to cry because he thought his ribs were broken in a fall and he did not want to appear a crybaby at school. He complained that he was starving and had not eaten since breakfast and needed a glass of water or preferably a hot drink. When he realized that I verbalized rather than gratified his longings to be fed and made more comfortable, he began to bring food and drink to the sessions and consume it with relish and exaggerated pleasure. Although he strongly denied my interpretation that this self-provision concealed his dissatisfaction and anger with me for not doing enough for him, the subsequent transference material confirmed my view. He began to linger on after sessions as though to invite me to throw him out in favor of others. He became intensely interested in and rivalrous with other patients. He wanted to hang up a "marvelous drawing" in the consulting room for everyone to admire. When he discovered that an older boy had a session after his, he asked me for a gun. He explained that he meant a toy gun, of course, and justified the demand by saying it was hard for him to ask for such things, but one had to be honest in analysis. While he could barely hide his anger with me for not providing the gun, he tried to strike up a friendship with the other patient rather than reveal his murderous impulses. One had to work painstakingly on his defenses—denial, reversal, and reaction formations—to demonstrate to David what he was covering up and why.

We learned that David's anger with his mother for depriving him of his fair share had early roots. It appeared to stem from a time when he felt envious of the attention and care his handicapped brother received from her. His initial identification with Darren, based on this envy, probably preceded his recognition of Darren's handicap. Later Darren's affliction, and certainly his death, mobilized fears that such misfortune could also strike him.

A pervasive preoccupation with injury, and death was ever present in David. A boy in his school had died of leukemia and as a memorial the school made an appeal to parents to become blood donors. Of course, his mother volunteered, and took him to see a film about research into the illness. Another boy was killed in a road accident while riding a bicycle, and this tragedy was reported with complaints that his parents did not let him ride his bicycle in London. There was hardly a session in which he did not mention his dead brother in some context or another, and he began to remember some of Darren's accidents.

Occasionally he would wear a new shirt, pullover, or jacket and ostensibly display it, inviting my response. When I verbalized his wish that I notice his new clothes, he explained that it was not new and was really Darren's. When I wondered whether he minded the fact that his clothes were hand-me-downs, he assured me that he loved wearing garments that reminded him of Darren. He loved his brother and he hoped he would never forget him. In any case he could not possibly forget him because everyone at home was always talking about him anyway.

I gradually learned that David now slept in Darren's former room, which was still referred to by the family as Darren's room. Darren's toys had remained in the room and David had "inherited" them.

There were many references to family celebrations when Darren was lovingly remembered. His birthday and death were always commemorated. When David reported that Darren and Dora shared a common birthday, he said, "I used to hate this when I was little because I felt left out. Now I hate it because I always have to think of Darren who might feel left out."

Darren had clearly remained a presence in the family, and the parents' mourning process still continued; but, for David, Darren seemed to live on in a very concrete way. He could be quite philosophical when discussing death. What was death? Life could not just end when the heart stopped beating or the brain stopped working. Darren's brain was damaged before his death. Even now, 3½ years later, he could not believe that Darren was no longer around. Sometimes when he walked about the house at night, he thought of meeting Darren behind a door. He believed firmly in life after death and he had seen two ghosts: the first ghost appeared when he slept in a hotel which was a converted eerie old castle known to be haunted by an angry ancestor. The second ghost he saw at home, where he was particularly frightened because he was sure it was Darren coming to have a look around and see "what was going on." I reminded David that he had told me that he slept in Darren's room, wore his clothes, played with his toys, and that he well might feel that Darren would not like to see what was going on and might want to take his revenge. For once David readily agreed and added that this was exactly what he would do if he were in Darren's place and someone had stolen his things.

At this point David also began to wonder whether his tormentors at the school were attacking him because they felt envious of his being a bit more clever than they were. He spoke of being teased about getting good marks, knowing the answers in class, and talking in a posh accent. The teasing was no longer confined to his poor performance in sport. When these feelings were worked through in terms of his "survivor guilt," he experienced some relief—his level of anxiety decreased, and with it the excessively stringent control of any form of aggressive expression.

In the sessions David began to move about with increased freedom, displayed some pleasurable excitement, and permitted himself to make a token attack on me. He made and tested paper darts, and enjoyed it when they narrowly missed me. When eventually one hit me, he became anxious, apologized profusely, and almost at once slipped on the floor and knocked his arm against my desk. He rubbed his elbow as he examined my desk for any possible damage. This was one of many incidents in which he demonstrated his fear that phallic sexual/aggressive attacks would cause permanent damage or destroy the object, and therefore had to be inhibited or turned against himself. Indeed, these became habitual modes of defense.

His complaints about school now shifted away from bully boys. His music teacher, formerly much admired, was felt to be unfair in his criticism of David and in his failure to give him adequate recognition. Whereas, hitherto, active involvement in the music department had been relatively conflict-free and a sought-after refuge from the stresses encountered in the playground, David now spent his sessions working out schemes of revenge. He would not make sacrifices and give up free time to come to rehearsal; he would try to organize strike action of all orchestra members so that the teacher would beg him to play in the concert; he would write a protest about the undemocratic way the orchestra was run; and he would complain to the head of the school. It was quite clear that David provoked the teacher's hostility and criticism, but it took time to discover that David's resentment stemmed from a thwarted desire to lead the orchestra. It emerged that previously his teacher had been liberal in his praise and had told him that he had considerable musical talent. "And now," David blurted out, "he won't let me be leader of the orchestra because he wants his pet daughter instead." It was unfair and he resented it.

David began to talk about rows at home with his father. They had always had rows because his father lost his temper more easily than his mother and shouted at him. His father had always been strict and not always fair to him. When, as a small boy, he was naughty, his father spanked only him and not the others. Darren did not get spanked because he was handicapped and Dora escaped because she was a girl. Now his father teased David a lot and made him angry. Perhaps, he said pensively, he got angry more often than his father and he was the one who shouted. Usually he tried to leave the room to cool off but did not always make it. But his example was interesting. His father had been very nice recently, helping to build airplane models. They had fun working on a model together last Sunday. Soon afterwards his father walked behind him on the stairs and put his hands affectionately round his neck. David screamed in rage and swore at his father, who apologized for startling him. David felt awful and was ashamed to have tea with the family. I suggested that he screamed in fear rather than in rage—perhaps he feared his father might strangle him in retaliation for some of the things David sometimes wanted to do to him.

That night David had what he described as "a very painful dream." He was in a group of unknown people in a disused airfield. The people were hostile, ordered him about, and bullied him. When they chased him around, shouted at him, and finally locked him in a little hut, he felt angry rather than frightened. In the hut was a machine gun. He picked it up, stepped outside, and "mowed everyone down." He added, "and I didn't have a very nice feeling after I had done that." I said that feeling guilty was very painful even if these people in the dream had made him very angry so that he felt like killing them all. With a laugh, David added, "Like I feel at home when my Dad makes me angry." The associations to the disused airfield led him to talk about his wish to join the air cadets. He had obtained a leaflet and shown it to his parents, but they said that the meeting times clashed with his sessions and he would not be able to join. All his life he had been interested in planes and now he wanted to learn to fly. It was an interest he shared with his father who would have become a pilot in his youth had he not failed his medical. But, he, David, was fit and healthy and would not be put off joining the air cadets for more than a term, whatever I or his parents said.

His masculine strivings showed in other ways as well. He planned to build up his body: it was the only way to deal with bullies. Once he was able to show that he could take them on in a fight, he would gain the respect of the group. He put himself on a diet, he walked to school to get exercise, and decided to spend more time in the gymnasium and the swimming pool. At home he started using a chest expander.

At about this time David saw the film *Jaws*, which mobilized his sadistic fantasies as well as his castration anxiety. David's defenses against his sadistic wishes had so far only permitted their emergence into consciousness in relatively tame and modulated fantasies of revenge. Now he described Jaws in every gory detail and proclaimed that it was the best film he ever saw. With a considerable degree of anxious excitement he described the "marvelous scene" where the sea was colored "bright red from the blood with bits of the dead boy floating about." The scene he found most enjoyable and exciting, however, was the one in which the shark bit off a man's leg. He completely denied that this film might have made him feel anxious as well as excited, saying that he knew it was not real and that the sharks were only expensive models constructed in film studios. But that night he awoke from a dream so frightened that he dared not go to sleep again. In the session that followed he looked pale and shaken, and could not recall details of the dream until I had wondered whether it had a connection with the previous day's material.

In the dream he was in a boat with an adult man. It was not anyone he knew. Suddenly a shark knocked the boat over. They fell in the water and the man disappeared. But he and a friend were in the water and both boys were trying to get away from the shark. The shark got hold of his friend and David failed in his attempt to rescue him. He was reluctant to remember the rest of the dream and brushed it aside with a remark that it ended in a typical dream chase where one tries and tries but can't make the shore. He woke up, frightened and sweating, and didn't dare go to his parents' room. In his associations he was afraid his father might not be there; perhaps he had been the man who drowned in the dream.

David had more difficulty understanding the second part; he thought of Darren whom he once rescued when he fell over in the swimming pool. Even though it was in the shallow end, it was difficult to pull him out. His mother managed it, but Darren was winded and couldn't get his breath. David thought he was dead. Darren was the only dead person he ever saw. He died in the hospital, but he saw him in his coffin before the funeral. His parents did not want him to come along, but he insisted. He looked so pale and peaceful David could not forget the sight. It was like the ghost face he once saw in the house when he woke at night. Now he recalled the rest of the dream. "When we reached the shore it was more like a swimming pool with high walls and I couldn't pull myself up to get out of the water. When, in the end, I managed, it was too late, the shark had bitten off my leg too." He readily accepted my interpretation that both castration wishes toward father and fears of his own castration had been mobilized while watching the film.

That was why he had pushed them out of his mind the day before; but they could not be kept away in the dream.

The thought of the swimming pool with high walls led to a memory of a time when he was 3 or 4 years old. His sister could swim already. This helped him to master his fear of going into the water. She could also pull herself up by the side of the pool and climb out that way, but he couldn't do so, and his swimming teacher made him swim all alone to the stairs in the deep end.

Up to this point in treatment he had described his older sister as kind, helpful, and motherly toward him. Now he reported that they had arguments over TV programs. When he did not give way, she attacked him. He recalled a fight they had had soon after Darren's death. She hit him really hard and sat on his chest so that he couldn't breathe. She was frightened when he went white in the face. His parents were very upset when he accused her of trying to kill him, and his mother started crying. We talked about the many other occasions on which Dora must have made him feel angry, inadequate, and helpless like in the dream when he couldn't manage to climb out and had to face the dangers of the deep water by himself. He smiled and said he always felt girls had all the privileges. They were spoiled, especially by their father; while boys were made to fetch and carry, give up the best seats, and get blamed and punished. To top it all, when it came to washing up, Dora believed in the equality of the sexes!

Yet, even such relatively mild expressions of anger and hostility toward his sister were followed by fears that she might suffer an accident or even meet with death. A few days later, David arrived at his session in a state of great anxiety. He was carrying a sealed letter for his mother. The school secretary had told him not to forget to give it to her right away. When I wondered what he thought the urgent message contained, he said that it might be a complaint about him, but it might also be a note to tell mother that Dora had met with an accident at school.

In this connection David recalled an accident he himself had had at junior school. He recalled that he had been quite a naughty child and was always fighting with other children at that time. Once he ran away from a boy whom he had hit in the playground, and slipped and damaged his front teeth. There was a lot of blood, he was rushed to the hospital, and now he had a crown on one front tooth. This accident was fraught with anxiety not only because it represented a symbolic castration in punishment for an aggressive attack, but also because his mother could not be reached. When he was rushed to the hospital, he felt unsupported in his ordeal.

The floodgates had been opened, and many childhood memories began to emerge. David experienced considerable relief. He became happier and more joyful every day, and better able to handle aggressive conflicts.

His enjoyment of all his activities gave opportunities for creative self-expression. Drama class was fun. The boys were paired off and asked to act a spontaneous funny scene. He and his friend chose one in which he was the doctor carrying out an operation on his patient. The patient asked, "Doctor, are you giving me gas or an anesthetic?" and David turned to an imaginary nurse and asked for a hammer. He added laughingly that he had the audience in fits as he pretended to knock his patient over the head with the hammer. Accidentally, he did, in fact, punch his patient during the so-called operation, but he just apologized in a whisper and no harm was done.

David recalled his enjoyment in fantasy games with his friends when he was little. In particular he recalled playing monster games with a special friend. They scared each other and then looked over their shoulder to check whether the monsters were chasing them. This led to the recollection that he did not like it when his friends asked questions about Darren who usually came with his mother to fetch him from school. His friend playfully called Darren a monster. He did not mind his friend saying that, but he protested when other children called Darren names and said he was mad.

Any such communication had to be followed by reassurances that Darren was really quite intelligent and if he made strange noises, it was because he was a handicapped boy and couldn't help it. Sometimes David got cross with children who teased Darren and that was why he had so many fights. It became clear that he used to be able to fight to defend Darren while he was alive, but later identified with the helpless brother when the bullies attacked him.

He recalled getting cross with Darren when friends visited him. He disrupted their games. When Darren was told to go away, he screamed, and his mother got cross with him for being unkind. Darren was unsteady on his feet and always fell over. He could not get up and one never knew how badly he was injured because he yelled so much. As David recalled these episodes, he said that he often felt sorry for Darren, but sometimes Darren made him very angry and upset and he sometimes wished that he would "hit the bucket."

It was only after we had worked for some time on his loving as well as his hostile feelings for Darren that David began to talk about his mother's sadness. He was once taken together with Darren to a children's concert and his mother became very upset when they had to leave because Darren behaved so badly. David did not much care for concerts then, but he minded when he saw his mother crying. He used to listen to his parents talking about Darren and once heard his father say, "He is not like us, you can't expect it of him."

David's parents had been adamant that Darren's anticipated death had never been discussed with the children before he actually died. After a visit to a cousin, who was expecting her third baby, David reported that the parents did not really want another baby, but birth control did not always work. He thought most parents only wanted two children and that his parents had not really wanted him. It was a lot of work for his mother to look after a handicapped child as well as two others. When I carefully explored whether he thought he was born to replace his brother, he hotly denied this, saying no one knew that Darren was going to die, but they always worried about him. "And now I worry about who is going to die next in our family, that's why I was happy when I had my fourteenth birthday and nothing happened." David had not even mentioned this anxiety to me until the birthday had passed. The relief of having survived was liberating, however, and from that time on he began to talk about no longer needing analysis.

It seems to me that David's story illustrates very vividly the impact a handicapped child can have on his siblings' development. David was a potentially healthy and well-endowed child who grew up under the shadow of Darren's affliction—one which affected the whole family. He might have escaped the full impact of the fate of the "replacement child" because his parents' distress and anxiety were still focused on Darren. Nevertheless, in his early teens David complained bitterly about his parents' excessive concern about his safety, which he experienced as infantilizing and restricting.

Darren's handicap made David feel unable to express even age-appropriate aggression throughout his development. Even as a small toddler he appeared to have learned that knocking his own head was better than knocking Darren. This restriction on aggressive expression later led to strong reaction formations, talion fears, and a strict superego. In David's eyes, Darren received far more attention and much more indulgence from his mother; and his early longings to be in Darren's shoes formed a prototype for an identification with his rival for the mother's love. Later this identification must have mobilized considerable fears that he too would suffer Darren's fate. More positively it allowed him to empathize with his afflicted brother as well as to identify with his mother's protectiveness. From the analytic material it would seem that he never really understood the nature of Darren's affliction. The parents probably found it difficult to talk about it and preferred to use the umbrella term, "He is handicapped." This may have contributed to David's inability to come to terms with it and give his fantasies free reign.

David's intensified conflicts about death wishes and the expression of aggression must have increased the difficulty of negotiating the oedipal situation. His childhood recollections suggested, however, that he retained his ability to fight and defend himself and his brother against other children during the latency period.

Although, according to the parents, David coped better than the rest of the family with Darren's death, it heightened his anxieties and death became a formidable danger. Perhaps it was not so much the change of school which aroused his conflicts but the reinforced instinctual pressures of prepuberty which mobilized sexual and aggressive wishes and necessitated crippling defensive maneuvers.

It is, however, also possible to see some positive influences of this sibling relationship, even though the clinical material cited emphasized the negative ones. Indeed, it could be argued that these positive influences were of material help in the treatment process itself; and some of his character traits, capacity for concern, empathy, and insightfulness could, at appropriate points, be pressed into the service of the analysis.

It is, of course, impossible to predict the future of this child. Will he succumb to hypochondriacal symptoms or concerns? Will he be vulnerable to pervasive anxieties, especially those connected with illness or death? Will his relationships in his own future family be put in jeopardy and echo some of the miseries encountered in the past? Or will compassion and the character traits already well established lead to a medical career, the caring profession, a future defender of the needy or a crusader for the handicapped?

Note

* Presented as the Third Annual Marianne Kris Memorial Lecture at the Meeting of the Association for Child Psychoanalysis, Chicago, March 1984.

References

Barnes, M. J. (1964). Reactions to the death of a mother. *Psychoanalytic Study of the Child, 19*: 334–57.

Bergmann, T. & Wolfe, S. (1971). Observations of the reactions of healthy children to their chronically ill siblings. *Bulletin of the Philadelphia Association for Psychoanalysis, 21*: 145–61.

Binger, C. M. (1973). Childhood leukemia: Emotional impact on siblings. In: E.J. Anthony & C. Koupernik (Eds.), *The Child in His Family* (pp. 2: 195–211). New York: Wiley.

Bowlby, J. (1963). Pathological mourning and childhood mourning. *Journal of the American Psychoanalytic Association, 11*: 500–41.

Cain, A. C. & Cain, B. S. (1964). On replacing a child. *Journal of the American Academy of Child Psychiatry, 3*: 443–56.

Cain, A. C., Cain. S. Fast, I., & Erickson, M. B. (1964). Children's disturbed reactions to the death of a sibling. *American Journal of Orthopsychiatry, 34*: 741–52.

Colonna, A. B. & Newman, L. M. (1983). The psychoanalytic literature on siblings. *Psychoanalytic Study of the Child, 38*: 285–310.

Furman, E. (1974). *A Child's Parent Dies*. New Haven & London: Yale Univ. Press.

Furman, R. A. (1964a). Death and the young child. *Psychoanalytic Study of the Child, 19*: 321–33.

Furman, R. A. (1964b). Death of a six-year-old's mother during his analysis. *Psychoanalytic Study of the Child, 19*: 377–97.

Lament, C. & Wineman, I. (1984). A psychoanalytic study of nonidentical twins. *Psychoanalytic Study of the Child, 39*: 331–70.

McKeever, P. (1983). Siblings of chronically ill children. *American Journal of Orthopsychiatry, 53*: 209–29.

Model, E. (1984). Failure to thrive. *Bulletin of the Hampstead Clinic, 7*: 127–32.

Pollock, G. H. (1962). Childhood parent and sibling loss in adult patients. *Archives of General Psychiatry, 7*: 295–305.

Pollock, G. H. (1978). Childhood sibling loss and creativity. *Annual of Psychoanalysis, 6*: 443–81.

Rosenblatt, B. (1969). A young boy's reaction to the death of his sister. *Journal of the American Academy of Child Psychiatry, 8*: 321–35.

Solnit, A. J. & Stark, M. H. (1961). Mourning and the birth of a defective child. *Psychoanalytic Study of the Child, 16*: 523–37.

Trevino, F. (1979). Siblings of handicapped children. *Journal of Contemporary Social Work, 60*: 488–93.

Wann, B. (1978). The family and the handicapped child. In: E.J. Anthony & C. Chiland (Eds.), *The Child and His Family* (pp. 81–8). New York: Wiley.

CHAPTER FOURTEEN

Trauma in Childhood: Signs and Sequelae as Seen in the Analysis of an Adolescent*

Hansi Kennedy 1986

Peter's analysis lasted for 6 years and started at the age of 13. Early traumatic and disturbing events played a striking part in his pathology and were vividly reexperienced in treatment. This short paper describes some of these reenactments and gives reasons why the experiences from which they derived might properly be called "traumatic."

In spite of Peter's long and, in many ways, successful analysis, he remained a rather depressed young man, dominated by pervasive feelings of inadequacy and resentment from which he tried to escape by sexual activities.

During treatment, his compulsive masturbation, accompanied by sadomasochistic fantasies, and his tendency to enactment, increasingly forced me to think of his disturbance in terms of sexual perversion.

During his masturbatory practices, he needed to create, simultaneously or in quick succession, sexual excitement, pain, and anxiety. He masturbated from early childhood, but in adolescence he enhanced his orgasmic pleasure by tying a plastic bag over his head.

In this way his fantasy that a female partner was castrating and suffocating him was given an added dimension of reality.

A connection can readily be made between these sexual fantasies and practices and experiences in his third year of life, when he suffered intermittently from painful infections of the penis. These involved his mother in repeated examinations and manipulations of his genitals. Phimosis eventually required circumcision at 2 years, 8 months. His mother stayed with him in the hospital but could only report his bad reaction to the anesthetic. In analysis Peter claimed to have a memory of mother driving him to the hospital for the operation, but this memory lacked any affective coloring.

There can be no doubt from Peter's analytic material that these events were crucial in the formation of his psychopathology and that, at least retroactively, they were experienced as vengeful attacks and punishments by his mother. By the time he entered analysis, his masturbation conflicts were firmly linked with his feelings about his damaged penis and the conviction that he was an inadequate person in every respect. This narcissistic vulnerability and depleted self-esteem had, of course, earlier roots.

Peter was a disappointment to his mother from the day he was born. She was an inexperienced, anxious, rigid mother who was quite unable to cope with an infant whose behavior failed to match her exact expectations. The pregnancy proceeded according to plan until Peter arrived 12 days too early and had to be extracted by forceps. He cried a great deal during the first few months, which upset his parents' regimental household and lifestyle. He did not feed according to his mother's schedule, and her worry about his poor weight gain and stow physical growth led her "to force food into him." She probably became even less responsive to Peter's needs when she became pregnant, for a second time, when he was only 8 months old. All these circumstances reflect an unsatisfactory early interaction between mother and child, and the inadequate and curtailed symbiotic phase formed the core of Peter's disturbed self and object relationship.

In the second year of life, Peter's interaction with mother was dominated by what she described as "their great battle over toilet training." A battle which started when he was only 1 year old went on until well into his third year of life, when daytime bladder control was finally achieved. Contributory factors to this long delay included a stressful 2-week separation from mother and home at the time of the brother's birth, and the onset, some months later, of the phimosis.

The mother's narcissistic hurt and guilt in relation to Peter's imperfections may well have been compensated by her pleasure and pride in the new baby who seemed to thrive both physically and psychologically. Both parents described this younger brother as more satisfactory in every way. Not surprisingly, Peter's development began to lag, and according to the mother, his younger brother talked before he did. Irrespective of the accuracy of this information, it does suggest that Peter could not express his feelings in words at the time of the circumcision.

The unfavorable comparison which began on the day his brother was born became a bane of Peter's life. He felt that his brother was not only better loved but was superior in every respect. Two years before his referral for treatment, which ostensibly was for learning difficulties in spite of his good intelligence (IQ 120+), Peter had suffered the ultimate humiliation of his younger brother's advance to a class above him at school.

He envied but also idealized this brother, casting him in the role of a genius—a second Einstein—whom he could never emulate. His revengeful hatred of the brother, an ever recurring theme in the analysis, was understood as a displacement of feelings he harbored toward his mother for producing the brother and for favoring him. Later in treatment this also appeared as an oedipal displacement from the father who "possessed" the mother.

I have discussed elsewhere the transference developments in Peter's analysis (1980). They led to a very clever recasting of his pathology in terms of a double identification: with the clever Jews who were nevertheless discriminated against and circumcised, and with the powerful, sadistic, yet morally despicable Nazis. This expressed both the ambivalent investment of self and object and the sadomasochistic object relationship. It provided immense opportunities not only for the development of the analytic process, but also for resistance and stagnation in the analytic work when he used the treatment to gratify his sadomasochism. Even the most careful monitoring of countertransference cannot prevent a sadomasochistic patient from exploiting the analytic situation for perverse gratification. At all times Peter worked hard to get himself into a state of sexual excitement which served to ward off his depressive feeling states.

I hope that this brief overview will provide sufficient background to give perspective to the analytic material which follows. This is unavoidably selective, but I hope it indicates the significance of Peter's experiences around the phimosis and circumcision.

Both anxiety and guilt helped to make Peter a secretive boy who, throughout the first year of analysis, deliberately withheld and distorted material. But at the beginning of treatment the anxiety was so pervasive that he could hardly communicate verbally. When he talked at all, his speech was difficult to understand and he was reduced to muttering under his breath such comments as "What is going to happen?" or "I haven't told you anything about my sins." I felt at the time that he was reacting to the analytic situation as if it represented the Day of Judgment. In retrospect it is not difficult to see that the intimacy of the analytic setting, of being alone in the room with a woman who was immediately cast in the role of dangerous castrator, was both terrifying and seductive. Affectively, it seemed to have revived the traumatic childhood experiences in the most dramatic way.

In the early weeks of treatment he would silently draw maps of the London Underground system and respond to any comment I made by blotting them out. He would do so with such ferocity that big holes were all that were left on the paper. Thus, while my attempts to establish contact through verbalization always mobilized fears that I might discover what he was deliberately trying to keep hidden, his sexual preoccupations were betrayed by his actions and concomitant affect.

Intense anxiety about his damaged penis was evident from the way he treated the felt-pens he used for drawing. He often handled them roughly and then anxiously looked at the tips for damage.

As if to underline his derisive rejection of my cautious and carefully worded interpretations, he also rejected my felt pens and brought his own from home. This led to a strange enactment in the third week of treatment. He selected a red pen and found that the protective cap was stuck so that he could not use it. He began to pull and push the cap with mounting excitement and anxiety. Once or twice he held it out to me, apparently to elicit my participation, but then mistrustfully withdrew it. His face was flushed and his hands were covered with red paint when he finally succeeded in pulling off the cap. He anxiously inspected the tip, hitherto protected, to see if it was damaged; and he disparagingly declared that it was now useless and that his mother would jolly well have to provide a new one. While this material opened up the analytic work on his masturbation conflicts, and his view of the mother as responsible for his damaged penis, the full significance of his enactment in terms of his childhood experiences when his penis was sore and he had difficulty in urinating was recognized only some months later in connection with another, more dramatic, enactment.

Following his brother's visit home from boarding school (week 36) we had an unusually good session. For once Peter seemed in touch with his unhappiness and was able to talk about his anger and resentment with his parents for being interested only in his brother. He complained that the whole weekend was spent in praise of his brother's good examination results and in making plans for his brother's future privileged education. He had experienced all this as a deliberate humiliation and reproach from his parents and throughout the weekend had felt an unwanted outsider in his own family. I had commented on the long-standing nature of such feelings and how they must have contributed to his pervasively low self-esteem. Peter replied that the brother was the cause of all his trouble and that he wished him dead or, better still, that he had never been born. Right at the end of this session it emerged that the weekend had also been the occasion for the celebration of the brother's birthday.

He arrived the next day in a completely different state of mind. He was regressed; his communications were again nonverbal; his nose was blocked by an attack of hayfever, and he was desperate about the discomfort. He considered phoning his mother for advice, but reproachfully demanded instead that I do something about his agony and provide him at least with tissues. This I did. He started to attack his nose in a most sadistic manner. He placed a paper tissue on his lap, leaned over it, and tried to force mucus out of his nose. He pulled, pushed, poked, and blew, using both hands for these manipulations. He was totally self-absorbed in this frenetic activity which went on for quite some time until I intervened. I suggested that his concern about, and vicious treatment of, his nose really referred to his penis and that he might be remembering something of what happened to it when he was a small boy and had phimosis. I tried to put into words some of the discomfort and pain he must have suffered at the time, especially when urinating or when his penis was touched by his mother. Peter listened attentively and smilingly said that I saw sex in everything. But he at once stopped attacking his nose and showed no further signs of discomfort from the hay fever.

Similar material reappeared on many subsequent occasions; it was particularly telling when we explored his compulsive need to masturbate. He explained that every time he failed to ejaculate he would have to try again. As this sometimes happened 10 or 12 times a day, it made his penis so sore that he feared permanent damage. In this way he was also attacking himself, while in his fantasies he was raping a girl.

The equation of ejaculation and urination, as a means of attack on the female object, persisted from his toilet-training battle with mother. This battle was the background to his somatic and psychological experiences at the time of the phimosis and circumcision. This was also the psychological content of enactments during the early months of treatment, when he wanted to use his felt-pens on me, tried to squirt drops at me with his nasal dispenser, and left little pools of water all over the floor of my room. Later, when verbalization replaced acting, he would just threaten to piss on me when he felt he needed to counterattack. There was a mounting excitement and triumph at the height of the attack, but this was at once followed by fear of retaliation. But eventually we learned that an important motive for the attack had been the wish to engage the object—even if it was only in battle.

This sadomasochistic mode of relating was evident in all of Peter's relationships outside the analysis as well. He provoked others to counterattack through his nonverbal attacks and abuse.

With his mother, he still achieved closeness through his body. While she was quite impervious to his psychological needs, she always appeared concerned about his physical ailments and imperfections. The slightest complaint of pains in his neck or back secured the mother's immediate attention, and she would start to massage him. She repeatedly drew attention to a minor impairment in the movement of his left arm for which she gave him physiotherapy. She often dragged him to doctors, e.g., for a verruca which she thought should be excised rather than treated medically as the doctor suggested. There were endless battles about cleanliness and about the need for Peter's hair to be "trimmed" (a term he also used to describe circumcision).

In this way the mother reinforced Peter's castration anxiety, and she communicated her view of him as imperfect. But her physical ministrations sexually excited her adolescent son and in this way she perpetuated and compounded his difficulties. When the doctor suggested prophylactic injections for the hay fever, the mother persuaded him to let her give Peter the course of injections herself. This both excited Peter and increased his anxieties. Although he feared that she might hurt or even kill him, he submitted to her without protest. In the analysis he spoke of using the experience as a stimulus for new variations of his sexual fantasies.

I can see with hindsight that this material was also enacted in the transference, long before the full implications were understood. In the eighth week of treatment he developed a sudden pain in his back and wanted me to do something about it. Instead of exploring with me what the "something" could mean, he quite literally stripped to the waist, ostensibly to see what his mother could have put in his vest to cause the pain.

There can be little doubt that the somatic and psychological experiences occasioned by the phimosis and circumcision were experienced by Peter as abuse and victimization. Child abuse by mothers and medical experiments by Nazi doctors on the sexual organs of concentration camp victims were recurring topics in the analysis. He always emphasized that such brutalities left the victims physically mutilated, mentally retarded, or even dead. He, of course, saw himself both as physically mutilated and mentally retarded.

It would seem that the traumatogenic experiences in his second and third year of life also unleashed massive aggression which his disciplinarian parents met with condemnation, physical beatings, and further assaults and abuse. Peter's "sins" and "guilty crimes," to which he alluded at the beginning of treatment, referred to quite violent, aggressive attacks on animals and children. He "accidentally" killed a kitten; he hit a boy over the head so that he needed six stitches; and he almost drowned a girl in the swimming pool. These episodes must have occurred between the ages of 4 and 8. He was riddled with guilt about these murderous attacks. After his banishment to boarding school, his behavior was reversed. Though, in more subtle ways, he may well have invited sexual attacks and humiliations, he himself soon became the butt and victim of others.

Primitive aggression threatens to destroy the object and the self and mobilizes massive anxiety. It may well be that for Peter the anesthetic concretized and dramatized self destruction, death, and suffocation. The mother had told us that Peter reacted badly to the *anesthetic*, but was unable to remember anything else about the circumcision. It may be speculative to suggest that Peter brought into analysis somatic memories of the panic he experienced when given the anesthetic, but the idea was prompted by the following events.

From time to time Peter froze into a motionless state and sat for several minutes with fixed staring eyes and a masklike facial expression. He would emerge from this trancelike state, either spontaneously or in response to my intervention, only after a violent jerking movement of his head, which was suggestive of a deliberate effort to rid himself of something compelling and terrifying. In discussion various hypotheses were suggested to account for these puzzling episodes. Did they indicate petit mal caused by organic impairment? Did they suggest a kind of hysterical twilight state or even some kind of hallucinatory experience? Did they represent attempts to immobilize his body in order to control sexual excitement and terrifying fantasies?

As soon as Peter's fear of treatment lessened and he could begin to permit himself to convey his feelings and fantasies, these trancelike states disappeared and an organic basis seemed unlikely. But a defensive "withdrawal into fantasy" in the face of anxiety, or painful affect mobilized by any kind of internal or external impingement, remained. At such times Peter was always difficult to reach.

It is of interest that in the third year of treatment the trancelike state made a brief reappearance in one of the sessions. I noted that it was a dramatization of the early states because by that time Peter's self-observing capacities were sufficiently developed to prevent precipitation into panic. He could also acknowledge what had happened and explore it a little. He recalled the frequency of such panic states in and out of analysis and thought of them collectively as "my madness." He thought now that it was his way of "shutting off" the outside world and concentrating exclusively on a fantasy. I was doubtful whether he really had this degree of voluntary control. We were able to link the heightened state of anxiety in this particular session to a transference fantasy that his sadistic attacks would really destroy me, bring treatment to an end, and leave him totally abandoned. It was this "painful" realization he must have tried to "shut out."

I have always harbored the fantasy that the anesthetic was given with a mask and bottle. If this were so, it would bring the anesthetic experience close to suffocation. This would make sense of Peter's perception of death as suffocation, and his use of a plastic bag, in later adolescence, to support his fantasies of castration and suffocation by a big woman. It is a fact that fantasies of being victimized, passively overwhelmed, and cruelly punished to the point of death were sexually exciting just because the aggression was turned against the self and alleviated guilt.

Discussion

The events surrounding the phimosis, the concomitant interventions, and subsequent operation profoundly affected Peter's development. Self and object representations were crystallized around these experiences, and the relationship locked in a sadomasochistic battle for survival. The perception of his mother as malicious attacker, whose longed-for attention and concern could be attained only by suffering pain and by relinquishing his penis, absorbed, restructured, and organized a whole range of earlier experiences and conflicts.

His unrequited longing to be loved, his envy of the brother as usurper of his rightful place, the dangers stemming from his heightened aggression—nurtured by unmet early needs, forced feeding, and rigid toilet training—all became organized around the experiences engendered by the phimosis and circumcision. The anal phase battle for power and control acquired a particularly potent input from hurting and being hurt and became focused on the penis. The mother became all important as the provider of pain and sexual excitement—a sadistic attacker and seducer—and a powerful model for identification.

All this colored the way Peter came to experience his rivalry with the feared and powerful oedipal father, his highly ambivalent relationship to his brother, his banishment from home at the age of 8, and his relationships to teachers and peers at boarding school. What was so striking in Peter's analysis was the way in which all the avenues pursued analytically ultimately led to the experiences surrounding the circumcision.

How do we conceptualize the nature of such an "organizing experience" (Yorke, 1986) which not only shapes what Herzog (1985) has called "the developmental line of personal meaning" but also propels the psychosexual development along a deviant path and generally constricts ego functioning?

Of course, the analysis only gradually and laboriously unraveled the various layers and developmental transformations of Peter's masturbation fantasies and conflicts. But how do we explain the emergence of specific and apparently encapsulated memories, through the most primitive, symbolic, and concretized enactments at the beginning of the analysis?

Do these unconscious enactments of the manipulations of his penis, the difficulties in urinating, and the experiences of the anesthetic reflect the "traumatic" impact of these events? Affectively they were all highly charged with an admixture of excitement, pain, and panic. Are we to interpret them as signs of "trauma" in the classical sense, that they mobilized a degree of affective excitation which overwhelmed vulnerable ego functions; could not be dealt with at the time, became encapsulated as primitive memory structures, until they were reworked and raised to a higher level of integration in the course of the analysis?

There were also some technical implications concerning reconstruction, which arise when working with a patient like Peter. I found it useful to organize my reconstructions around the "trauma of the circumcision" because this was most meaningful in terms of Peter's current experience. But in the view taken of an intrapsychic "organizing experience," reconstructions of this kind may also be more meaningful in terms of the childhood past. Reconstructions must be intrapsychically meaningful rather than be historically or developmentally accurate.

Note

* Presented at the International Scientific Colloquium on "Repeating: Enactment and Verbalization in Different Stages of Development" held at the Anna Freud Centre, November 1985.

References

Herzog, J. M. (1985). Early somatic illness and pain. Presented at the Anna Freud Centre Colloquium. Unpublished.

Kennedy, H. & Yorke, C. (1980). Childhood neurosis vs. developmental deviations: Two clinical case histories. *Dialogue: Journal of Psychoanalytic Perspectives, 4*: 21–33.

Yorke, C. (1986). Reflections on the problem of psychic trauma. *Psychoanalytic Study of the Child, 41*: 221–36.

CHAPTER FIFTEEN

Reflections on the Aim of Child Analysis*

Hansi Kennedy and George Moran 1991

Abstract

Childhood disturbances can best be studied in a developmental frame of reference. Following Anna Freud, the authors distinguish between outcome aism and intermediary aims. They present the analyses of a child and an adolescent to demonstrate how these aims affect the nature and progression of treatment.

In developing the psychoanalytic method, Freud brought a physician's approach to the treatment of the neuroses. He focused his observations on the patient's symptoms, deduced the nature of the underlying psychopathological processes, and formulated treatment aims directed toward elucidating the cause of the disturbance and gaining relief from suffering. With further developments in psychoanalytic theory and technique, the aims of treatment became more specific and also addressed issues of how changes were brought about. Thus in the topographical era of psychoanalysis

Freud stressed "the process of bringing into consciousness that which has been unconscious" as the means to achieve a satisfactory outcome. In 1933, in line with the structural frame of reference, he reformulated his statement and said, "Where id was, there ego shall be" (p. 80). Discussing character disorders in 1937, he stated that "Our aim will not be to rub off every peculiarity of human character for the sake of a schematic 'normality', nor yet to demand that the person who has been 'thoroughly analysed' shall feel no passions and develop no internal conflicts. The business of the analysis is to secure the best possible psychological conditions for the functions of the ego; with that it has discharged its task" (p. 250).

Since then, in what is often referred to as the "widening scope of psychoanalysis," the question of broader aims had to be addressed. Psychoanalysts began to reformulate the criteria for mental health and attempted to define what was meant by normality, maturity, and even happiness.

In a survey of analytic views about the goals of psychoanalysis, Wallerstein (1965) pointed to various dimensions or polarities that needed to be explored and brought together. First, there was an apparent paradox between *goallessness* as a technical stance adopted to allow the analytic work to proceed properly, and the *far-reaching goals* of fundamental changes in the personality to which psychoanalysis aspired. Second, he drew attention to the distinction between the outcome sought for and reflected in observable behavior, for example, in the patient's better relationships and more effective living, and the means by which these aims were realized, conceptualized in metapsychological terms, for example, the evolution of the transference neurosis or the acquisition of new insights. The latter implicitly posits a theory of how analysis brings about change and reaches the intended outcome. Wallerstein also pointed to the distinction "between the more limited and the more ambitious, the more pessimistic and the more optimistic view of how much of this sought-for change can actually be accomplished" (p. 768).

In more recent years a broader model of development has influenced our conception of process and outcome in psychoanalysis, and the contributions stemming from child analysis have profoundly influenced this developmental approach. Childhood disturbances can best be studied and elucidated within a developmental frame of reference. Anna Freud's succinct formulation of the aim of child psychoanalysis as "restoring the child to the path of normal development" has found ready acceptance.

In formulating her theory and technique of child analysis Anna Freud put great emphasis on the concept of normality and on assessing pathology in terms of deviation from a hypothetical norm. Implicit in her theory of development was the concept of a psychobiologically based thrust that impels the child in a progressive direction. Therapeutic interventions aim to "remove the obstacles" on that developmental path. Child analysis is not preventive in the sense that new "obstacles" can still be encountered at later developmental stages. These are fundamental concepts underlying the clinical approach and assessment procedures adopted at the beginning and end of analytic treatments by the Anna Freud Centre. The aim of "restoring the child to the path of normal development" is an integral concept in evaluating therapeutic gain and for making tentative prognostic predictions.

The distinction between the outcome the therapist aims at, and the process by which he hopes to reach it, was one also adopted by Anna Freud. In discussing short-term aims and long-term aims, she suggested that analysts should make a clear distinction between aim and method. The analyst reaches his aim only if he concentrates on the analytic process. "It is very much like driving somewhere. Your aim is to arrive, and if instead of looking at the road, you think how nice it will be when you arrive, you will probably have an accident. Concentrating on the driving process implies steering the car" (in Sandler, Kennedy & Tyson, 1980, p. 251).

It was not until a Study Group on Psychoanalytic Concepts at the Anna Freud Centre began to address the question of aims that, somewhat uncomfortably, we found we had to question a formulation that had been clinically useful over a good many years. What did we really mean by "restoring the child to the path of normal development?" And how was this global aim related to the more specific aims usually suggested at the diagnostic stage when, for a particular child, analysis was recommended? Furthermore, we had to consider how aims arrived at on the basis of a full and detailed diagnostic assessment would affect the way the analysis was conducted. We were led to the recognition that it was not as easy as it looked to draw clear distinctions between aim and method.

Goallessness as a technical stance, where the analyst's free-floating attention responds only to the patient's free associations, cannot be directly applied to child analysis where the analyst has to respond far more actively to the enactments or other forms of expression brought by the child to his session. Nevertheless the child analyst's aim of following the patient's material wherever it leads remains an essential part of technique, even though this general aim will be impeded by a number of other technical considerations. Apart from the obvious fact that, at a very rudimentary level, the analyst's wish "to follow the material wherever it leads" will be impaired by the limits of what he can understand at any given point, other considerations enter into the choice of material to be interpreted. Intermediary aims will be formulated which relate, for example, to establishing and maintaining the treatment alliance; to the need to take into account the relative immaturity of the child's ego as well as any developmental imbalances a particular child might reveal. These intermediary aims will change as the analysis progresses.

Even where the child's symptoms are dystonic (e.g., in phobias, nightmares or distress at an inability to do what other children can do) and the wish for relief of suffering can be mobilized to establish a treatment alliance, such an alliance will not be easily sustained with young children who readily externalize repudiated wishes or superego injunctions. When, for example, aggressive wishes toward a newly arrived sibling, blatantly expressed in the child's play, are interpreted too directly, the child may become afraid of coming to his session if he perceives the analyst as an embodiment of his own aggression, if he expects the analyst to condemn or punish him, or if, in the transference, he fears retribution. Thus, to deal with such threats to the treatment alliance, the child analyst may first aim to foster the child's view of him as a trusted and helpful adult. Fostering such a relationship in the early stages of treatment was seen by Anna Freud as a *means* of establishing and maintaining the analysis in the face of resistance.

Verbalizing and interpreting aggressive wishes toward a newly arrived sibling may be perceived by a young child as permission to enact them and lead to an attack on the baby. One will then have to formulate interpretations couched in terms of conflict and defense. When we are dealing with a more structured neurotic disturbance, however, interpreting a death wish may intensify the child's intrapsychic conflict and lead to increased anxiety or nightmares. Here too, though for different reasons, interpretation of aggressive wishes will have to be complemented by interpretation of conflict and defense. Insight gained in this way may lead to greater tolerance for what was previously unacceptable and warded off. Interpretation will then serve the process of integration.

Intermediate aims affect technique and depend on accurate assessment of the nature of conflict and the nature of defense, as well as the level of ego maturity and/or developmental lags. Only a relatively small group of our patients suffer from clear-cut childhood neuroses. Where the disturbance is due not only to internal conflict but also to developmental psychopathology deriving from a mixture of early neglect and damage, lost opportunities for development, unavailable or inconsistent objects, and other sorts of adverse environmental influences, the analyst will have to recognize that a purely interpretative approach may not achieve the desired aim. It is difficult to *restore* something to the child that was missed in his early development. At best, the therapist can help him to make adaptations to such deficits and the consequent distortion of development. This work is based on psychoanalytic knowledge of developmental needs and involves an admixture of interpretation and ego-supportive elements within the context of a one-to-one relationship. At the Anna Freud Centre we have come to refer to this as "developmental help" and this kind of treatment approach will be illustrated with a clinical vignette.[1]

Adam was an intelligent 4-year-old boy, well advanced for his age in cognitive and language development and conceptual thinking. A sturdily built child with a habitually solemn expression, he appeared to be self-absorbed and distracted by the pervasiveness of his anxiety.

Adam's concern about lack of safety was at once apparent when treatment began. He was not an easy child to engage and tended to roam about the treatment room, keeping up a loud and continuous monologue which the therapist experienced as a kind of bombardment. He was conspicuously preoccupied with danger and clearly courted it. He would frantically climb on furniture, saying anxiously, "I might fall down and hurt myself," and then trip or lose his balance as he scrambled along. As his functioning deteriorated under the impact of anxiety, making him much more clumsy and increasing the likelihood that his fears of hurting himself would be realized, the therapist intervened. She decided what was safe for him to do and what was not and at times showed him how to make things safer for himself. Adam's initial response to this stance was one of surprise. "Mummy would let me fall," he said. On another occasion he told her that "Daddy let me fall off the swing." With further evidence that Adam was uncertain of the object's investment in his safety and well-being, the provision of a consistently containing and protective environment became an important feature of treatment.

His compulsive enactments of the dangers he feared were accompanied by poorly controlled aggressive and destructive behavior which necessitated the setting of firm limits, and again Adam responded with surprise: "Mummy lets me do naughty things and then she gets cross." Adam's anxiety was heightened by his feeling that no one could or would check his omnipotently aggressive wishes, which threatened the very objects he depended on. As he put it: how could the therapist stop him hurting himself if she was dead?

He threw building bricks at her, tried to scribble on the walls or spill water all over the floor, but this was usually followed by attempts to make reparations. His behavior suggested frantic attempts to cope with anal aggressive and destructive wishes and talion fears.

Adam's parents separated in his second year of life and since his mother began to work full-time both parents became less available to him. While he had been used to baby-minders from an early stage, these arrangements also broke down due to his provocative and difficult behavior. The relative physical absence of the parents was matched by their psychological unavailability. At the time of Adam's referral for treatment they seemed an unusually depressing and defeated couple, oppressed by a sense of gloom and guilt about themselves, both as people in general and as parents in particular. Within these limitations they were loving and caring toward Adam, but their desire to do well by him was seriously impeded by inappropriate and inconsistent handling. The mother was prone to quite severe mood swings. She veered between excessive permissiveness and, when she felt provoked by Adam beyond endurance, harsh intolerance. The father was even less convinced than the mother about the whole concept of limit setting, fearing that it would discourage Adam's spontaneity. The father often used his 4-year-old son as a confidant and burdened him with his problems.

Once Adam became able to play in the sessions, his preoccupation with loss tended to have anal connections. He hoarded plasticine, endlessly tied up toys in little bags, and threatened to throw his therapist out as rubbish. Whenever there were tensions at home, he responded by withholding feces. In the sessions he constructed guns with clamps to stop the bullets coming out and killing everyone! He defended against the anxiety mobilized by such fantasies by delivering lectures on how guns worked or on the sewage system which was designed to clean and reuse water. The notion of recycling to avoid loss had special appeal and also made him self-sufficient. Once, when faced with a separation from the therapist, he said, "I'll drink my own spit and eat my own food."

Many of these conflicts were later explored through play with a baby doll whose nappies needed continual changing. Adam repetitively cellotaped up the nappies so that there would be no leakage or loss. This activity became pronounced at the end of sessions and led to his verbalizing that the baby would cry because we had abandoned it and shut it in the locker. This could then be linked with his own anger and sadness about being sent away by therapist and mother.

This was followed by a shift of focus onto the theme of fire, of which he developed a considerable fear. He would arrive at sessions already talking about stoves and fireplaces; he thought he could smell bonfires or see sparks of flame. He was anxious about the central heating and the hot water pipes and though he attempted to master these fears, the anxiety invariably spread. The notion of fire came to contain his central conflicts about his instinctual wishes and his object relationships. In the broad sense the fire which was all-pervasive represented his lack of safety, his feeling of being out of control and overwhelmed by anxiety. In its most acute form it seemed to amount to a fear of annihilation, but this was comparatively rare. Once when he was running around the room saying he could see flames, he shut himself in the cupboard. Very soon he shouted out, saying that the flames had got inside the cupboard too. He did not really believe the therapist could help him. He told her that other people expected him to be able to put out the fire, but he was not sure that he could do so. He seemed to be enacting the sensation of being out of control and unsupported by his environment.

He gradually came to see that the flames derived from his own feelings. This prompted him to attempt other solutions. "I know," he said, "I'll just forget about the feelings." But he couldn't forget. His compulsive attraction to fire did nothing to contain his fears and indeed suggested a sexualization of anxiety. Adam was able to describe how his fear of fire began. When visiting friends, with his mother, he had suddenly been frightened by the loud noise of coals being put on the fire; Adam thought Father Christmas might be coming down the chimney. Later on, he elaborated on this, pointing to his fear that Father Christmas would get burned if he did so.

Adam's fears and excitement about anal aggression and object loss were contributants to this fantasy. A good deal of his material about fire seemed to symbolize his excitement and anxiety about withholding and expelling body products. He spoke of hot coals crammed into the fireplaces that he built with bricks. He was preoccupied with chimneys, air vents, and smoke. Fire also represented excitement and fear about his sadistic phallic wishes, particularly urethral ones. He was drawn to fire extinguishers and hoses and wanted to squirt water; he thought hot water would burn or kill people.

It was not until Adam's anxiety was somewhat reduced by interpretations of his fear that his exciting wishes and fantasies might incur damage to or loss of his objects that he began to be able to make use of other defenses and thus gain some distance from the immediacy of his conflicts. Hitherto Adam had not been able to engage in role play as he could not tolerate his therapist assuming a "pretend" role. Now he became able to initiate a game of parent and child which brought him great relief. The therapist became the child who was burdened and unsupported by the adult.

They played games of barbecues. Adam suggested that the therapist, who played the role of baby, was frightened by fire. When she voiced her doubts about the safety of the fire, Adam portrayed his version of the parent: "I'll try to look after you. I'll do my best." He would explain repeatedly how safe the fire was, but would somehow undo this by adding anxiety-provoking remarks: "Of course it's safe; there are no flames, only glowing embers; if you fall in there, I'll get an ambulance."

While this was a reflection of Adam's own wish to hurt, he also conveyed something of the flavor of his parents' way of handling him. By their own account, both parents constantly fed Adam's anxiety. The father, in particular, felt that he would be deceiving Adam if he gave him false reassurance. For instance, when Adam asked his father whether the house would fall down, the father felt he had to admit the possibility of this happening. Adam's immaturity made him unable to cope with all the possibilities of danger with which he was presented. In a sense, the father attempted to deal with Adam's anxiety as he dealt with his own—by providing him with detailed information. Thus, at the height of Adam's pervasive fear of fire, the father introduced the notion of spontaneous combustion. It seemed likely that hostility to his son underlay the father's repeated fueling of Adam's anxiety. But Adam attempted to elicit similar responses in the transference and tried to make his therapist feed his anxiety. For example, he clamored to know why the therapist would not let him go out on the windowsill; was the therapist worried about what might happen to him? Was she worried? What could happen? And so on.

He began to experience a loyalty conflict as he realized the therapist had a different response to his question. It was important to him to have confirmation that his father's information was correct, and yet he felt reassured by the therapist's stance that dangers did not lurk everywhere.

On one occasion he commented on how it had been raining when he came to his session and how the umbrella had not been big enough. Had his therapist also been caught in the rain? Later on, the source of his anxiety became clearer when he began to relate what his father had told him about acid rain and how it could kill trees and people. The therapist said she knew he was worried by some of the things the grown-ups told him; talking about these things had made him think he and she could get hurt walking in the rain, although he really knew they would come to no harm.

Treatment during the first year was dominated by the pervasiveness of Adam's anxiety and by his inadequate and often unadaptive ways of coping with it. Although Adam's anxiety was anchored in conflicts over aggression and talion fears, his feelings of lack of safety derived from his parents' inappropriate and inconsistent handling. Perhaps the most disruptive influence on his development was their alternating investment in him, so that at one moment he was the exclusive focus of attention and at another was ignored by a parent intolerant of his needs. His expectation of external danger and fear of loss of the object must be seen in the light of the intermittent unavailability of his depressed parents.

In treatment the provision of a safe, consistent environment was of prime importance as a first step in alleviating his anxiety. In time he ceased to fight the provision of safety and began to participate in it. With the development of a more positive and trusting relationship to the therapist, the analytic work could proceed more readily.

No child analyst would of course permit a 4-year-old to expose himself to physical injury in the treatment room, but technical approaches vary. Adam's therapist recognized that her patient's almost total preoccupation with danger and the fashion in which he courted it contained a challenge for her to respond. She inferred that Adam was uncertain of his object's investment in his safety and well-being and decided that in addition to her interpretative approach, she needed to provide a consistently containing and protective treatment environment. In fact, she pinpointed a developmental deficit, caused by early unmet needs, and formulated intermediary aims to facilitate developmental processes. These interventions became closely interwoven with the analytic work. Developmental and therapeutic processes were complementary. The analytic task of interpreting Adam's aggressive and destructive wishes and talion fears was ardently pursued. It led to the emergence of material around more primitive levels of anxiety, conflict over object loss, feelings of self-depletion, and vulnerable narcissistic supplies. All these were defended against in Adam's "recycling fantasies."

Adam's initial surprised response of "Mummy would let me fall," to the analyst's consistent stance of keeping him safe and setting limits, might arouse doubts about a technical intervention that seemingly casts the analyst in the role of "new object" and consequently might interfere with the development of transference. This did not happen: the analytic material unfolded in an orderly fashion. Conflicts over separation evolved around the beginning and ending of sessions and weekend breaks, and could readily be linked to problems related to the parents' separation and the unpredictable care he received, both past and present. Later in treatment Adam attempted to elicit a transference situation where the therapist would feed his anxiety, as his parents always did. This suggested that these pathological features were already internalized in Adam and only currently reinforced by his parents' pathology as reflected in the way they handled him.

It would seem that Adam could not readily identify with the analyst who provided safety, although the relief of some of his anxiety enabled him to widen his defensive repertoire. The switch from being the anxious child to becoming the anxiety-promoting parent, so evident in the fantasy role play with the analyst, indicated a new flexibility. Initially unable to tolerate the analyst's taking on a "pretend" role, he could now reverse roles. However, if the therapist diverted from his scenario, he experienced a loyalty conflict and would, for example, anxiously inquire why the therapist did not agree with his father's views. This material seems to confirm J. Sandler's view of transference as an actualization of an internal dialogue with the parental introject, in this case an anxiety-promoting dialogue, and yet one that the patient clings to.

All this raises interesting questions about the changes we hope to bring about in child analysis. The young child's internal and external worlds are not yet firmly separated and "new object" experiences may therefore have more impact on his intrapsychic world. Conversely the young child is more vulnerable to pathological input, and we need to be more concerned about how analytic gains can be consolidated and sustained in the face of massive pathological parental influence. Work with parents then becomes an essential part of the young child's treatment and will represent another set of intermediary aims and aims of outcome that the child analyst has to take into account. It will not be surprising that the work with Adam's parents achieved only limited success.

Phase-specific developmental considerations will also provide criteria for formulating treatment aims, in terms of both outcome and intermediate ways which affect technique. In young children, with developmental delays, the advance to the oedipal level itself, which presupposes important developmental achievements in drive organization, object relationships, and ego functioning, may be seen as a satisfactory therapeutic outcome, although analysts usually prefer to help the child negotiate oedipal conflicts as well. The move into latency and the concomitant establishment of the repression barrier create some developmentally appropriate resistances which sometimes make the child unwilling to continue the analytic work. However, developmental consideration may lead the analyst to consider that a latency child needs distance from his conflicts in order to integrate and consolidate his personality structure and defensive organization. To this end, the analyst may side with the resistances that manifest themselves in the child's wish to terminate treatment. A child who terminates with good feelings about his analysis may be able to return to treatment in adolescence to sort out some of the sexual conflicts which the analyst anticipated would occur, but which could not be dealt with in latency.

It is more important perhaps to consider *how* developmental phase-specific considerations affect technique. To interpret oedipal conflict to a child who is in the process of negotiating this phase for the first time, at a more or less age-appropriate time, will be different from revisiting these conflicts with an older child or an adolescent. In order to synchronize the therapeutic and developmental processes in the oedipal phase it may be helpful to formulate interpretations of conflict in a way that will facilitate adaptive resolutions. For example, one might say, "Of course it feels terrible to want to get rid of daddy because you also love him and want to be like him."

In preadolescence or early adolescence, it may be advantageous to interpret the defensive aspects of a boy's passive wishes rather than to focus on the passive feminine content of those wishes. So instead of saying, "You sometimes want to be a woman because you wonder what it feels like," the analyst might choose to say, "Being a man feels dangerous and you may sometimes think that women get a better deal." Where there is conflict between active and passive tendencies, interpretations may be formulated which support the boy's active masculine strivings. The aim here would be to support the developmental move in puberty in the direction of heterosexuality.

With many older adolescents, the analytic work may be impeded by focusing too much on transference aspects of the material. The need to break away from dependence on parental protection and the wish to consolidate a relationship with a new sexual object may be promoted by extratransference interpretations of conflict which focus on the parents as experienced in the present as well as in the past, and by making links to wishes and fears in relation to peers in the here and now. This does not exclude transference interpretations where these are appropriate and necessary. Some resistances cannot be overcome without them.

However, not all technical parameters in the treatment of adolescents relate to phase-specific developmental issues alone. Many of our patients' neurotic solutions are rooted and enmeshed in early developmental deficits or distortions and when these are recognized, they may require interventions which affect technique.

Marilyn, aged 17, referred herself for treatment.[2] She said that she was uncertain about seeking help but had agreed to come at the behest of her father. In the initial months of treatment she usually dressed scantily in pastel shades, seeming seductively eager to please. She described her mother as demanding, critical, and unspeakably selfish. She lived with her father in the north of England for some years following the parents' divorce and spoke of him as caring and concerned. However, she was so distressed by his recent remarriage that she returned to live with her mother.

Marilyn's parents were married as teenagers following her mother's decision not to abort her unplanned pregnancy with Marilyn. She brought many memories of a time when she was a young child and her parents took her along with them to raucous parties where she felt she was the center of attention. From her accounts of her early childhood it appeared that she was uncommonly capable of attracting the interest and admiration of adults, the most important reward for which she felt was physical affection. Throughout latency she maintained herself at the top of her class in a selective school. She continued to have an apparently problem-free childhood despite a background of an increasingly turbulent parental relationship. Overt extramarital relationships and frequent episodes of violence culminated in an acrimonious divorce.

Marilyn maintained a tenuous commitment to treatment during the first year. She had chosen her analyst from a list of five persons for the sole reason that he was the only man. She behaved with him in the sexually suggestive manner in which she described her behavior with all men, and she seemed reassured when he acknowledged this without responding to it. However much she wished to please the analyst, she did not take readily to the role of patient. She fluctuated in the frequency with which she agreed to attend sessions, made difficulties over times, and interrupted the treatment twice by taking prolonged holidays. With every step forward in the analytic work, she became increasingly disappointed and angry, complaining that her analyst did not care about her but only about getting her well.

Her accounts of everyday life and relationships were shallow and inordinately sexualized. In the evenings she drank alcohol, took drugs, and danced at night dubs. She recounted with glee countless episodes of being picked up by "dirty old men," and plied with alcohol and presents. More often than not she managed to find ways of avoiding intercourse with these men. Frequently, however, she found herself in bed with men whom she hardly knew. While her exhibitionism led her to such extremes as dancing for groups of men in bars, she was embarrassed if seen naked, was sexually passive, and derived no pleasure from genital sexuality. In contrast to her pleasure in recounting her adventures, she became increasingly miserable, depressed, and ashamed. With difficulty she spoke of her wish to take an overdose.

Marilyn's superficial compliance in the analysis and the quality of her seductive behavior gave a clear indication of her need to please in order to feel safe and loved. It was equally apparent that she experienced her compliant response to the demands of others as a potentially devastating threat to her fragile sense of her self. Her life as she recounted it was a desperate oscillation between tentative attempts at being a person in her own right, rebellious and uncontrollable, and harsh self-condemnation for failing to live up to her ego ideals. To be loved, she believed she had to do what others demanded of her, yet to comply with those demands led her to feel taken over, empty, and worthless. For Marilyn, a central difficulty concerned her conflicts over control. She once said, "If you don't try to control me, I feel you don't love me; if I do what you suggest, I feel empty and like nothing is mine."

Marilyn's dilemma revealed serious developmental distortions of her sense of self. Throughout her childhood, her traumatic circumstances forced her to adapt to an environment over which she had no control and which was unresponsive to her needs. Paradoxically, she could exploit her fragile sense of self in the service of gaining admiration through her success in taking on the roles prescribed by others. Her mother's mixed feelings about having a child, the history of violence between the parents, and the high social and academic standards expected of her, all contributed to, and sustained, harsh and violent features of her superego. In puberty, she was thus in conflict about her sexuality, and her self-injurious behavior and reckless life-style served masochistic ends.

During the first year of analysis, her sexual encounters were initially interpreted in terms of recognizing neediness in others and wishing to please them in order to feel loved. Increasingly, conflicts over her promiscuity began to characterize the material. Gradually, transference links could then be made, though transference interpretations were often restricted to her feelings of neediness and the fear that the analyst did not care enough about her. For example, Marilyn described one of her sexual exploits with a man she found to be "stupid, repulsive, and yet so desperate" that she could not get rid of him, and found herself inviting him to spend the night with her. She felt so disgusted with her actions the following morning that she took repeated baths and compulsively cleaned the house. Her analyst commented on this and on similar situations, "I think you could see and respond to the neediness in that man because you find it so difficult to experience your own neediness here or anywhere else." Some months later, in one Monday session, Marilyn said she had found herself half-drunk in bed with two boys she had met at a party. Her analyst said, "I think it is very hard for you to feel that there may have been someone that you needed over the weekend who wasn't there, and the only way you could find to meet that need was do what you saw your mother do after the divorce—when she had one man after another in her bed and you felt so left out."

Still later in the analysis, when Marilyn became affectively aware of the neediness that determined her behavior, she was able to curb her promiscuity and self-destructive tendencies, except in holiday breaks. She also prepared for and passed her exams, took on a routine job, and dressed in an attractive and nonprovocative way. Thus the transference could be seen to have developed in the direction of pleasing her analyst as she had tried to please her father throughout her childhood when he was her primary caregiver.

During the second and third year of treatment it became possible to talk to Marilyn about her sexual excesses during analytic holidays in terms of her need to obliterate her sense of desolation at being abandoned yet again, and despite her efforts to please her analyst while she was coming to treatment. For example, before a break in treatment, she revealed her plan to submit to the sexual demands of a man, a doctor, with whom she had an affair over the previous holiday. She spoke of "being stripped and screwed" by him and likened it to feeling beaten. Her analyst recalled that the man with whom she had had an affair before the one with the doctor had the same first name as the analyst, adding that she had an affair with a doctor and a George. There was only one name left. She smiled and said that there was a Doctor Moran at work, but he was just too old. Her analyst linked her reactions to the holiday break to the rage that she had felt when her father left both her and her mother. Now she felt compelled to hide these feelings by arranging for others to express her rage through their physical and mental abuse of her. She replied that she supposed incest must be truly horrific, but added that she thought it must be pleasurable as well. It was then possible for her analyst to bring her attention back to her pleasure in her father's physical care of her as a child, and to reconstruct her anger at the limitations on physical love which he imposed. This interpretation allowed her to reflect somehow less passionately on her anger with her father for discouraging her from sitting on his lap when she was 14, and she was able for the first time to express anger with her analyst for not making a pass at her.

In a short vignette one cannot provide sufficient context for a full understanding of the case. Nevertheless, we feel the analyst was justified in adopting an unusual flexibility in his technique over an extended period. While initially the analyst was forced to comply with Marilyn's dictates concerning her attendance, as is often the case with adolescents, an understanding of her special needs in this regard became a crucial intermediary aim.

From the beginning and for most of the first year of treatment, the analyst allowed himself to be seen to respond to Marilyn's neediness but not to her sexual provocation. For example, he allowed her unusual flexibility in the frequency and times of her sessions and in the duration of her holidays. Her external circumstances from the age of 10 were such that they endorsed her feeling of being dependent and neglected. By allowing her some control over the treatment setting, he was better able to address her inner neediness and its defensive elaboration in her sexual activities.

With adequate analytic understanding of her fears of dependency on the analyst and her destructive enactments aimed to obliterate her neediness, the analyst could begin to work with Marilyn on the importance of establishing a daily routine which could promote the progress of her analysis, boost her self-esteem, and ultimately make her future life more effectively adaptive. There was a turning point when, after one year of treatment, Marilyn decided "to move" to Portugal and "start life afresh as a barmaid." The analyst interpreted the resistance and registered his doubts about her solution, but also said that he would make every effort to find her a place with him again if she decided to return. When she came back, after 3 months, Marilyn was able to agree to regular daily attendance, and used the analysis effectively to organize her external life. On one occasion she asked her analyst to help her negotiate with both parents an allowance to enable her to share a flat with a girlfriend and to help her establish herself in a job.

Resolving her unsupported external situation made Marilyn feel less guilty about her dependence. This in turn made it possible for her to tolerate the emergence and interpretation of her sexual conflicts in the transference, including reconstruction.

Summary

In exploring the concept of aims in child analysis we have followed a developmental approach and tried to distinguish between outcome aims and intermediary aims. Intermediary aims change as the analysis progresses, and they affect technique. The pursuit of intermediary aims requires the analyst to assess within a psychoanalytic frame of reference why the child acts and talks as he does and to address these issues.

At the start of the analysis the intermediary aims will focus on getting the child to attend, form a treatment alliance— which includes developing a wish to come even in the face of resistance—and to work in analysis. The analyst needs to use a technique that will facilitate the child's wish to attend. In some cases the analyst will have to guard against rushing in with interpretations which may frighten the child; with others, quick and meaningful interpretations are immediately necessary to make the child feel understood and, on this basis, develop a readiness to engage in the analysis. Parental support for treatment, beyond bringing the child to his session, is often needed for auxiliary support, especially with younger children.

Intermediary aims are also influenced by the child's phase-specific developmental status. In the treatment of children under 5, issues of cognitive capacity, reality testing, the capacity for impulse control, and so forth, will have to be taken into account. In the treatment of latency children the analyst needs to be aware of the fact that the analytic process runs counter to the developmental process. This situation is reversed in preadolescence or early adolescence when the emergence of instinctual forces and the associated conflicts can be exploited to facilitate the analytic work.

In the treatment of children with marked developmental delays or deficits, we must formulate intermediary aims which may lead to interventions that try to address developmental needs in addition to conflict and defense analysis. An example of this was given in the case of Adam where the provision of safety and the setting of consistent limits accompanied the interpretative work, especially during the first year of analysis. Likewise, in the case of Marilyn, the analysis of transference was initially restricted because of the pervasiveness of her neediness and the deficiency in her self-organization. These features were understood to be important determinants of her promiscuity and recklessness and led her analyst to formulate the intermediary aim of helping her to recognize her neediness, not only through interpretation, but by responding to it in token ways.

In the treatment of borderline or severe narcissistic disorders such interventions often play a central part in the therapeutic work. But closer scrutiny of our technique may show that such interventions enter, to varying degrees, into our therapeutic work with many child patients. In this context we consider that the notion of intermediary aims may represent a more flexible, fluid, and dynamic concept than Eissler's (1953) parameters of technique.

What about *outcome aims* and our wish to clarify the meaning of Anna Freud's global formulation of the aim of child analysis as "restoring the child to the path of normal development"? The analyst will conceptualize her aims in terms of intrapsychic structural change. In Arlow's (1988) terms, psychic structure refers to the manner in which the individual organizes or constructs experience. By structures we are not referring to the id/ego/superego agencies but to what Gill (1963) referred to as microstructures. Structural change implies enduring modification of mental organization.

We take the view that a child's capacity to regulate his inner world, and to understand the world outside, depends upon increasingly elaborate internal organizations, and that the use of earlier, more primitive, structural organizations is abandoned when they are at odds with more highly developed levels of functioning. However, earlier psychic organizations always remain and can potentially be reactivated under the impact of regressive shifts.

In the course of a child's analysis preconscious and unconscious representations of events, deriving from earlier levels of organization, emerge as affectively significant organizers in the material. Abrams describes therapeutic action in terms of the revival in the psychoanalytic process of earlier pathogens and their reintegration into higher levels of developmental organization.

The outcome aimed at in child analysis is reached when previous pathogenic organizations and solutions cease to be applied automatically to deal with conflict. From a developmental point of view the outcome aimed at is the building up of suitable structural organizations which optimize the potential for development, within the limitations set by the child's constitutional, maturational, and environmental givens.

Notes

* An earlier version of this paper was given at the Anna Freud Centre 10th International Scientific Colloquium: "The Impact of Developmental Considerations on the Aim of Child and Adult Psychoanalysis." This paper brings together the results of some of the eliberations of the study group on Psychoanalytic Concepts whose members are J. Sandler (chair), A. Gavshon, H. Kennedy, M. McCutcheon, J. Miller, and G. Moran. The authors are indebted to the group members for their numerous helpful contributions.

1. This case was treated by E. Phipps-Buchan and supervised by H. Kennedy.
2. Marilyn was treated by G. Moran.

References

Abrams, S. (1988). The psychoanalytic process in adults and children. *Psychoanalytic Study of the Child*, 43: 245–61.

Arlow, J. A. (1988). Summary commentary. *Journal of the American Psychoanalytic Association, 36*: 283–94.

Eissler, K. R. (1953). The effect of the structure of the ego on psychoanalytic technique. *Journal of the American Psychoanalytic Association, 1*: 104–43.

Freud, A. (1965). *Normality and Pathology in Childhood.* New York: Int. Univ. Press.

Freud, S. (1933). New introductory lectures on psycho-analysis. *Standard Edition, 22.*

Freud, S. (1937). Analysis terminable and interminable. *Standard Edition, 23.*

Gill, M. M. (1963). *Topography and Systems in Psychoanalytic Theory.* Psychology Issues Monograph 10. New York: Int. Univ. Press.

Sandler, J. (1976). Countertransference and role-responsiveness. *International Journal of Psychoanalysis, 3*: 43–7.

Sandler, J., Kennedy, H., & Tyson, R. L. (1980). *The Technique of Child Analysis: Discussions with Anna Freud.* Cambridge: Harvard Univ. Press.

Wallerstein, R. S. (1965). The goals of psychoanalysis. *Journal of the American Psychoanalytic Association, 13*: 748–70.

PART FOUR

ANALYTIC TECHNIQUE WITH PRE-LATENCY CHILDREN

Introduction

In hindsight it is apparent why Kennedy's focus was so often on the pre-latency child. It is during this time of life that the two divergent pathways for personality development begin and the two types of disturbances can most readily be assessed. After the oedipal phase of development, the intertwining of both forms of pathology and other developmental considerations make it more difficult to see them in "pure form". Through Kennedy's interest in delineating neurotic conflict and developmental disturbances, and in contributing to the clarification of developmental help, she was able to refine the analytic technique of working with very young children.

Kennedy's paper "The technique of psychoanalysis with the pre-latency child", written in 1988, was a discussion of a number of analyses of young children presented at the 1988 Annual Meeting of the Association for Child Psychoanalysis. She used these analyses to illustrate her ideas on child analytic technique. The children Kennedy discussed suffered from developmental disturbances, not necessarily due to parental pathology but to medical interventions and traumas. As in all of her work, she emphasized technique based on developmental considerations that changed based on the child's age, developmental level, and the particular disturbance. Rather than focusing on earlier arguments of child versus adult technique, Kennedy directed her attention to the question of the psychoanalytic method with children, especially those suffering from delays and severe distortions. She drew together and expanded her earlier theories of technique, looking at the analytic relationship and the ways in which conflict and developmental needs are addressed.

Kennedy's final major work evolved not only from her many years of clinical experience with young children, but also from the examination of the extensive case reports of over seven hundred children and adolescents treated at the Anna Freud Centre ("Psychoanalytic work with under-fives: Forty years' experience", 1991). Kennedy and Mary Target undertook the work presented here as part of a larger effort to create a prospective study of analytic cases at the Centre. They had a number of goals, of which one was to consider those contexts and problems where child psychoanalysis was most effective and those where its value was limited. Kennedy provided commentary on the pre-latency analyses conducted at the Centre, focusing on such technical issues as parental involvement in the child's treatment, the young child's modes of bringing material into the analysis, the analyst's role in facilitating the child's self-understanding, and transference-countertransference aspects of pre-latency analysis. Once again she pointed to the role of analytic work in aiding the child not only to deal with conflict but also in promoting the consolidation of structural development.

CHAPTER SIXTEEN

The Technique of Psychoanalysis with the Pre-Latency Child*

Hansi Kennedy 1988

A review of the literature on technique suggests that child analysts are moving away from the mere delineation of differences and similarities between adult and child psychoanalysis. They are developing a theory of technique based on developmental considerations. There is nothing surprising about this: it reflects a general trend in psychoanalytic theory vividly illustrated by the contributions of A. Freud, Hartmann, Kris, Mahler, and others who gave new and wider perspectives from which to view normal and pathological development. Today, our efforts are more concerned with defining the limits of the psychoanalytic method and with considerations of those therapeutic interventions that aim to redress delays or severe distortions in child development.

A study of some more recent contributions on technique which focus on these issues—for example, those of Kestenberg (1969), Maenchen (1970), Olch (1971), Neubauer (1972), Solnit (1975), Glenn (1978), Ritvo (1978), Sandler, Kennedy and Tyson (1980), and Harley (1986)—reflects a consensus of opinion regarding the essential features of clinical child analysis. In fact, M. Harley's Marianne Kris lecture (1985) at Chapel Hill looked at these questions from a historical perspective with a clarity that I will not even try to emulate. Instead, I will address some of the more controversial issues in the analyst/child/parent interaction which, I believe, assume special significance in work with pre-latency children.

If ready agreement can be reached among authors on a comprehensive but global definition that child psychoanalytic technique is signified by the analyst's interpretive approach to the child's intrapsychic life with due consideration to his developmental status, disagreement and controversy arise as soon as the meaning of the three components of this statement are narrowed down.

What is referred to as "the analyst's interpretive approach" can encompass wide-ranging differences of technique. An application of technique which is geared to the needs of the individual patient and his level and mode of functioning can be firmly based on the bedrock of psychoanalytic theory; however, adherence to a more rigidly defined, strictly interpretive stance may require the analyst to remain personally distant and aloof in his interactions with the child. Both approaches may work if not carried to extremes, but it is my personal belief that every child analyst practices within a technical framework allowing adaptation to the child's needs and level of functioning even if he or she does not theorize about it. This will be most needed in the treatment of pre-latency children, who confront the analyst with different tasks and different problems than older children.

Anna Freud's general dictum that the aim of child analysis is to restore the child to the path of normal development is particularly relevant in terms of the developmental status of the pre-latency child's intrapsychic world. A significant landmark on his developmental path will be the negotiation of the oedipal phase, an ontogenetic point of demarcation at which the child's intrapsychic world attains a crucial degree of structural autonomy. We postulate that substantial structural changes occur with entry into latency. Massive repression leads to the "infantile amnesia," perhaps insufficiently talked about nowadays, resulting in a more effective "censorship" or "repression barrier" (Kennedy et al., 1985). We associate this major occurrence with concomitant changes in the structure of the superego and a more definite compartmentalization in the mind between unconscious and preconscious systems. In addition, Piaget's work has alerted us to important changes in cognitive functions which occur at this same time and which have important implications for psychoanalytic technique (A-M. Sandler, 1975; Rees, 1978).

Developmentally, the preoedipal (and even the oedipal) child's "intrapsychic world" is still in a relatively fluid state, and to some extent his internal and external worlds remain open systems. Frustrations, prohibitions, and conflicts, even though they may originate internally, are experienced predominantly in relation to the external world. Even after parental prohibitions have become internalized, the primitive defenses at the child's disposal will tend to relocate conflicts as if they were still between himself and the external world.

Such defensive maneuvers, aimed at reducing tension and maintaining feelings of well-being, also have a bearing on the child's object relationships, both internally and interpersonally. The stability of self and object representations is constantly undermined by a lack of synthesis of contradictory images of the object, kept alive by unresolved ambivalence and fueled, in turn, by the impact and intrusion of the external world. Until "good self" and "benign object" representations are firmly established and provide internal sources of support and protection, the child is much more dependent on external feedback to maintain internal equilibrium. And likewise, external experiences in interaction with the primary objects (and perhaps their extensions in the transference) will have a more profound effect on the building up of stable, cohesive, and benign self- and object-representation.

In the treatment of pre-latency children, the ready availability of id content in the clinical material is particularly helpful to the analyst. Feelings, wishes, and fantasies are more openly and freely expressed; and this eases the task of understanding the underlying content that is not consciously known to the child but is not truly repressed in a dynamic sense. This advantage, however, has to be weighed against the young child's greater vulnerability: his internal controls are insufficiently stabilized to safeguard him against overwhelming feelings and wishes. This vulnerability is a frequent source of resistance and can undermine the effectiveness of interpretations whenever these are experienced as too dangerous or painful for the child to bear. The analyst's interpretations, ostensibly aimed at strengthening the ego, may threaten ego functions that are precariously established, and not just impulse control, although this is a very prominent technical problem in our work with under-fives. Interpretations, if not carefully worded and adapted to the child's level of functioning, can be misconstrued by him and threaten his reality testing, his self-esteem, and even his capacity to maintain object differentiation. A three-year-old, for example, who made a slip and called his therapist "mummy," could not allow himself to hear the therapist's appropriate transference interpretation because he felt humiliated by his inability to maintain proper object boundaries.

In extreme forms such difficulties are encountered only in children with specific delays in ego development, but they are met with, in lesser degree, in work with all preoedipal children. The advance to the oedipal level itself presupposes important developmental achievements in drive organization, object relationship, and ego functioning. These provide the ego with new flexibilities in dealing with wishes, fears, and internalized prohibitions and with more scope to react appropriately to interpretations of defense, resistance, and transference.

The importance of the move into the oedipal phase stressed in each of the cases presented here, but the developmental issues to which I referred in these introductory remarks and their important implications for technique, touch significantly on the assessment of whether our patients have re the oedipal level and regressively retreated from it or whether this important developmental progression is negotiated for the first time during the analysis. Equally, we must consider differences in the nature of oedipal transference in children are in the process of negotiating the oedipal phase and in who are regressively reliving oedipal relationships and conflict analysis.

Although the very interesting cases present a variety of referral problems, including differences of age (from two nine months to four years, six months), of developmental stage reached at the beginning of treatment, and of length of respective analyses (from five months to four years), they have a striking feature in common: They have all been subject to the impact of a physical condition or illness on their early development. Five of the children had medical histories, and the mother of the sixth had a physical illness. Dr van Dam's case suffered from SIDS (Sudden Infant Death Syndrome), needed to be on a monitor the first year of her life, and experienced many life-threatening episodes. The same conditions prevailed for her brother, when she was two and a half years old, and thus relived by the family and herself when she began treatment at two nine months. Dr Epstein's case (not included in this volume) was born with a congenital hypospadius and Dr Gavalya's with a congenital urinary tract defect; both children were exposed to many exciting and anxiety-provoking examinations and painful surgical interventions. Dr Haber's (not included in this volume; see Haber, 1991) patient's chronic ear infection from the age of six months as well as the regular injections for allergies against which he fought vehemently were still continuing when he entered analysis at three years, nine months. Dr Nover's patient Jenny had an organically based eye defect, diagnosed also at six months. It led to her good eye being patched for a large part of her waking hours, and she too protested and struggled against it with vehemence. Dr Tyson's patient Johnny had no impingement of a personal physical condition, but a tragic impingement of his mother's illness. She had a brain tumor, removed surgically six months into her pregnancy with Johnny, and although still alive in his infancy she could not care or relate to him and died when he was two years old. As a result, he had multiple caretakers and suffered many separations and object losses in his early years.

It is not difficult to draw some general conclusions about the impact of such major and prolonged physical problems on the whole family. They color the child's perception of his world as potentially frightening, painful, and hostile, contaminate the mother-infant relationship, and mobilize undue aggressive investment in self- and object-representation. All are preconditions for complicating the separation-individuation process, irrespective of the more individually determined dangers of preoedipal libidinal fixations.

Most of the children showed considerable unevenness in their ego development, being precocious in some aspects such as verbal or reasoning capacities, yet prone to express themselves in an action mode because of lack of impulse control and aggressive conflicts.

Important reasons for recommending analysis usually were the pervasive difficulties affecting most areas of the child's life and the primitive inflexible defenses leading to stalemates in the mother-child relationship and defeat of the parents. In spite of these severe problems, in several cases it was difficult to gain parental support for the analysis, and this, in turn, had repercussions on the analytic work.

We cannot dispense with parental cooperation in child analysis, least of all in work with pre-latency children. The degree and nature of the analyst's involvement with the parents is the subject of much discussion in the literature on technique and is an area of considerable controversy. What is the parents' role in their child's analysis and how can it be accommodated? If we exclude the parents too much we create serious difficulties for the preschool child in engaging in the analytic work. The parents may wittingly or unwittingly accentuate the child's loyalty conflicts or extend punitive, denigrating, or hostile attitudes toward the child in the analyst's direction. But parental intrusiveness in the child-analyst relationship can be equally detrimental, encroaching on the child's budding needs for autonomy and undermining therapeutic expectations that the therapist is available for the child and will keep his confidences. For the analyst there is a danger that too little contact with the parents may blur his view of the child's overall functioning (for example, the analysis is going well, but the child's adjustment is deteriorating everywhere else) and, conversely that too much external information may contaminate his view of the analytic material.

For the parents, in addition to the external strains related to time and money, their child's analysis will touch on many of their internal concerns. In the mother, the need for her young child's treatment mobilizes guilt and fears of having failed or damaged the child; and her narcissistic hurt and feeling of inadequacy will be heightened by having to hand over her child to a therapist, who conveys that he understands her child better than she does (Furman, 1969). This will be even more painful if the analyst succeeds in engaging the child quite soon in an intimate and close relationship on whatever basis.

If the child is currently engaged in an openly defiant, hostile, or sadomasochistic relationship to the mother, he may grasp immediately the opportunity to engage positively with the analyst because this represents an attack on the mother. When the child's aggression toward her is defended against by excessive clinging or controlling, the opposite may occur. The child may insist that the mother stay in the room or make constant visits to the waiting room or insist on her symbolic presence in the consulting room by keeping hold of her handbag or her chair, and so on.

One could say that the new relationship to the analyst is so intimately linked with current as well as past interactions in parent-child relationships that, psychologically speaking, in the treatment of pre-latency children, the mother or father or both are always present in the consulting room.

This implies that, as therapists, we all feel more comfortable if the parental presence in the consulting room is metaphoric rather than actual, but the recognition may have some bearing on the tenacity and speed with which we pursue our efforts to bring about a physical separation.

The youngest child, Betty (age two years, nine months), could be separated in the first session from her psychoanalytically enlightened mother, with whom a separation strategy had been carefully discussed in a preliminary interview But one could not fail to be impressed with the skillfully handled first contact with the child, partly through nonverbal actions, partly through verbalization, which enabled the child to move from sitting on mother's lap unbuttoning her blouse and averting eye contact with her therapist to playing with him while mother left, ostensibly to feed the parking meter. To quote Dr van Dam, "I felt that it was important to separate mother and child during treatment sessions as soon as practicable for the sake of the unfolding of the therapeutic process to afford the child separation and privacy from the parent and to foster her ability to reveal herself with more ease."

By contrast, Dr Epstein had to conduct the analysis of his patient (age three years, two months) with the mother in the consulting room for more than two years, and not as a passive observer but an active participant in a highly eroticized relationship with her son aimed at excluding the analyst. She not only colluded with the boy's enactment of his defensive fantasies of having omnipotent and exclusive possession of her, but also responded with excitement in playing this role. Every effort was made to work this through in the shared sessions as well as in sessions with mother alone.

In order to maximize the benefit that analysis can provide for the pre-latency child, parents need to be actively involved in the analytic work with a young child. It is not enough to meet the analyst to give information or to discuss conflicting feelings about the continuation of the treatment. The child's developmental needs also have to be met by the parents. Regular work with them offers unique opportunities to facilitate their understanding of the child's current feelings and conflicts and will lead to better handling of the child.

In this way it is possible to create an environment for our patients which genuinely supports the analysis and enables the parents to retain confidence in their parenting roles. Even more important, it may also create a home milieu that can support the patient's gains after the treatment is over.

There are various ways to work with parents toward these ends. Sometimes they need to be present in the consulting room for shorter or longer periods and be part-recipients of the analyst's interpretations, tempered as they may have to be for both mother and child. Additional individual sessions with the mother are even more important in this situation, to work through her reactions and her feelings and enable her to respond appropriately to the analyst's handling of the separation issue. Sessions with the parents, however, are best not traded off against the child's treatment time, which would be diminished as a result.

Whatever contact the child analyst has with the parent must be regarded as a part of the work with the child. When, for example, Rachel (age four years, six months) had a temper tantrum when her mother announced in the waiting room before her session that "we almost fell asleep on the way here," Dr Gavalya told the mother that Rachel wanted to speak for herself about her own sleep.

The child must always remain the primary patient, and this implies that he must be kept in the picture regarding any contact with the parents, who soon learn to put this into practice as well. Of course, the child analyst will not give details of the child's fantasy material to the parents, but the danger of making a child feel threatened by possible breaches of confidence through contact with the parents is, I believe, often exaggerated with young children. While omnipotent thinking is still dominant, children are not surprised that parents know what they are thinking or feeling and indeed sometimes feel relieved by this knowledge. Their concept of secrets is usually first built up around "family secrets" that should not be talked about to outsiders. The so-called secrets that emerge in analysis are revelations that the young patient does not want to know about himself; and this maybe even more important than having the parents know about them. There are different levels of knowing, and it is particularly important to bear in mind the fact that the superego is still largely dependent on parental approval or disapproval. When forbidden wishes are not taken up in the context of a conflict in the analysis, a young child may have to resort to complaining to the parents about the naughty things the analyst is telling her to do or gauge the parents' reaction in seeking their protection in the consulting room.

Parental secrets, which must not be conveyed to the child, are unwelcome burdens for the child analyst and hamper his freedom to interpret. This is quite different, I believe, from obtaining extra-analytic information about the child which can be kept as a potential resource and used when appropriate. It is interesting but not really surprising that, under favorable when the analysis and the work with the parents go well, there is remarkable overlap between the child's and the parents' material on a week-to-week basis; this does not occur to anything like the same extent with older children or if different therapists work with child and parents.

I want to move from the direct analyst/parent relationship to the analyst/child one. The young child only gradually develops the capacity to contain the analytic material session; he has a tendency to carry the product of the work into the home even if the analyst tries to curb this tendency through the symbolic action of keeping toys, drawings, and so on in the consulting room. But the child's tendency to "spill over" or to "act out" in this way affects the interactions with his parents and, in turn, adds to the analyst's distinguishing between current reality defense, or transference in the child's material. These problems are underlined by the child's mode of communication. The pre-latency child's verbal statements are still partly tied to primary process thinking. The analyst will have to learn to understand the child's language and also to "tune in" to the meaning of his nonverbal communications. This includes observing the child's behavior and giving meaning to it. For example, in the first session obeying Betty's demand to sharpen pencils, Dr van Dam explained that he was there to help her not only with the pencils, but also with many other things, like her feelings and thoughts about her mother and her brother. Betty then made scribbles and asked the analyst to erase them. The meaning of such symbolic actions could be open to different interpretations.

Containment in the session of the child's enactments, his "acting in," faces us with even greater difficulties than his acting out. When a child is prone to wrecking the consulting room or to attacking the analyst physically in sudden eruptions of rage or panic, attention tends to be diverted from the analyzing function. Such outbursts frequently arise in response to the child's frustrated attempts to control the therapist and failure to coerce the therapist into acting a specific role (as in Dr Nover's case).

So-called role-play is an important part of the analytic work with young children but may challenge the analyst's wish to adhere to a rigid set of technical rules. The main consideration in determining whether and for how long the therapist should comply with the patient's demand actively to play a role in his scenario must always depend on what the therapist's involvement will mean to the child and what purpose it is serving in the analytic work. A fine balance has to be kept between eliciting fantasy material in a mode natural to the child's level of functioning and self-expression and providing too much gratification or excitement in doing the analytic work itself. We aim in child analysis to facilitate a move from action to verbalization, ostensibly to help the child gain better ego control. But we may sometimes overlook the young child's cognitive need to experience or to "replay experiences" in a concrete, action-based modality which may enhance his capacity to gain mastery and better integration.

In several of the cases presented, the trauma of surgery or of other medical interventions was reenacted with the analyst in circumstances in which passive was turned into active. One child gave shots to his analyst in a doctor's game; another child stuck an embroidery needle into her therapist's finger with obvious delight, accompanied by reassurances that it would not hurt. The children carried out imaginary surgery resulting in either death or recuperation. We know that this kind of play in the service of mastery occurs in and outside analysis. When it is brought into the analysis by the child as a reflection of his current concern, the analyst, through verbalizations and interpretations, transforms the action play into a meaningful communication. In this way an analytic process becomes established in the form of a dialogue between patient and analyst. In the course of the dialogue the fantasies, past and present, associated with the surgery will appear in the analytic material in different forms and contexts. The analyst's interpretations allow the child to view the effects of his past traumatic experiences from a new perspective. The language of this dialogue between child and analyst is communication through both play actions and words.

Fantasy play with toys permits a degree of distancing and displacement which is often preferred by the analyst to action play. When Betty wanted her therapist to give her a bath and started to undress, the analyst, for obvious reasons, diverted her by encouraging her to bathe the doll instead. She accepted this and gave the doll a bath with only minimal assistance from her analyst. Sometimes Betty assigned to the analyst the role of being her baby brother on the monitor, so that his fate was in her hands. She would then either "fix" the monitor or pull out the plug on him. In this context the analyst could interpret her wish to stop her brother's breathing and her resulting fear as one of the reasons for her bedtime difficulties, to which Betty retorted, "I know that."

Some children need to maintain a rigid distinction between pretend play and real-life experiences. They have to protest if the therapist steps out of the role of play and interprets. The therapist may have to concede and formulate his interpretations within the framework of the play scenario to keep the analytic work going (Kelly, 1970). While this may be a quite acceptable technique in the early stages of treatment, the analytic aim would still be the direct address of the patient's feelings, fantasies, and conflicts. We assume that the capacities for self-awareness and insightful understanding are increased by acknowledgment of full proprietarial ownership.

What should not be overlooked in adjusting technical interventions to the appropriate cognitive level of the child is that play interaction may be an important or even necessary adjunct to interpretation and working through if the ego mode is action based and still tied to concrete experience.

Thirteen months into Rachel's treatment a termination date was set. It prompted Rachel to become very bossy and provided opportunity to talk about her intense need for control in the past. She listened intently to Dr Gavalya's interpretations, who also playacted for Rachel the scenes in the car and at home when she had temper tantrums if mother acknowledged her as Rachel instead of a make-believe character. To this Rachel responded with great delight, saying, "I can hardly believe it, I can hardly believe it, but I remember, it is true."

Apart from making important links between separation anxiety and her defensive need to control, this clearly helped Rachel to organize her experiences in a time sequence, to look for motivation, cause and effect, all in the service of improved self-awareness. This form of reconstruction enables the child to gain a new perspective of current feelings, from the vantage point of recent ego achievements (Kennedy, 1972).

This was illustrated also In Dr Haber's case (Haber, 1991): "Stanley appreciated genetic interpretations as long as the word 'baby' was included. He appreciated the time relationships, because his narcissism was not injured by the implication that now he was older and smarter."

I have used action and play as synonyms because in the context of the analytic material they are both enactments of a sort. In one of the cases the child referred to her activities in the session as work, without, I think, reference to the analyst's endeavor. Playing can be a serious activity for the young child, and its illusory quality may encompass features in the child's fantasy lift with which we can work in analysis.

I have so far omitted any reference to transference in describing these child/analyst interactions. In a shorthand way, we may describe all these aspects of the interpersonal relationship as "transference," and this would be simple enough. But there are many complexities in an issue such as this (Scharfmann, 1978; Tyson and Tyson, 1986).

How do we categorize role-play in which the analyst is assigned the role of mother, brother, doctor, or the child himself and related to effectively within a scenario which appears to be based on fantasied or real experiences in his current or past life? Some of the role casting is quite enduring and is probably based on a splitting of ambivalence; but some more fleeting images of a good, caring, neglectful, or frightening mother suggest an externalization or unintegrated object representations linked with memories of the past. In several cases the child's positive attachment to the analyst was linked to the temporary absence of the parents; in other cases fluctuations between positive and negative feelings corresponded to similar swings in the child's relationship to the parents. All these could be described as spillovers or extensions of the child's current relationship to the parents where, strictly speaking, the parent of the present is also the transference object of the past. This statement emphasizes what I have said earlier, namely, that the preoedipal and oedipal child's current conflicts, whether external or externalized, still involve the primary objects, and that earlier conflicts continue as live issues or, in modified form, as part of these relationships.

Sometimes children also externalize aspects of their intersystemic conflicts as, for example, described by Rachel's therapist. "She not only projected onto me her sense of being unclean, but also made me do all the things she wished to do but feared doing. I understood this game to be an expression in the transference of her need to deal with those parts of herself which were not acceptable to her parents." And one could add, "Because they were not acceptable to her parents, they were also not acceptable to her budding superego."

Transference evolves as part of the analytic process, and this will result, on occasion, in the child experiencing transferences to the analyst with greater intensity than the corresponding relationships with the parents. This is not at all unusual in the transition to the oedipal phase, which may unfold first, and quite intensively, in relation to the therapist and from there "extend" to the parents. But this is still different from the revival of preformed object related fantasies when these are freed from repression and reexperienced in relation to the analyst.

Such conceptual refinements need not trouble us too much in our clinical work. One conclusion we should draw from it is that the pre-latency child's "transference material" should not be interpreted only in relation to the analyst and the parent of the past, but also in relation to the here and now feelings toward the parents.

Although there was hardly any mention of countertransference in the case reports, some authors (Kohrman et al., 1971) have drawn attention to a ready intensification of countertransference reactions in child analysis Child analysts are prone to overidentify with their child patients or to have rescue fantasies often mobilized by their direct contact with parents. Phyllis Tyson referred to her considerable technical difficulties of "juggling Johnny's positive transference and his stepmother's negative transference in a way that remained therapeutic and enabled the analysis to continue," but she did not spell out the counter-transference involvement in dealing with these difficulties.

Like transference, countertransference has undergone considerable conceptual expansion (Marcus, 1980; R. Tyson, 1986) since Freud's original formulations, so much so that nowadays one sometimes listens to case reports in which the analyst's feelings are the main criteria for interpretation of the patient's material. While our understanding of the analytic material is obviously not entirely based on our empathic identification with the child, the need to be "in tune" with our young patients is underscored by having to rely quite heavily on observing and interpreting behavior and other nonverbal material. We also have to monitor carefully our reactions to the child's destructive and aggressive enactments and provide "containment" for both ourself and for the child, as ego auxiliary support.

What the Sandlers (J. Sandler, 1976; J. and A-M. Sandler, 1978) have described as "free floating responsiveness" to the patient's wish to actualize his unconscious fantasies focuses on another aspect of the extended meaning of countertransference, one that may have special relevance for what we have been discussing. They describe how fantasies involving self and object interaction in the patient's intrapsychic life tend to be actualized in relationships with external objects, especially in the transference. It is not unlike the way we viewed the child's scenario for his role-play, except that the adult has to find more subtle ways of imposing role responses from his analyst, and that the child's scenario is more transparent. Countertransference, in this sense, can indeed become an aid in the analysis of the pre-latency child provided the child analyst carefully monitors his spontaneous contributions to the role-play.

Ritvo (1978, 298) questions the degree to which young children can enter fully into the analytic process. "The analyst uses his conceptualizations of the analytic process and his understanding of the phenomena of transference, resistance, defense, etc., to initiate, guide and intensify the process." As a result, the child's conflicts find more direct expression of repetitions of past experience in the transference, but the analyst's role as the knowing and informing one will not readily give way to self-exploration and insight.

Mangham (1981) traces the origin of pleasurable affects associated with insight to affective experiences in the mother-child interaction in infancy. I expressed similar ideas (Kennedy, 1984) when I suggested that the genesis of affective awareness and self-understanding has to be sought in the experience of being and feeling understood. The infantile prototype of the later feeling of being understood by the analyst originated in the infant's affective experience of his mother's appropriate responses through her more sophisticated understanding to his needs. This analogy can be taken further; just as the mother understood what the infant needed before he could do so, so the child analyst's insights into his patient's wishes, fantasies, and conflicts usually precedes the patient's "higher level of knowing." This should remind us that, in the initial phases of treatment, some children perceive our interpretations merely as "friendly noises" and also highlight the experiential components of the interaction between the child and the analyst. Quite a number of our child patients need the affective experience of "feeling understood" before they can feel safe enough to participate in the often painful endeavor to increase self-understanding.

Many will find my approach to the technical problems in the analysis of pre-latency children quite controversial. Indeed, it may once again raise doubt about whether this work is truly analysis. For this reason I was interested to read Dr Kestenberg's reply to the same question raised at the end of a panel discussion on "Technical Problems in the Analysis of the Preoedipal and Preschool Child" some eighteen years ago (Olch, 1971). A. Maenchen, who was chairman of the panel, agreed with Dr Kestenberg's statement that "since we analyze the developing ego and superego, the defenses and wishes, and help the child to remember and integrate, we can call it analysis" (p. 550). We can be even more positive in answering this question today. The required technical adaptations discussed are necessitated by the developmental status of the pre-latency child and can readily be encompassed in our earlier definition of child psychoanalytic technique.

Therapeutic results are potentially far-reaching and often obtained much quicker. This is due to the fact that the analytic work not only helps the child in dealing with conflicts and finding new solutions and adaptations but also promotes the consolidation of structural development itself: This is especially significant in the treatment of the preoedipal child, in whom the therapeutic efficacy linked with the assistance that can be given to developmental processes that are still in a state of flux is substantial.

A. Freud (1965, 229) drew attention to the fact that the child makes his own selection for therapeutic use from the full range of possibilities that are contained in the child analytic setting.

I have said earlier that our efforts today are more concerned with defining the limits of the psychoanalytic method and with considerations of therapeutic interventions that aim to redress developmental disturbances.

The cases presented at this symposium could all be classified as developmental disturbances and in some instances as accumulative traumatization. The impact of major and prolonged physical conditions or illnesses in their early life profoundly affected these children's development and complicated the separation individuation processes. Parental conflicts often reinforced these difficulties.

Anna Freud (1974) suggested that the ego can change only what it has done and not what has been done to it. She referred here to her frequent attempts to distinguish between neurotic conflict and developmental disturbances. In the former, "interpretation of the repressed, of transference and resistance, enables the child's ego to replace pathological conflict solutions by more adaptive ones." In the latter, the child will at best learn "to cope better with the after-effects of what has happened to him. But child analysts. . . are reluctant to accept the humiliating fact that the developmental damage which they understand so well and reconstruct so efficiently, can be beyond their power to cure, by truly analytic means" (1976, 259).

This would explain some of the difficulties encountered in the analysis of some of these patients, the need for extending the treatment over several years, and some reservations on the analyst's part about the successful conclusion of the analysis. Perhaps it is precisely in cases such as these that applied psychoanalysis and psychoanalytic treatment become one and the same thing.

Note

* Presented at the Annual Scientific Meeting of the Association for Child Psychoanalysis, New Orlearns, LA, 1988.

References

Furman, E. (1969). Treatment via the mother. In: R. Furman and A. Katan (Eds.), *The Therapeutic Nursery School* (pp. 64–123). New York: Int. Univ. Press.

Freud, A. (1974). A psychoanalytic view of developmental psychopathology. In *The Writings of Anna Freud, 8* (pp. 57–73). New York: Int. Univ. Press.

Glenn, J. (1978). The psychoanalysis of pre-latency children. In: J. Glenn (Ed.), *Child Analysis and Therapy* (pp. 163–205). New York: Aronson.

Haber, C.H. (1991). A three-year-nine-month boy with a gender identity disorder. *Journal of the American Psychoanalytic Association, 39*: 107–30.

Harley, M. (1986). Child-analysis 1947–1984. *Psychoanalytic Study of the Child, 41*: 129–54.

Kelly, K. (1970). A precocious child in analysis. *Psychoanalytic Study of the Child, 25*: 122–45.

Kennedy, H. (1972). Problems in the reconstruction in child analysis. *Psychoanalytic Study of the Child, 26*: 386–402.

Kennedy, H. (1984). The "baby at the breast" experience: Memory or fantasy? Some further thoughts on reconstruction. *Bulletin of the Hampstead Clinic, 7*: 15–24.

Kennedy, H., Moran, G., Wiseberg, S., & Yorke, C. (1985). Both sides of the barrier: Some reflections on childhood fantasy. *Psychoanalytic Study of the Child, 40*: 275–83).

Kestenberg, J. (1969). Problems of technique of child analysis in relation to the various developmental stages: Pre-latency. *Psychoanalytic Study of the Child, 24*: 358–83.

Kohrman R., Fineberg, H., Gelman, R., & Weiss, S. (1971). Technique of child analysis: Problems of countertransference. *Internal Journal of Psychoanalysis, 52*: 487–97.

Maenchen, A. (1970). On the technique of child analysis in relation to stages of development. *Psychoanalytic Study of the Child, 25*: 175–208.

Mangham, C. (1981). Insight: Pleasurable affects associated with insight and their origins in infancy. *Psychoanalytic Study of the Child, 36*: 271–7.

Marcus, I. (1980). Countertransference and the psychoanalytic process in children and adults. *Psychoanalytic Study of the Child, 35*: 285–98.

Neubauer, P. (1972). Psychoanalysis of the pre-school child. In: B. Wolman (Ed.), *Handbook of Child Psychoanalysis* (pp. 221–53). New York: Van Nostrand Reinhold.

Olch, G. (1971). Reporter 1971 Panel: Technical problems in the analysis of the preoedipal and the preschool child. *Journal of the American Psychoanalytic Association, 19*: 543–51.

Rees, K. (1978). The child's understanding of the past: Cognitive factors in reconstruction with children. *Psychoanalytic Study of the Child, 33*: 37–59.

Ritvo, S. (1978). The psychoanalytic process in childhood. *Psychoanalytic Study of the Child, 33*: 295–305.

Sandler, A-M. (1975). Piaget and psychoanalysis. *International Review of Psychoanalysis, 3*: 43–8.

Sandler, J., Kennedy, H., & Tyson, R. (1980). *The Technique of Child Psychoanalysis: Discussions with Anna Freud.* Cambridge: Harvard Univ.

Sandler, J. & Sandler, A-M. (1978). On the development of object relationships and affect. *International Journal of Psychoanalysis, 59*: 285–96.

Scharfman, M. (1978). Transference and the transference neurosis in child analysis. In: J. Glenn (Ed.), *Child Analysis and Therapy* (pp. 275–307). New York: Aronson.

Solnit, A. (1975). *Psychoanalytic Study of the Child,* Monograph Series, 5. *Studies in Child Psychoanalysis: Pure and Applied* (pp. 1–13). New Haven: Yale Univ. Press.

Tyson, R. (1986). Countertansference evolution in theory and practice. *Journal of the American Psychoanalytic Association, 34*: 251–74.

Tyson, R. & Tyson, P. (1986). The concept of transference in child analysis. *Journal of the American Association of Child Psychiatry, 25*: 30–9.

CHAPTER SEVENTEEN

Psychoanalytic Work with the Under-fives: Forty Years' Experience

Mary Target and Hansi Kennedy 1991

Introduction

It may be useful, in order to place these reports in context, to outline here briefly the major programme of research on the process and outcome of child analysis currently being undertaken at the Anna Freud Centre.

It was felt that there was a need to investigate and establish the contexts and problems for which child psychoanalysis is especially effective and other circumstances where its value is limited. We were aware that there has been very little research on intensive treatments for either children or adults, with the important exception of Wallerstein's (1986) work[1] on the assessment of the outcome of analytic treatment of forty-two adult patients. We were also aware that we were well placed to undertake such research since we hold the well-documented case records of several hundred children and adolescents in analytic treatment, and further we have a uniquely high number of experienced therapists and of children currently being assessed and treated in child analysis. Our work in these respects over the past two years has recently been bolstered by an invitation to participate in the collaborative multi-site programme of psychoanalytic therapy research being organized by Professor Robert Wallerstein under the auspices of the American Psychoanalytic Association.

Our long term goal is to establish a prospective study of the process and outcome of child analytic treatment. To achieve this goal a number of intermediate steps need to be taken. It is important that our psychoanalytic diagnoses of children should be aligned with psychiatric research nosology, so that children treated analytically treatment, types of intervention which have, for the most part, already been the subject of a good deal of research. However, it is equally important that our research should go beyond currently available empirical measures of describing psychopathology, so that problems presented and their modification during treatment can be assessed according to uncompromised psychoanalytic criteria.

There are many considerations in establishing a prospective study of therapeutic outcome for which a retrospective look at the successes and failures of the treatment concerned are invaluable. These include most of the fundamental questions of design and procedure, such as where to direct the focus of the investigation (e.g. the age group to be included); how to assess the effects of treatment; how to describe the nature of the treatment; which characteristics of the patients and families should be measured, and how; which variables may predict important aspects of outcome, and therefore need to be controlled for within the research design, etc. We have tried to answer a number of these questions by conducting a retrospective study of the 777 cases already treated in child analysis or non-intensive therapy at the Centre. This is allowing us to see more clearly the general shape of the population and patterns of treatment, to acquire a preliminary idea of the predictive variables, and to find out to what extent the necessary information is already being recorded, or may need special measures. Some information which is very likely to be important, such as detailed recording of life events, assessment of parental attitudes to treatment, and so on, could not be included in the retrospective study, but will certainly need to be measured in standardized ways as part of the prospective investigation. The material available to us, however, has proved to be of immense value in designing the necessary instruments. Alongside the retrospective study, good progress is being made in writing a manual of child analytic treatment, and in a further study we are looking at ways of judging the quality of analysis (independently of outcome).

The results presented at the WAIPAD conference and published here provide an outline of the work done with under-fives at the Centre since 1950. They represent a small part of the data collected so far in the retrospective study; and, even on the small database presented here, more work is being done to identify variables which seem to be important predictors of outcome. The contribution by Hansi Kennedy is intended as a first effort to integrate the wealth of clinical experience at the Anna Freud Centre with this most recent empirical initiative.

Retrospective Study of Case Records

We have records of 143 cases of children treated who were under five at the time of referral. These children were all seen individually, the great majority in full analysis.

Demographic Details

Over half of the children in this age-group were more than four years old by the time treatment started; the youngest was 2 years and 1 month. Two-thirds of the under-fives were boys, one-third girls; this is a rather higher proportion of boys than in the older age-groups (62% of 5–11-year-olds, 52% of 12 and over).

Families of Origin

59% of parents were British or Irish, many of the remainder were Europeans who arrived as refugees. Over half were Jewish. The majority of parents were middle-class (76% of fathers were in Social Classes I and II), many of them in professional occupations. (The proportion of middle-class parents has risen since 1950 from 64% to 78%.) 98% of fathers and 21% of mothers were in employment at the time of the child's assessment; three-quarters of the working mothers were employed part-time.

78% of children lived with both natural parents, while 14% were living with mother only. The number of intact families falls steadily over the four decades from 1950 to 1990, particularly in the '70s (see Figure 1). These figures reflect the population trend towards more frequent marriage breakdown and single parenting over the years. The percentage of intact families is consistently lower in these patients than in the general population, but almost certainly higher than in (other) child psychiatric settings.

Among the broken families, the majority had divorced or separated parents, one quarter had single mothers, and in a substantial minority of cases the father had died (see Figure 2).

Child's Position in the Family

Among the under-fives, almost three-quarters of the children coming into treatment were first-born children. By comparison, the percentage of first children in the older age-groups was just over half, as shown in Figure 3. Of the second and later-born children in the under-five group, half had an older sibling already in treatment at the Centre. Mrs Kennedy comments on these findings in her paper.

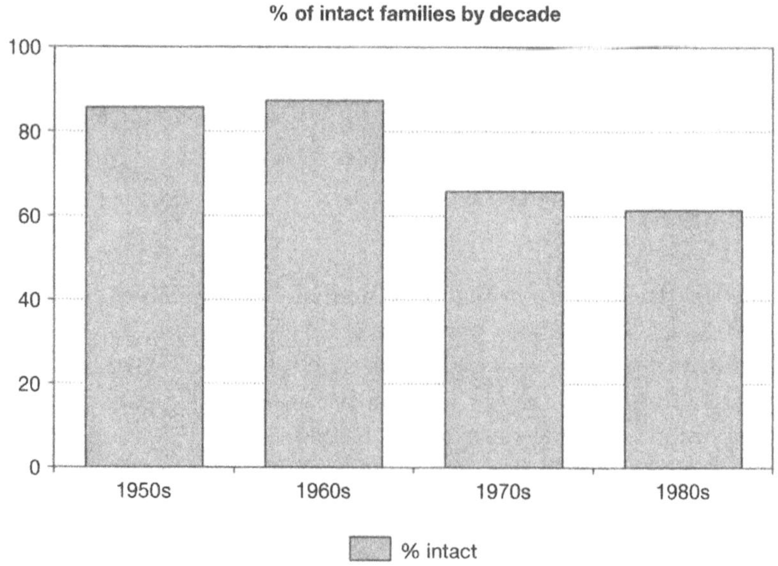

Figure 1

Referral Sources

Under-fives were less likely to be referred by their parents than older children; only 30% of under-five referrals were from parents (see

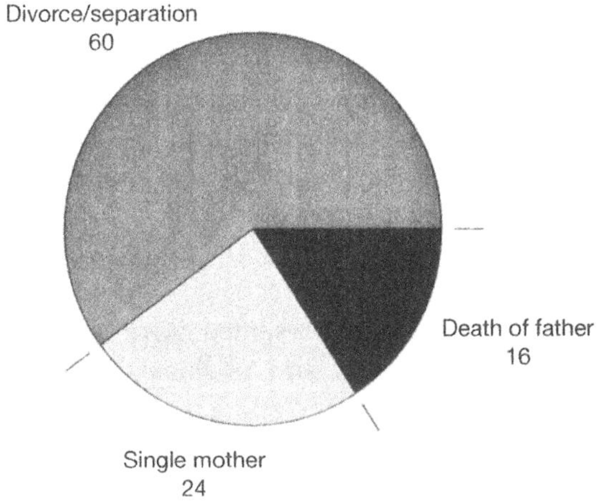

Figure 2

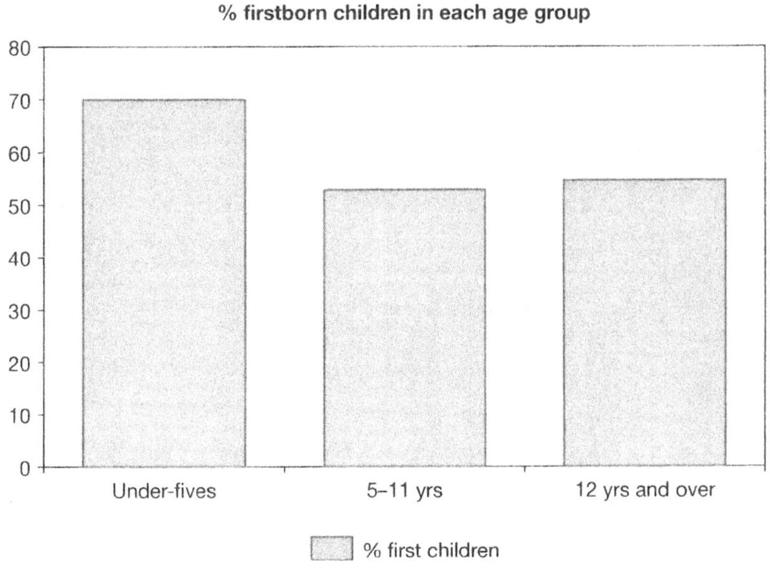

Figure 3

Figure 4). The difference seems to be due to the number of under-fives referred from within the Anna Freud Centre: from the Nursery School, Well-Baby Clinic, Toddler Group and Baby Observation (20% altogether). Other sources included doctors, paediatricians, child psychiatrists and social services. Looking at changes in referral pattern over the years, the number of children (including under-fives) taken on for treatment each year is about half the number in the 1950s and 1960s. Previously a substantial minority of these referrals came from outside doctors; this has now largely been replaced by internal referrals (Nursery School and Well-Baby Clinic).

Symptoms Leading to Referral

The most common problems presented were anxiety symptoms (especially separation anxiety and phobias), aggressive, defiant behaviour and sleep difficulties. Wetting and soiling were common referral symptoms in 4-year-olds, usually in the context of more general anxiety or provocative behaviour. There was a small group of borderline or psychotic children. Children referred from within

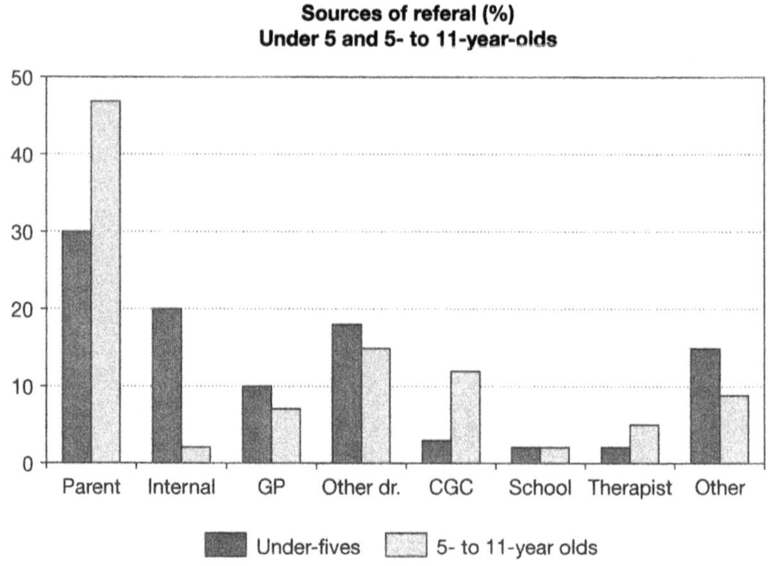

Figure 4

the Anna Freud Centre were often showing signs of slow or very uneven development, withdrawal, or problematic family relationships, without necessarily having more specific symptoms.

Diagnostic Categories

Miss Freud developed a system of five diagnostic categories for classifying children's psychopathology: Category 1: essentially normal; Category 2: transient symptomatology or developmental strain; Category 3: neurotic, with "permanent regressions, fixations and symptom formation"; Category 4: atypical, distorted personality development; and Category 5: destructive processes disrupting mental growth (examples would be organic or psychotic illnesses). Figure 5 shows the distribution of those children assigned to a category as part of the diagnostic procedure. The Category 5 children were almost all taken on for treatment in the 1970s, after which it was decided that analytic treatment was not the best way of helping them.

Psychiatric Diagnoses

Diagnoses were retrospectively assigned to each child where appropriate, using both the DSM-III-R and ICD-10 diagnostic systems.

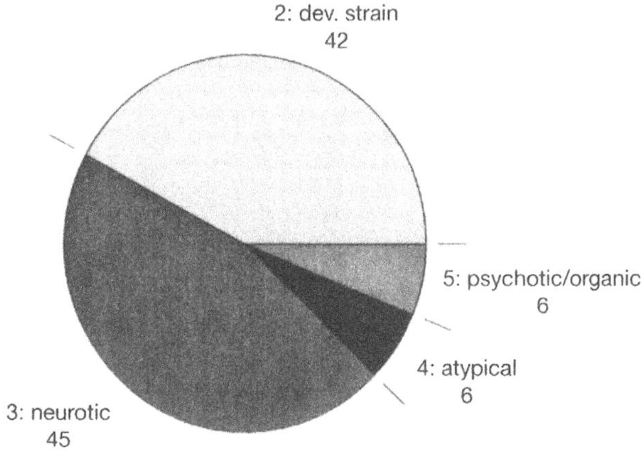

Figure 5

These are the two major systems of classification of psychiatric disorders, which use explicit diagnostic criteria in order to categorize syndromes with high levels of reliability and validity. Diagnoses were assigned on the basis of the child's state at the time of assessment and at termination. 71% of children met the criteria for at least one diagnosis when assessed for treatment (many could be given several); 25% did not meet the criteria for any specific diagnosis, and in 4% of cases there was insufficient information to make a judgment. The most common diagnoses are shown in Figure 6 (DSM-III-R categories only), together with their frequencies at assessment and termination. One can see that the "Axis II" disorders (developmental disturbances) more often persisted to the end of treatment.

CGAS scores: Overall level of impairment

We used the Children's Global Assessment Scale (devised by Shaffer et al., an adaptation of Endicott's GAF scale for adults) to describe the overall level of psychological impairment in the children who

Psychiatric diagnosis of under-fives
% of group; diagnoses for under 2% excluded

	Assessment	Termination
Oppositional defiant disorder	17	4
Separation anxiety disorder	16	1
Nightmares/night terrors	16	0
Overanxious disorder	9	3
Primary insominia/dyssomnia	7	0
Avoidant disorder	5	1
Simple phobias	5	0
Functional encopresis	4	1
Pervasive development disorder	4	4
Adjustment disorders	4	0
Development expressive language disorder	3	1
Functional enuresis	2	1
Autistic disorder	2	2
Anxiety disorder n.o.s.	2	0
Posttraumatic stress disorder	2	0
Attention def. hyperactivity disorder	2	1
Development articulation disorder	2	1
Psychological factors affecting physical condition	2	1

Figure 6

had been treated at the Centre. This scale gives a single figure from 1–100, which indicates the overall severity of symptomatology. Scores above 70 are considered to be within the normal range. CGAS scores at assessment ranged from 32 (usually psychotic or autistic symptoms) to 75 (mild and limited disturbance, within normal limits). The average score was 56, which indicates a moderate degree of interference in functioning in most social areas, or severe impairment in one area.

Medical Conditions and History of Hospitalization

A substantial number of the under-fives had medical conditions or a history of hospitalization and separation which often formed an important part of the reason for referral. 21% had a chronic medical condition (for example, impaired vision or hearing, or severe and chronic eczema), at least 11% had experienced surgery, and 8% of the patients had been hospitalized with acute illnesses. 6% of these children had experienced accidents requiring in-patient treatment, usually for a period of weeks.

16% of the Centre's under-five-year-old patients had been separated from their parents while being treated in hospital, for between a few days and several months. Mrs Kennedy will be discussing the impact of these events both on the child's development, and on the parents' willingness to bring a child for analytic treatment.

Psychiatric Symptomatology in the Parents

The case records contained far more information on psychiatric symptoms and treatment of mothers than of fathers. It is difficult to know how far this reflects a higher level of disturbance in mothers, a belief in the greater influence of the mother's pathology, or simply more contact with the mothers of patients. The parents of under-fives appeared to have more psychiatric symptoms and to have received more treatment than those of older children; this might again reflect a reporting bias rather than a real difference. Figures 7 and 8 show the frequency of psychiatric symptoms among the parents of the under-fives at the time of the child's referral, and earlier in each parent's life. Symptoms are divided into serious, moderate and mild. Serious symptoms include most psychotic

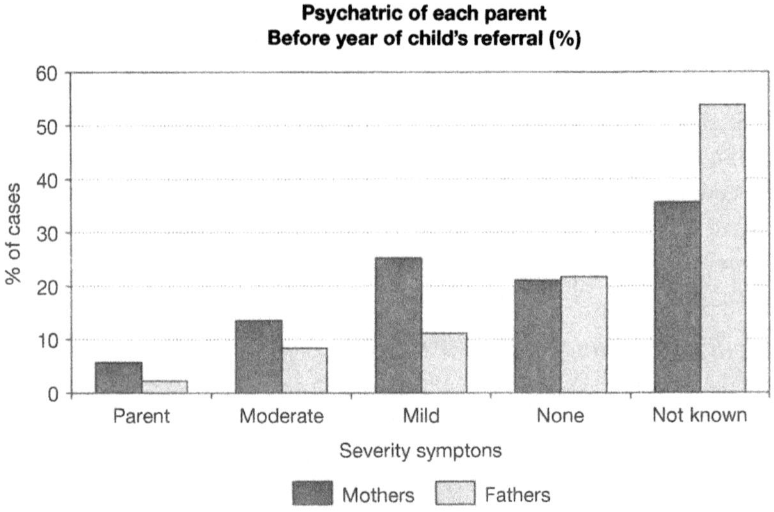

Figure 7

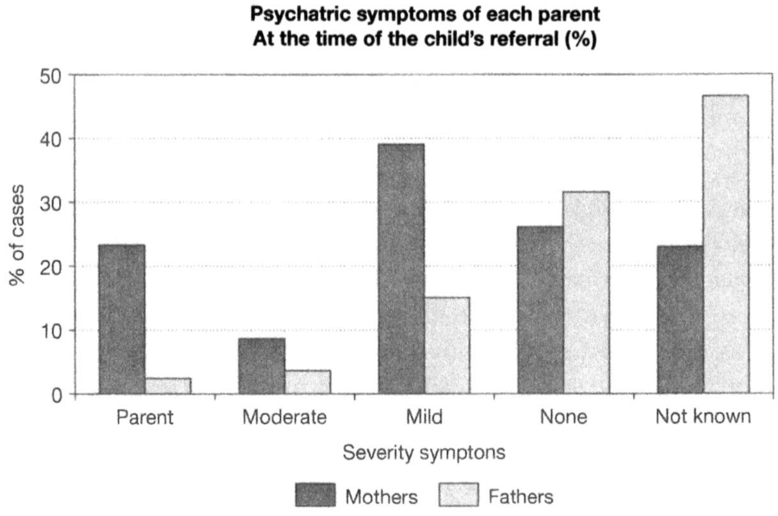

Figure 8

illnesses, and other disorders likely to lead to compulsory treatment, e.g. endangering the life of oneself or others (this group included one father who had murdered his wife as a result of delusional jealousy, and one who had attempted to murder the whole family, as well as several serious suicide attempts).

Moderate symptoms generally required in-patient or intensive out-patient treatment: most were affective illnesses, but there were some disabling neurotic or personality disorders. Mild disorders were similar in kind to moderate, except that they could be managed with less professional support, and would not necessarily prevent the parent from functioning adequately in some situations, at work for example. These would include chronic mild depression and sexual and personality disorders, some of which would of course be far from mild in their effects on family relationships.

It can be seen that although there was insufficient information to make a psychiatric judgment in many cases (for over half the fathers, in particular), nearly half of all mothers of under-fives were psychiatrically disturbed to some degree, both at the time of referral and previously (generally within the child's lifetime). The figure for fathers was around 21% in each case. Most of these disorders were rated as mild, particularly those present at assessment, but they would be likely to have a significant impact on the parent-child relationship, as Mrs Kennedy will be discussing in her paper.

Quite a high proportion of parents were known to have experienced psychiatric treatment, psychotherapy or psychoanalysis, as might be expected from the prevalence of psychiatric symptoms, the family backgrounds and area of London. Figures 9 and 10 show the frequency of different forms of psychiatric and psychotherapeutic treatment for each parent. (Given the paucity of information on some parents, especially fathers, our figures are certainly conservative estimates.) Note that 22% of mothers and 13% of fathers had been in psychotherapy or analysis, and a further 11% of mothers and 3% of fathers were taken into treatment through the Anna Freud Centre (see below, under *Work with Parents*).

Treatment Outlines

Figure 11 shows the distribution of session frequency within the under-five group. One can see that 81% of the under-five-year-olds

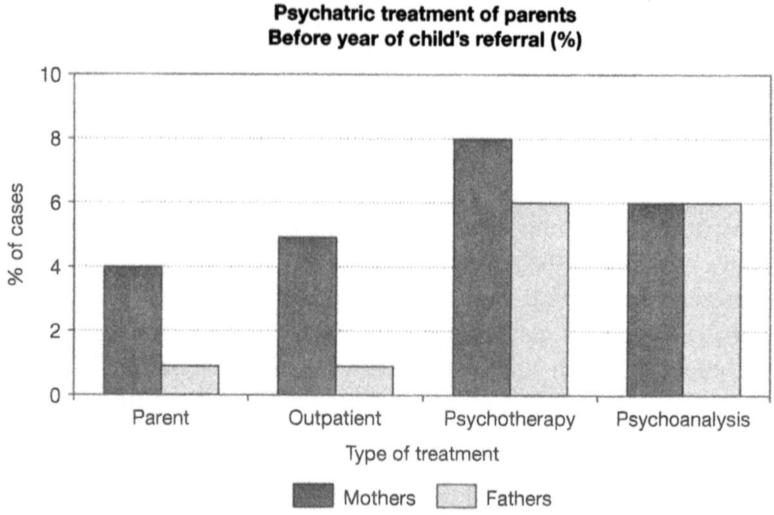

Figure 9

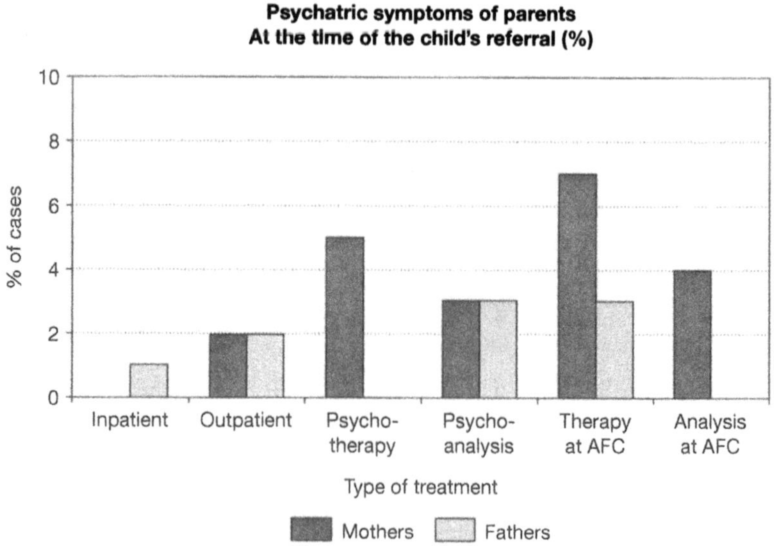

Figure 10

were in intensive treatment (4 or 5 times per week). This compares with 73% of 5- to 11-year-olds and 66% of children 12 years and over. Children in Category 3 (established neurotic symptoms) were the most likely to be in intensive treatment (95%). The other obvious influence on frequency of sessions was that most of the children who lived outside London (12% of the total) were seen non-intensively.

The average length of treatment was 1 year and 9 months, including cases terminated prematurely for a variety of reasons. Figure 12 shows the distribution of lengths of treatment for the under-five group, compared with the 5- to 11-year-olds. It is clear that treatment tended to be shorter in the younger age-group.

Where treatment was terminated by agreement and regarded as completed, the average length was 2.5 years. Figure 13 shows the distribution of length of completed treatment, again showing the 5- to 1 l-year-olds for comparison. The average length of completed treatment rises with starting age up to about 13 or 14 years of age (average length 4.5 years), after which it falls again to around 3 years for late adolescents. The particularly long treatments among the

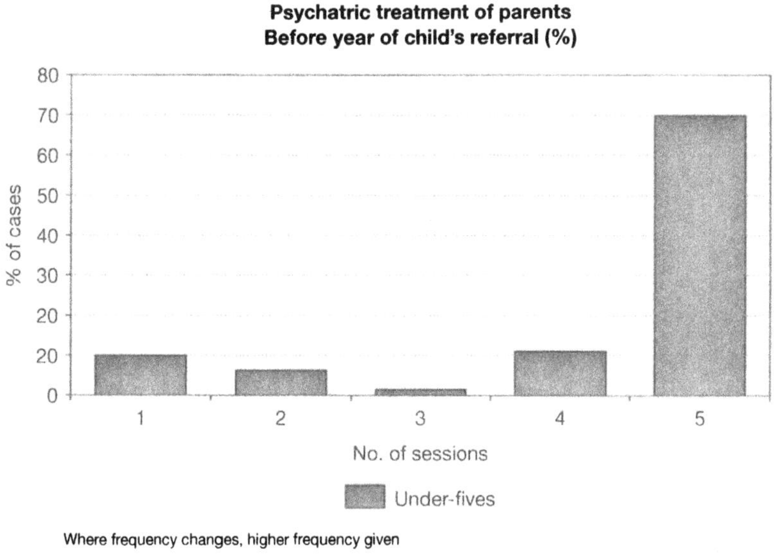

Figure 11

under—fives (three children, all girls, were in analysis for between 5 and 11 years) were all of cases where there was a combination of early environmental deprivation and long-standing mental disturbance in the mother. There was a strong tendency for intensive

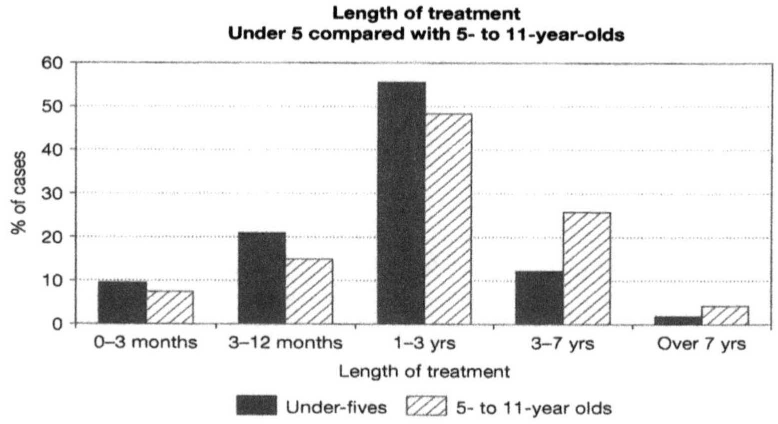

Figure 12

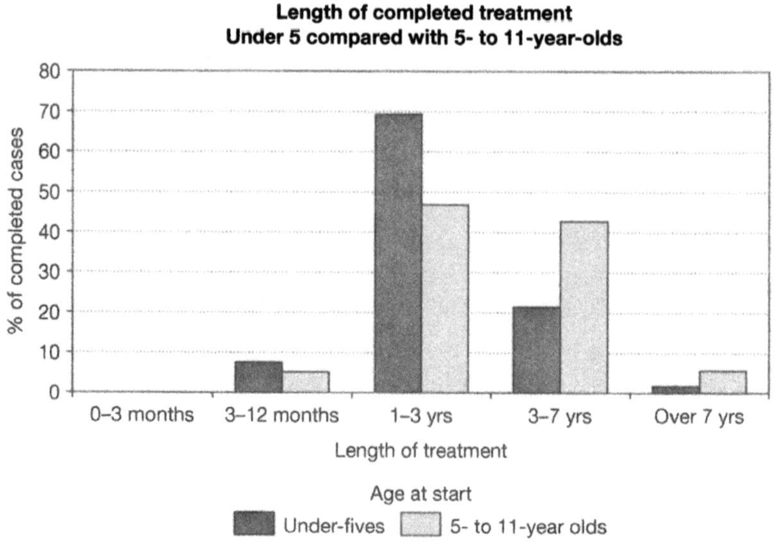

Figure 13

treatment to last longer than non-intensive; this seemed to be largely accounted for by the more frequent premature termination of non-intensive treatment (i.e. withdrawal of the child by the parents without a compelling external reason, and against advice).

Premature Termination by Parents

Since inconvenience is one of the most common reasons given by parents for dropping out of treatment, it is perhaps surprising that in fact children were more commonly withdrawn from non-intensive treatment (42%, vs. 24% from 4–5 sessions per week). The same trend is evident in the older age-groups, but is less marked.

Boys were more often withdrawn prematurely than girls (27% of boys, 18% of girls). Figure 14 shows the distribution of different reasons for ending treatment in boys and in girls.

Patients regarded as falling primarily into Category 2 of Miss Freud's five categories ("transient symptomatology or developmental strain") were also more commonly withdrawn (44%). This links with a very common finding on these "drop-out" cases, that parents

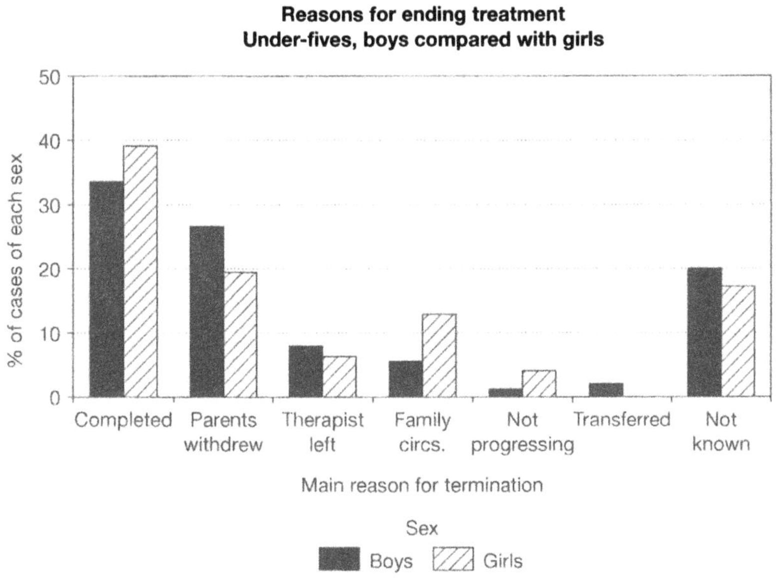

Figure 14

frequently withdrew children when the referral symptoms had improved, although the importance of overall emotional development (not just symptomatology) had been put to them. This happened most often in Category 2. Once the referral symptoms had been relieved, the burden and stigma of bringing the child for treatment were felt to constitute more pressing problems for the family, especially if the child started school. Other common influences seemed to be resentment or fear of the child's attachment to the therapist, feelings of competition with a "better parent", dislike of changes in the child, or disapproval of the technique of analysis when the parent stayed in the treatment room with the child (this is discussed later). Examples would be disapproval of the therapist's tolerance of messy play, or of interpretations, particularly sexual ones. Occasionally, work with one parent seemed to enable him or her to support the treatment, but the other became increasingly hostile.

A further factor which sometimes prevented the parents from continuing their child's treatment was when one or both parents became aware of their own pathology or contribution to the child's difficulties, and took flight from a painful conflict about accepting help with this. In the great majority of cases, the parents could be helped to change, and if necessary to find treatment for themselves, but this was not always achieved.

This brings us on to the issues of working with the parents and of parental presence in the child's sessions.

Work with Parents

Around 90% of the parents of children in treatment were seen regularly to discuss the child and the therapy. Usually this was done by the child's therapist. Some parents were also taken into treatment through the Centre during their child's therapy. This occurred when the parent's pathology was thought to be closely linked to that of the child, or when sessions with a parent (usually the mother) became increasingly concerned with material about her own difficulties, relationships, childhood and so on. 4% of the mothers of under-fives were taken into simultaneous analysis in the Centre, and a further 7% of mothers and 3% of fathers were helped to arrange psychotherapy. As well as recording diagnoses and symptoms of each parent, we also indicated the overall level of psychological functioning in the parents, using the GAF scale which parallels the CGAS measure used with children. As one would expect, the GAF scores of parents receiving treatment were lower than the average; more interestingly, we found that those children whose mothers had relatively low GAF scores, and were in psychotherapy or analysis, showed a substantially larger improvement in their CGAS score than did those whose mothers were not being treated (see Figure 15). Note that although it is generally true that treating the mother helped the child to benefit more from his analysis, there were variations according to the mother's level of functioning. The more impaired the mother was overall, the more the child seemed to be helped by her being treated, but where, the mother was functioning at a normal level, this trend was reversed. The same pattern emerged even more clearly when we looked at mothers who had been in therapy in the past.

Parental Presence in Treatment Sessions

One-third of the children in this age-group separated from their parents from the first session. (Some were brought from the Nursery

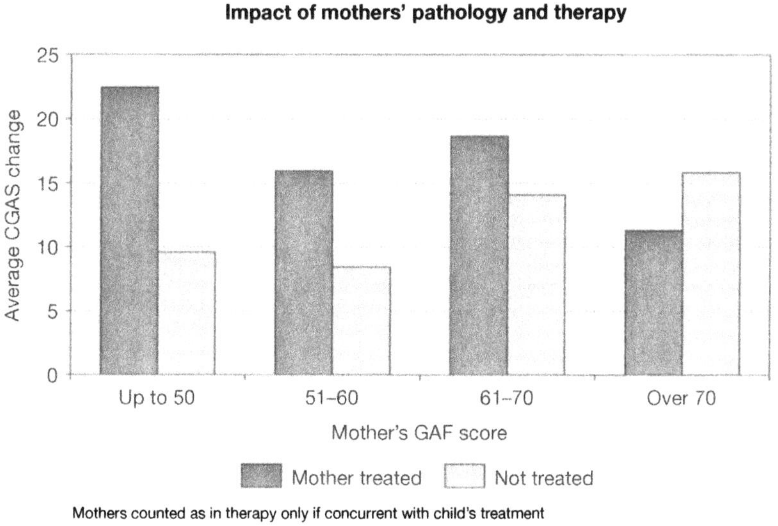

Figure 15

School, so that the issue of separation from parents was not directly tackled, although there were sometimes problems in separating from the Nursery or its staff.) The remaining children had a parent (Or teacher) in the treatment room for up to 90 sessions. Figure 16 shows the distribution of sessions required before the child could be seen separately. In several cases, the child would succeed in leaving the parent for a number of sessions, but would then want her to come with him again when disturbing material arose in the treatment. As might be expected, the children who needed parents to stay tended to be under 4 years old, and to have referral symptoms of either overt separation anxiety or anxious provocative behaviour to the parent. In some cases the mother showed great anxiety about leaving the child with the therapist than the child did, and this needed to be worked on with the mother before separation was successful.

The Outcome of Treatment

We are currently considering standardized ways of measuring the outcome of child therapy in psychoanalytic terms. For the present we have looked at psychiatric diagnoses at the beginning and end of therapy, together with CGAS scores, which are an indication of

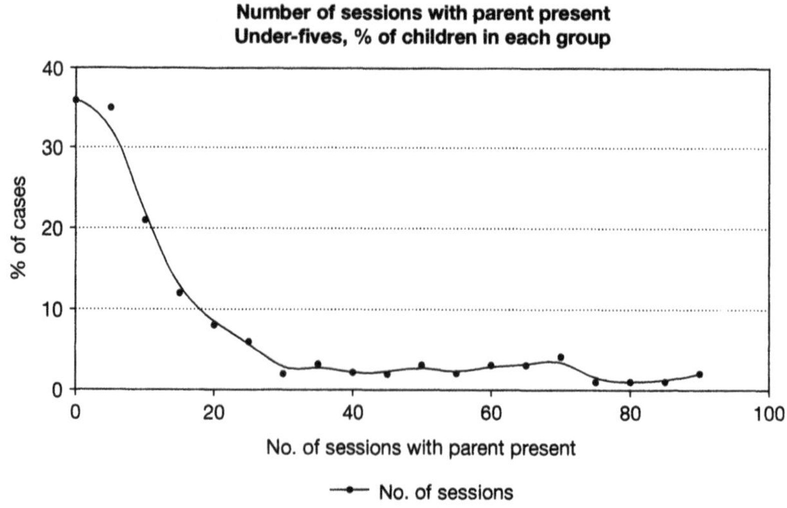

Figure 16

the overall level of psychological functioning on a scale from 0–100. 17% of the children referred under five were psychiatrically diagnosable at the end of treatment, compared with 75% at the beginning. (In a further 29% of cases, no judgment could be made on diagnosis because of poor information at termination. On looking at this group of cases it is likely that most of them had a good outcome; notes, reports and letters were kept more fully when problems persisted or the child needed to go on for further treatment.) Most of the diagnosis made at the end of treatment were of specific or pervasive developmental disorders or of unchanged referral symptoms in children withdrawn very early. The average change in CGAS score at the end of treatment was a rise of 14 points, bringing the average score at termination to the lower end of the normal range (no impairment or only minor difficulties). This average of course covers a very wide range of outcomes—autistic children who remained grossly handicapped, severely neurotic children many of whom showed very large improvements, children who were withdrawn too early for change to occur, and so on. As would be expected, children in Categories 4 and 5 showed smaller improvements than those in Categories 2 and 3. In all the age-groups including those referred under five, we have found a steady increase in CGAS change with length of treatment, i.e. the longer the analysis the greater the improvement in overall emotional adjustment.

Figure 17 shows this in the under-five age-group.

It is not yet possible to be sure, without comparison groups, to what extent this improvement over time might have occurred without treatment, or with different methods of treatment.

Subsequent treatment

25% of these children received further treatment after the termination of their analysis. Just over half of these were children who had been well at the end of treatment, but had developed new symptoms later in childhood and were seen for a further period of non-intensive treatment. The general pattern was for such a child to return for a few months of once-weekly sessions, usually with the same therapist. A further group (one quarter of those requiring later treatment) were severely disturbed children who went on to special units (for example, residential schools for autistic children) at or

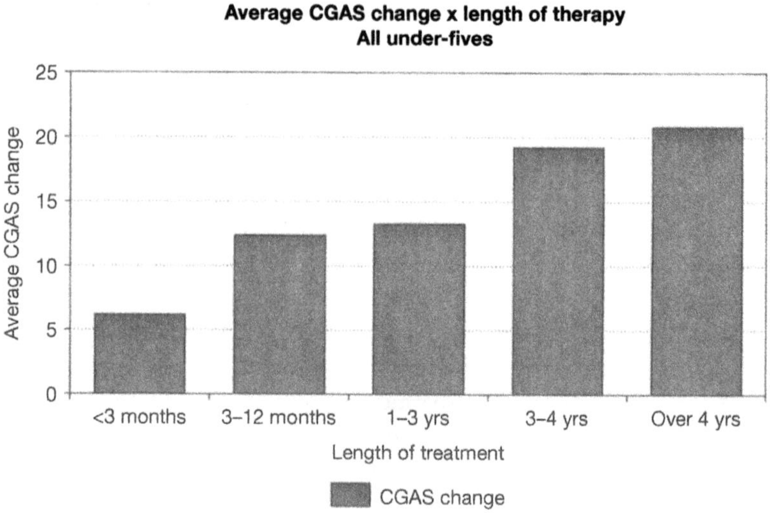

Figure 17

before termination. The remaining children (4% of the total) had been withdrawn from treatment prematurely, and sought help elsewhere some years later.

Mary Target

* * *

An Appraisal of the Study from a Clinical Viewpoint

In view of the importance for future mental health that we attach to early childhood development, it is somewhat surprising that the total number of cases of under-fives treated during the 40 years of the Centre's existence (143 cases out of 777) is relatively low, despite the widely-held view that treatment results with under-fives are often more far-reaching and obtained in less time than at later developmental stages. It would appear that there is even greater reluctance to refer young children for treatment than to refer older children, and that all too frequently problems are not taken seriously enough and are dismissed in the belief that the child "will grow out of" them. Transient symptoms, of course, often appear in early childhood as indicators of so-called "normal" developmental conflict but this does not mean that the transiency of a symptom can be taken as evidence that the underlying disturbance that produced it has also disappeared. Reaction to medical interventions, painful illnesses or hospitalizations may serve to illustrate this point.

A well-supported young child may be helped to grasp the significance of medical events, recognize the role of doctor or nurse as a beneficent one, or accept the necessity for having injections or complying with dietary or motor restrictions. But this will not prevent the child from being swamped by fantasies of mutilation or castration or violent assault or oral deprivation in response to such experiences. Anger and hostility are likely to be reinforced, and parents who permitted such things to happen, whether in their presence or absence, may cease to be protective figures for the child. It may be much more difficult for parents to understand these conflicts when they are hidden behind a relatively contained surface picture, although the child's relationship towards them may change from trust to mistrust, from feeling loved and cherished to feeling rejected and worthless.

Mary Target has reported that a high proportion of under-fives treated at the Centre had chronic medical conditions and/or histories of hospitalization for acute life-threatening illnesses surgery etc. There may be obvious and observable signs of disturbance at the time and parents may be alerted to the fact that the child needs help. But the deeper disturbance caused may also remain relatively "silent", clinically speaking, but still have long-lasting effects on the child's future development.

Chronic conditions and hospitalizations were not always the reasons for referral but they may point to increased awareness of the traumatogenic potential of such experiences for the child. It may also be easier for parent to acknowledge the damaging effects of "extraneous events on their young child, although unconsciously parents will feel responsible for their child's bodily and mental welfare. Even where unavoidable reality has contributed to the child's difficulties, parents will feel guilty for not having shielded the child better. While appropriate feelings of responsibility or guilt may make parents more ready to refer their children for assessment and may make them more co-operative in the treatment, on the other hand narcissistic hurt, and fears of having damage the child may mobilize parental defences towards denying the existence of problems. You may wonder why I raise such issues at all, when 30% of all under-fives were referred directly by parents. But since parents are the highest source of referral of all cases at the Centre it is interesting to note that the percentage of referrals by parents is higher for older children than for under-fives.

Other statistics may give a special slant to our consideration of effect of relationships on relationships notably that 70% of all under-fives treated were first-born or only children. Going far beyond explanation that parental relationships to their first-born child frequently are fraught by anxieties, by unrealistic and irrational expectations and by an intensity of affective involvement that may adversely affect the developing child, was the statistic relating to the incidence of psychological disturbance in the parents. These figures were strikingly high, and higher, we heard, than in parents of children in other age groups treated at the Centre.

A considerable number of parents had received psychiatric or psychotherapeutic treatment on the positive side, this may have the parents more insightful and more ready to secure treatment for the child. However, about one quarter of the under-fives had parents suffering from anxiety or depression of clinical severity at the time of the child's referral, and a similar number of parents had had episodes of psychiatric illness earlier in the child's life. Pervasive anxiety and depression in a parent will have a profound impact on the development of a young child, whether or not similar surface pathology will be manifested in the child. Amongst these cases, for example, were a three-year-old boy who dealt with his mother's withdrawal and sadness by trying to entertain her with excessive clowning, and a four-year-old girl whose precocious development enabled her to become the caretaker of her chronically depressed mother. She woke her mother and older brother every morning and prepared breakfast, and in this way tried to ensure that mother would be ready to drive the children to school and nursery respectively.

In formulating her theory and technique of child psychoanalysis, Anna Freud put great emphasis on the concept of normality and of assessing pathology in terms of deviation from a hypothetical norm. Implicit in her theory of development was the concept of a psycho-biologically based thrust that impels the child in a progressive direction. Therapeutic interventions aim to remove the obstacles' on that developmental path. Child analysis is not preventive, in that new "obstacles" can still be encountered at later developmental stages. These are fundamental concepts underlying the clinical approach; and the comprehensive assessment procedures are aimed at countering the tendency to look for single pathogenic determinants and to overemphasize isolated areas of the personality at the expense of the rest. An accurate assessment of the nature of conflict and the nature of defence as well as the level of ego maturity and/or of developmental lags will be essential before a recommendation for treatment will be made.

Mary Target has reported that 81% of all under-fives treated at the Centre during the last 40 years were in 4- or 5-times-weekly analysis. (We have also heard that this figure is high in relation to other age-groups, 73% of 5- to 11-year-olds and 66% of children of 12 and over.) It is a unique feature of the Anna Freud Centre that the bulk of treatment provided takes the form of full psychoanalysis, in which each child is seen individually, five times a week, for sessions of fifty minutes, over an extended period of time. We consider that daily contact with the child is desirable to gather the maximum amount of material and maintain the interpretative work, to keep the analytic material within the bounds of the consulting room, to deal with the anxieties mobilized and not to place too great a burden on the child's environment. We believe that daily treatment enhances the efficiency of the therapeutic work and this is especially true of the treatment of under-fives.

Now let me address a few specific issues about the treatment of these young children. Child analytic technique can be defined as the employment of an interpretative approach by the therapist to the child's intrapsychic life with due consideration to his/her developmental status. But the intrapsychic world of an under-five is still in a relatively fluid state where internal and external worlds are not firmly separated. Frustrations, prohibitions and conflicts, even though they may originate internally, are experienced predominantly in relation to the external world. The primitive defences at the child's disposal will tend to relocate conflicts as if they were still between himself and the external world.

Such defensive manoeuvres, aimed at reducing tension and maintaining feelings of well-being, also have bearing on the child's object relationships, both internally and interpersonally. The stability of self and object representations is readily undermined by contradictory images of the object, kept alive by unresolved ambivalence, and fuelled in turn by the impact and intrusion of the external parent. Until "good self" and "benign object" representations are firmly established and provide internal sources of support and protection, the child is much more dependent on external feedback to maintain internal equilibrium. And likewise, external experiences in interaction with the primary objects (and perhaps their extensions in the transference) will have a more profound effect on the building up of stable, cohesive and benign self and object representations. These considerations, relating to the developmental status of the pre-latency child, have implications also for treatment technique. In keeping with the topic of this symposium, I will restrict myself to comments on some of the more controversial issues in the therapist-child-parent interaction which, I believe, assume special significance in the treatment of under-fives.

For the parents, in addition to their external strains related to time and sometimes money, their child's analysis will touch on many of their internal concerns. Guilt, fears and narcissistic hurt will be heightened by having to hand over their child to a therapist who conveys that he understands their child better than they do. This will be even more painful if the therapist succeeds in engaging the child quite soon in an intimate and close relationship on whatever basis this will be.

The child will perceive such parental reactions and respond accordingly. For example, if he is currently engaged in an openly defiant or hostile relationship to the mother, he may grasp immediately the opportunity to engage positively with the therapist because this represents an attack on the mother. Where the child's aggression towards her is defended against by excessive clinging or controlling, the opposite may occur. The child may insist that the mother stay in the treatment room, or show marked reluctance to relate to the therapist. One could say that the child's new relationship to the therapist is so intimately linked with current, as well as past, interactions with a parent that, psychologically speaking, the mother and/or father are always present in the consulting room, in the treatment of the pre-latency child. This should not be taken to imply that, as therapists, we do not feel more comfortable if the parental presence in the consulting room is metaphoric rather than actual;

but the recognition may have some bearing on the tenacity and speed with which we pursue our efforts to bring about physical separation.

In order to maximize the benefit psychoanalysis can provide for a pre-latency child, parents need to be actively involved in the therapeutic work. It is not enough to meet with parents only when the continuation of the treatment is threatened. The child's developmental needs also have to be met by the parents. Regular work with them provides unique opportunities to facilitate their understanding of the child's current feelings and conflicts and will lead to better handling of the child. In this way it is possible to create an environment for our patients which genuinely supports the treatment and enables the parents to retain confidence in their parenting roles. Even more importantly, it may also create a home milieu that can support the young patient's gains after the treatment itself is over.

There are different ways of working with parents towards these ends. Sometimes the child needs to have the parent in the consulting room for shorter or longer periods and they then become part recipients of the analyst's interpretations, tempered as they may have to be for both parent and child. Additional individual sessions with the parent are even more important in this situation, in order to work through the parent's reactions and feelings and to enable the mother or father to respond appropriately to the therapist's handling of the separation issue.

But the child must always remain the primary patient, and that implies that he must be kept in the picture about any contact between therapist and parents. It is usual practice in the treatment of under-fives for the child's therapist also to work with the parents. We have found that when the five-times-weekly work with the child and the once-weekly work with the parent or parents goes well, there is a remarkable overlap between the child's and the parents' material on a week-to-week basis; this does not occur to anything like the same extent with older children or if different therapists work with child and parents.

Because young children have a limited capacity to contain the analytic material inside the session, there is often a "spillover" which observant parents will pick up. Even if we try to curb this kind of "acting out" through the symbolic action of keeping toys and drawings, etc., in the consulting room, the analytic work will affect the child's interaction with the parents and his preoccupations and behaviour at home in a much more direct and immediate way than with older patients. Containment in the session, of the young child's enactments his "acting in", presents the therapy with even greater difficulties than his "acting out". When a child is prone to wreck consulting room, or to attack the therapist physically in sudden eruptions of rage or panic, attention tends to be diverted from the "interpreting" role. But such outbursts frequently arise in response to the young child's frustrated attempt to control the therapist and his failure to coerce the therapist into acting a specific role.

So-called "role play" is an important part of the therapeutic work with young children the main consideration in determining whether and for how long the therapist should comply with the patient's demand actively to play a role in this scenario must always depend on what the therapist's involvement will mean to the child, and what purpose it is serving in the therapeutic work. A fine balance has to be kept between eliciting fantasy material in a mode natural to the child's level of functioning and self expression, and providing too much gratification or excitement in doing the analytic work itself we aim in child analysis to facilitate a move from action to verbalization ostensibly to help the child gain better ego control however with the young age-group in therapy, we must also adjust technical interventions to the appropriate cognitive level of the child, and recognition that play interaction may be an important or even necessary adjunct to interpretation and working through, if the child's ego mode is action-based and still tied to concrete experience.

How does this kind of role-play fit in with our concept of transference? The therapist is assigned the role of mother, brother, doctor, witch or the child himself and related to affectively within a scenario which appears to be based on fantasied or real experiences in the child's present or past life. It could be viewed as an extension of the child's current relationship; to the parents where strictly speaking, the parent of the present is also the transference object of the past. The view emphasizes that earlier conflicts continue to involve the primary objects, the parents as live issues or in modified form.

Transference evolves as part of the therapeutic process and this will result, on occasion in the under-five experiencing transferences the therapy with greater intensity than the intensity felt in the corresponding relationship with the parent. But this is still different from the revival of pre-formed object-related fantasies when these are freed from repression and re-experienced in relation to the analyst. Perhaps this should lead us to the conclusion that the pre-latency child's "transference material" should not be interpreted only relation to the therapist and the parent of the past, but also in relation to the here-and-now feelings towards the parent.

There is not time enough to go more fully into the complex theoretical issues of "countertransference" and counter-responsiveness in the treatment of under-fives, but I want to make just a few brief comments on this subject. While the therapist's understanding of the young patient is obviously not based on empathic identification alone, the need to be "in tune" with the young child is underscored by having to rely, quite heavily, on observing and interpreting behaviour and other non-verbal material. Many of our young patients need the affective experience of "feeling understood" before they can feel safe enough to participate in the often painful endeavour to increase self-understanding. Just as the mother understood what the infant needed before he could do so, so the therapist's insights into the child's wishes, fantasies and conflicts usually precede the patient's "higher level of knowing". This should remind us that, in the initial phases of treatment, many young children will perceive our interpretations merely as "friendly noises" and highlight the experiential components of the interaction between the young child and the therapist.

The developmental features of the under-fives which were briefly referred to in these comments, also contribute positively to therapeutic results. The therapeutic work not only helps the child in dealing with conflicts and finding new solutions and adaptations, but will promote the consolidation of structural development itself.

Hansi Kennedy

Note

1. R.S. Wallerstein (1986). Forty-two lives in treatment: A study of psvchoanalysis and psychotherapy. New York: Guilford Press.

COMPLETE BIBLIOGRAPHY OF HANSI KENNEDY'S PUBLICATIONS AND PRESENTATIONS

In order to more easily grasp the development of Kennedy's thinking, articles are ordered by year published, as opposed to author's name.

Publications

Kennedy, H.E. (1950). Cover memories in formation. *Psychoanalytic Study of the Child, 5*: 275–84.

Frankl, L. in collaboration with I. Harris, H. Kennedy and V. Thompson (1961). Some observations on the development and disturbances of integration in childhood. *Psychoanalytic Study of the Child, 16*: 146–63.

Joffe, W. and Sandler, J. in collaboration with S. Baker, R. Edgcumbe, M. Kawenoka, H. Kennedy, L. Neurath (1965). Some conceptual problems involved in the consideration of disorders of narcissism. *Journal of Child Psychotherapy, 2*: 56–66. Also in *Psyche Stuttgart, 21*: 152–65, 1967. Also in *Rivista de Psicoanalisis, Vol. XXV*, 1968.

Thomas, R. in collaboration with R. Edgcumbe, H. Kennedy, M. Kawenoka, L. Weitzner (1966). Comments on some aspects of self and object representation in a group of psychotic children. *Psychoanalytic Study of the Child, 21*: 527–80.

Kennedy, H. (1969). Film review: Young children in brief separation. *British Journal of Medical Psychology, 42*: 191–3.

Sandler, J.; Holder, A.; Kawenoka, M.; Kennedy, H.E., & Neurath, L. (1969). Notes on some theoretical and clinical aspects of transference. *International Journal of Psychoanalysis, 50*: 633–45. Also in (1967) *Psyche*: 10–11. Also in (1970) *La Psychiatrique de l'enfant, Vol. XIII*. Also Sandler, J. (1987) *From Safety to Superego* (pp. 264–84). London: Karnac.

Kennedy, H. (1971). Problems in reconstruction in child analysis. *Psychoanalytic Study of the Child, 26*: 386–402.

Kennedy, H. (1972). Film review: Young children in brief separation—Revisited. *British Journal of Medical Psychology.*

Berger, M. & Kennedy, H. (1975). Pseudobackwardness in children: Maternal attitudes as an etiological factor. *Psychoanalytic Study of the Child, 30*: 279–306.

Sandler, J.: Kennedy, H. & Tyson, R. (1975). Discussion on transference: The treatment situation and technique in child analysis. *Psychoanalytic Study of the Child 30*: 409–41.

Kennedy, H. (1976). Young children in brief separation: A critical review of five films by James Robertson and Joyce Robertson. *International Journal of Psychoanalysis, 57*: 483–6.

Kennedy, H. (1977). The Hampstead Centre for the Psychoanalytic Study and Treatment of Children. In: B. Wolman (Ed.), *International Encyclopedia of Neurology, Psychiatry, Psychoanalysis and Psychology.* New York.

Kennedy, H. (1978a). The analytic treatment of two siblings: A foreword. *Bulletin of the Hampstead Clinic, 1*: 119–20.

Kennedy, H. (1978b). The Hampstead Centre for the Psychoanalytic Study and Treatment of Children. *Bulletin of the Hampstead Clinic, 1*: 7–10.

Edgcumbe, R.; Kennedy, H.; Sandler, J. & Yorke, C. (1978). Some reflections on infantile neurosis. *Bulletin of the Hampstead Clinic, 1*: 101–9.

Kennedy, H. (1979). The role of insight in child analysis: A developmental viewpoint. *Journal of the American Psychoanalytic Association, Supplement 27*: 9–28. Also in H. Blum (Ed.), *Psychoanalytic Explorations of Technique.* New York: Int. Univ. Press, 1980.

Kennedy, H. (1980a). Dorothy Burlingham, 1891–1979. *Psychoanalytic Quarterly, 49*: 508–511.

Kennedy, H. (1980b). Dorothy Burlingham: Funeral tributes. *Bulletin of the Hampstead Clinic, 3*: 71.

Kennedy, H. (1980c). Dorothy Burlingham: Hampstead Clinic memorial contributions. *Bulletin of the Hampstead Clinic, 3*: 78–9.

Kennedy, H. & Yorke, C. (1980). Childhood neurosis vs developmental deviations. *Dialogue: Journal of Psychoanalytic Perspectives, 4*: 21–33.

Burgner, M. & Kennedy, H. (1980). Different types of sado-masochistic behavior in children. *Dialogue: Journal of Psychoanalytic Perspectives, 4*: 49–59.

Sandler, J.; Kennedy, H. & Tyson, R. (1980). *The Technique of Child Psychoanalysis: Discussions with Anna Freud.* Cambridge: Harvard Univ. Press. Also in C. Yorke (Ed.), *The International Psycho-Analytic Library*, no. 110. London: Hogarth Press, 1980.

Yorke, C., Kennedy, H. & Wiseberg, S. (1980). Clinical and theoretical aspects of two developmental lines. In: S.I. Greenspan and G.H. Pollock (Eds.), *The Course of Life, 1*: 619–37. Washington: U.S. Department of Health and Human Services. [Revised and Reprinted as *The Course of Life: Middle and Late Childhood* (pp. 135–60). Madison, CT: Int. Univ. Press, 1991.]

Kennedy, H. (1981a). Die Bedeutung der Einsicht in der Kinderanalyse. In: G. Biermann (Ed.), *Handbuch der Kinderpsychotherapie*, Vol. 4.

Kennedy, H. (1981b). Reports by chairmen on the work of study groups at the Hampstead Clinic: Study group on developmental disturbances. *Bulletin of the Hampstead Clinic, 4*: 295.

Kennedy, H. (1981c). Vergangenheit und Gegenwart in der Sicht des Kindes: Folgerungen für die Kinderanalyse. *Studien zur Kinderpsychoanalyse*, Jahrbuch *1*.

Kennedy, H. (1982a). Die Hampstead Klinik: Ein historischer Überblick. *Studien zur Kinderpsychoanalyse*, Jahrbuch 2.

Kennedy, H. (1982b). El papel del insight. *Psicoanalisis, 51(1).*

Kennedy, H. (1982c). The Hampstead Clinic: A historical perspective. *Sigmund Freud Gesellschaft Bulletin, Anna Freud Memorial Issue.* Vienna.

Kennedy, H. (1982d). Questions soulevées par la reconstruction en analyse d'enfant. *La Psychiatrie de l'enfant, 25(2).*

Kennedy, H. & Yorke, C. (1982). Steps from outer to inner conflict viewed as superego precursors. *Psychoanalytic Study of the Child, 37*: 221–8.

Sandler, J.; Kennedy, H. & Tyson, R. (1982). *Kinderanalyse: Gespräche mit Anna Freud.* Frankfurt: S. Fischer Verlag.

Kennedy, H. (1983a). Anna Freud, 1895–1982. *Psychoanalytic Quarterly, 52*: 501–6.

Kennedy, H. (1983b). Anna Freud: Funeral tributes. *Bulletin of the Hampstead Clinic, 6*: 11–12.

Sandler, J., Kennedy, H., & Tyson, R. (1983). *La Tecnica Della Psicanalisi Infantile.* Italy: Bollati Boringhieri.

Yorke, C., Kennedy, H. & Wiseberg, S. (1983). Algunos aspectos clinicos y teoricos de dos lines de desarrollo. *Revista Psicoanalisis, 5(2).*

Kennedy, H. (1984). The "baby at the breast" experience: Memory or fantasy? Some further thoughts on reconstruction. *Bulletin of the Hampstead Clinic, 7*: 15–24.

Kennedy, H. & Moran, G. (1984). The developmental roots of self-injury and response to pain in a 4-year-old boy. *Psychoanalytic Study of the Child, 39*: 195–212.

Kennedy, H. (1985a). For or against child placement: A clinical illustration. *Bulletin of the Anna Freud Centre, 8*: 245–52.

Kennedy, H. (1985b). Growing up with a handicapped sibling. *Psychoanalytic Study of the Child, 40*: 255–74.

Kennedy, H.; Moran, G.; Wiseberg, S. & Yorke, C. (1985). Both sides of the barrier: Some reflections on childhood fantasy. *Psychoanalytic Study of the Child, 40*: 275–83. (Earlier version presented at the International Scientific Colloquium "The Role of Fantasy in the Adaptive Process" held at the Hampstead Clinic, October 1983. See *Bulletin of the Hampstead Clinic, 7*, 1984.)

Kennedy, H. (1986a). Memories of Anna Freud. *American Imago, 53*: 205–9.

Kennedy, H. (1986b). Trauma in childhood: Signs and sequelae as seen in the analysis of an adolescent. *Psychoanalytic Study of the Child, 41*: 209–19. (Earlier version presented at the International Scientific Colloquium "Repeating: Enactment and Verbalization in Different Stages of Development" held at the Anna Freud Centre, November 1985. See *Bulletin of the Anna Freud Centre, 9*, 1986.)

Yorke, C. in collaboration with Kennedy, H. (1987). On the concepts of fixation and regression: Their clinical relevance. *Bulletin of the Anna Freud Centre, 10*: 119–35.

Kennedy, H. (1988a). The pre-history of the Nursery School. *Bulletin of the Anna Freud Centre, 11*: 271–5.

Kennedy, H. (1988b). The technique of psychoanalysis with the pre-latency child. In: R. Tyson (Ed.), *Analysis of the Under-Five Child* (pp. 262–81). New Haven: Yale Univ. Press, 2001.

Kennedy, H. (1989a). Die Erfahrung als "Baby an der Brust": Erinnerung oder Phantasie? *Studien zur Kinderpsychoanalyse,* Jahrbuch 9.

Kennedy, H. (1989b). Sadomasochistische Perversion in der Adoleszenz. Eine entwicklungsgeschichtliche Betrachtung. *Zeitschrift für psychoanalytische Theorie und Praxis, 4*: 348–60.

Kennedy, H. & Moran, G. (1991). Reflections on the aim of child analysis. *Psychoanalytic Study of the Child, 46*: 181–98. (Earlier version presented at the International Scientific Colloquium "The Impact of Developmental Considerations on the Aim of Child and Adult Psychoanalysis" held at the Anna Freud Centre, October 1989. See *Bulletin of the Anna Freud Centre, 13,* 1990.)

Target, M. & Kennedy, H. (1991). Psychoanalytic work with under-fives: Forty years' experience. *Bulletin of the Anna Freud Centre, 14*: 5–29.

Kennedy, H. (1993). Developing resilience in high-risk Nursery School children. In: T. Cohen, M.H. Etezady and B. Pacella (Eds.), *The Vulnerable Child, Vol. 1.* Madison, CT: Int. Univ. Press.

Fonagy, P.; Moran, G.; Edgcumbe, R.; Kennedy, H. & Target, M. (1993). The roles of mental representations and mental processes in therapeutic action. *Psychoanalytic Study of the Child, 48*: 9–48. (Earlier version presented at the International Scientific Colloquium "Therapeutic Process in Child and Adult Psychoanalysis" held at the Anna Freud Centre, November 1991. See *Bulletin of the Anna Freud Centre, 15,* 1992.)

Kennedy, H. (1994a). Book review: Robert Coles, "Anna Freud: The dream of psychoanalysis". *Psychoanalytic Quarterly, 63*: 587–90.

Kennedy, H. (1994b). Doris Wills, 1908–1993: Memorial tributes. *Bulletin of the Anna Freud Centre, 17*: 57–62.

Fabricius, J. & Green, V. in collaboration with T. Baradon, J. Davids and H. Kennedy (1995). Termination in child analysis: A child-led process? *Psychoanalytic Study of the Child, 50*: 205–26. (Earlier version presented at the International Scientific Colloquium "Aims and Criteria for Termination of Adult and Child Psychoanalysis" held at the Anna Freud Centre, November 1993. See *Bulletin of the Anna Freud Centre, 17,* 1994.)

Presentations

(1956). *The Work of the Hampstead Clinic.* The Hampstead Clinic Freud Centenary Celebration. London, England.

(1961). *Development of the Hampstead Index of Psychoanalytic Material of Children's Cases.* International Psychoanalytical Association Pre-congress Meetings. London, England.

(1964). *Aspects of the psychology of borderline children.* World Health Association Meetings, Danish Society for Child Psychiatry and Clinical Psychology. Copenhagen, Denmark.

(1967). *The Imaginative life: The importance of play.* BBC radio talks. London, England.

(1969). *Seminars on Child Analysis, March–September.* Sigmund Freud Institute. Frankfurt, Germany.

(1969/1970). *Seminars on child analysis.* Hamburg Psychoanalytic Institute. Hamburg, Germany.

(1970). *Panel with Anna Freud and Joseph Sandler: The infantile neurosis.* English speaking members of European Societies. London, England

(1971). *Reconstruction in child analysis.* Association for Child Psychoanalysis. Williamsburg, VA.

(1971). *Clinical seminars with Samuel Ritvo.* Yale University Child Study Center. New Haven, CT.

(1972). *A boy with severe sado-masochistic fixations: A clinical report.* Hampstead Clinic 20th Anniversary Conference. London, England.

(1974). *Clinical and theoretical seminars: Transference and countertransference and other clinical issues in child analysis, March–May.* Dutch Psychoanalytic Society. Amsterdam, Netherlands.

(1975). *Reconstruction in child analysis.* Dutch Psychoanalytic Society. Amsterdam, Netherlands.

(1975). *Theoretical seminars: Latency development.* Centro Studi Psicologia. Padua, Italy.

(1976). *Theoretical seminars: School difficulties and learning problems.* Centro Studi Psicologia. Padua, Italy.

(1976). *Clinical seminars and presentations.* Über Lernstörungen. Zürich, Switzerland.

(1976). *Technical seminars.* Dutch Psychoanalytic Society. Amsterdam, Netherlands.

(1977). *Clinical seminars: The work of the child psychotherapist.* Centro di Studi Psicoterapia. Milano, Italy.

(1977). *Developmental seminars: Pathological influences on the development of the child.* Centro Studi Psicologia. Padua, Italy.

(1977). *The Hampstead Clinic Nursery School for disadvantaged children and Anna Freud's The Principal Task of Child Analysis.* The Hanna Perkins Center 10th Anniversary Conference. Cleveland, OH.

(1977). *Workshop Chair: The psychoanalytic process in different developmental phases.* Association for Child Psychoanalysis Meetings. Jerusalem, Israel.

(1977). *Technical seminars: Child analysis.* Dutch Psychoanalytic Society. Amsterdam, Netherlands.

(1977). *Welche Indikationen für welches Verfahren.* Institut für Psychogogie Hessen. Frankfurt, Germany.

(1978). *Clinical seminar: Adolescents.* Centro di Studi Psicoterapia. Milano, Italy.

(1978). *Seminars on disturbed development: Diagnosis and prognosis.* Centro Studi Psicologia. Padua, Italy.

(1978). *Insight in child psychoanalysis.* Psychoanalytic Institute of New England East. Cambridge, MA.

(1978). *Some thoughts on the role of insight in child analysis.* Michigan Psychoanalytic Institute. Ann Arbor, MI.

(1979). *Panel: The child and the family in a changing world.* Symposium celebrating 50 years of child guidance in Holland, sponsored by Dutch government. Amsterdam, Netherlands.

(1979). *Different types of sadomasochistic behavior in children* with Marion Burgner. San Francisco Psychoanalytic Institute extension division. San Francisco, CA.

(1979). *Two clinical case histories,* with Clifford Yorke. San Francisco Psychoanalytic Institute extension division. San Francisco, CA.

(1979). *Insight in children: A developmental view.* Langley Porter Psychiatric Institute and Children's Hospital, Stanford University. Palo Alto, CA.

(1979). *The role of insight in child analysis.* San Francisco Psychoanalytic Institute candidates and faculty. San Francisco, CA.

(1979). *Early developmental observations of a boy prior to analysis.* Centro Studi Psicologia. Padua, Italy.

(1979). *Panel: Insight in child and adult psychoanalysis.* Hampstead Clinic International Scientific Colloquium. London, England.

(1980). *Reconstruction and insight in child analysis.* Washington Psychoanalytic Institute. Washington, DC.

(1980). *Seminars for children and youth advisory group. Paper: Work at the Hampstead Clinic and its current research activities.* National Institute for Mental Health. Rockville, MD.

(1980). *Plenary discussant: What can we learn from pathology about normal development?* Association for Child Psychoanalysis. Amsterdam, Netherlands.

(1981). *Vergangenheit und Gegenwart in der Sicht des Kindes: Folgerungen für die Kinderanalyse.* Österreichische Studiengesellschaft für Kinderpsychoanalyse. Salzburg, Austria.

(1982). *30 Jahre Mitarbeit an der Hampstead Klinik.* Universitätsklinik für Neuropsychiatrie des Kindes- und Jugendalters. Vienna, Austria.

(1982). *Eine sadomasochistische Perversion aus einer entwicklungs-geschichtlichen Perspektive.* Wiener Psychoanalytische Vereinigug. Vienna, Austria.

(1982). *Panel: Clinical child analysis and developmental research.* Association for Child Psychoanalysis. Denver, CO.

(1982). *The child's view of past and present: Implications for psychoanalytic technique.* Swedish Psychoanalytic Society. Stockholm, Sweden.

(1982). *Panel: High risk parents and high risk children.* JACAPAC conference. Dublin, Ireland.

(1983). *Panel: The role of fantasy in the adaptive process.* Hampstead Clinic International Scientific Colloquium. London, England.

(1983). *Transference in child analysis: Comments on some conceptual and clinical problems.* Association for Child Psychotherapy. London, England.

(1983). *Developmental disturbances.* Downstate Medical Center Department of Psychiatry. New York, NY.

(1983). *Die Rolle der Übertragung in der Behandlung von Kindern.* Association for Child and Adolescent Psychotherapy. Vienna, Austria.

(1983). *Anna Freud's contribution to work with children.* Dutch Association for Psychoanalytic Therapy. Amsterdam, Netherlands.

(1984). *The treatment of an adolescent boy.* Canadian Association for Psychoanalytic Psychotherapists. Toronto, Canada.

(1984). *Marianna Kris Lecture: Growing up with a handicapped sibling.* Association for Child Psychoanalysis. Chicago, IL.

(1984). *Vulnerable child workshop: Intervention programs for blind from birth infants.* Association for Child Psychoanalysis. Chicago, IL.

(1984). *The developmental roots of self-injury and inadequate responses to pain.* Cleveland University Hospital. Cleveland, OH.

(1984). *A developmental view of a case of sadomasochistic perversion.* Washington Psychoanalytic Institute. Washington, DC.

(1984). *Das Leben und die Bedeutung von Anna Freud.* Balint Institute, Anna Freud Commemorative Meeting. Hamburg, Germany.

(1984). *Panel: Fantasy and body representations in physical disturbances.* Anna Freud Centre International Scientific Colloquium. London, England.

(1985). *Psychological and clinical issues in diabetes.* Middlesex Hospital. London, England.

(1985). *Vulnerable child workshop: The effects of a handicapped or chronically ill child on the family.* Association for Child Psychoanalysis. Chapel Hill, NC.

(1985). *Physical handicap and chronic illness in children: The effect on parents and siblings.* Chicago Psychoanalytic Institute. Chicago, IL.

(1985). *Growing up with a handicapped sibling.* Paddington Psychotherapy Centre. London, England.

(1985). *Panel: Repeating: Enactment and verbalization in different stages of development.* Anna Freud Centre International Scientific Colloquium. London, England.

(1986). *Clinical seminars.* Seattle Psychoanalytic Institute. Seattle, WA.

(1986). *Report on the analysis of a severely disturbed adolescent.* SAP (Jungian Society), Child section. London, England.

(1986). *Panel: On the concepts of fixation and regression, their clinical significance.* Anna Freud Commemorative Conference, University College London. London, England.

(1986). *Sadomasochistische Perversion in einem Adoleszenten.* Schweizerische Gesellschaft für Psychoanalyse. Zürich, Switzerland.

(1986). *Special problems in the treatment of adolescents.* Association for adolescent psychotherapy and psychiatry. Helsinki, Finland.

(1986). *Narcissistic problems in adolescence.* University of Oulu Psychiatric Clinic: Adolescent Psychotherapy Unit. Oulu, Finland.

(1986). *Developmental view of a case of sadomasochistic perversion.* University of Oulu Psychiatric Clinic: Adolescent Psychotherapy Unit. Oulu, Finland.

(1986). *Clinical seminars.* University of Oulu Psychiatric Clinic: Adolescent Psychotherapy Unit. Oulu, Finland.

(1987). *The work of the Anna Freud Centre.* Centre Alfred Binet. Paris, France.

(1988). *Panel: The technique of psychoanalytic work with the pre-latency child.* Association for Child Psychoanalysis. New Orleans, LA.

(1988). *Vulnerable child workshop: Analytic termination in high risk and high vulnerable young children.* Association for Child Psychoanalysis. New Orleans, LA.

(1988). *Special problems in the treatment of adolescents.* University of Mexico Psychology faculty. Mexico City, Mexico.

(1988). *The pre-history of the nursery school.* Celebration of 30 years of the Anna Freud Nursery School. London, England.

(1988). *Die Arbeit mit den Eltern während der Behandlung des Kindes.* Tagung der Schweizerischen Gesellschaft für Psychoanalyse. Zürich, Switzerland.

(1989). *Clinical seminars with Robin Anderson.* British Psychoanalytic Institute. London, England.

(1989). *Discussant: Ilse Hillman's follow-up studies of the War Nursery children.* The Anna Freud Centre. London, England.

(1989). *Panel: The Impact of Developmental Considerations on the Aim of Child and Adult Psychoanalysis.* Anna Freud Centre International Scientific Colloquium. London, England.

(1989). *Anna Freud Commemorative Lecture: Psychoanalytische Behandlung von Kindern in der Prä-Latenz-Periode.* Vienna Psychoanalytic Society. Vienna, Austria.

(1990). *Some thoughts on the aims of child analysis.* Los Angeles Psychoanalytic Society and Institute. Los Angeles, CA.

(1990). *Clinical seminars.* Los Angeles Psychoanalytic Society and Institute. Los Angeles, CA.

(1990). *The aims of child analysis.* San Francisco Psychoanalytic Institute. San Francisco, CA.

(1990). *Clinical seminars.* Sigmund Freud Institute. Frankfurt, Germany.

(1990). *Psychoanalytic work with under-fives: 40 years experience.* WAIPAD conference. London England.

(1991). *Clinical seminars.* Sigmund Freud Institute. Frankfurt, Germany.

(1991). *Reflektionen über das Ziel der Kinderanalyse.* Sigmund Freud Institute. Frankfurt, Germany.

(1992). *Clinical seminars.* Institute for Psychoanalytic Child and Adolescent Psychotherapy. Frankfurt, Germany.

(1992). *Vulnerable Child Workshop: Developing resilience in high-risk nursery school children.* Association for Child Psychoanalysis. Atlanta, GA.

(1992). *The aims of child analysis.* Baltimore-Washington Society for Psychoanalysis. Baltimore, MD.

(1992). *Clinical seminars.* Baltimore-Washington Society for Psychoanalysis. Baltimore, MD.

(1992). *Einige Gedanken über das Ziel der Kinderanalyse.* Schweizerische Gesellschaft für Psychoanalyse. Zürich, Switzerland.

(1992). *Treatment of under fives at the Anna Freud Centre: An overview.* Bologna Italy.

(1993). *A reconsideration of the aims in child analysis.* Sigmund Freud Institute. Frankfurt, Germany.

(1993). *Reminiscences of Anna Freud: 1895–1982.* Anna Freud Memorial Meeting. Mexico City, Mexico.

(1995). *Children in conflict: Anna Freud and the War Nurseries.* Anna Freud Centre and the Freud Museum 100th anniversary celebration of Anna Freud's birth. London, England.

(1995). *Panel: Anna Freud at Yale.* Western New England Institute for Psychoanalysis. New Haven, CT.

(1998). *Symposium: Problems in the analysis of under-fives.* Anna Freud Centre. London, England.

(1998). *The Life and work of Anna Freud: 1895–1982.* Yale University Child Study Centre. New Haven, CT.

BIBLIOGRAPHY

Essenhigh, C. (1995). Anna Freud Centenary Issue: Hansi Kennedy interviewed. *Journal of Child Psychotherapy, 21*: 347–53.

Freud, A. (1973). Tribute to Sara Rosenfeld. Memorial meeting at the Hampstead Child-Therapy Clinic. *Unpublished.*

Jessup, S. (2000). Emigration and the educative process: A case study. Submitted in partial fulfillment of MA (Ed.), University of Southampton. *Unpublished.*

Kennedy, H. (1973). Tribute to Sara Rosenfeld. Memorial meeting at the Hampstead Child-Therapy Clinic. *Unpublished.*

Kennedy, H. (1978). The Hampstead Centre for the Psychoanalytic Study and Treatment of Children. *Bulletin of the Hampstead Clinic, 1*: 7–10.

Kennedy, H. (1982). The child's view of past and present: Implications for child analytic technique. Presented in Stockholm, Sweden. *Unpublished.*

Kennedy, H. (1983). Anna Freud Memorial Issue. *Bulletin of the Hampstead Clinic, 6(1).*

Kennedy, H. (1988). The pre-history of the Nursery School. *Bulletin of the Anna Freud Centre, 11*: 271–5.

Kennedy, H. (1993). Reminiscences of Anna Freud (1895–1982). Presented at a commemoration meeting for Anna Freud, Mexico City. *Unpublished.*

Penman, A.B. (2004). In Memoriam: Hansi Kennedy. *Child Analysis, 15*: 189–90.

Yorke, C. & Wiseberg, S. (1976). A developmental view of anxiety: Some clinical and theoretical considerations. *Psychoanalytic Stucy of the Child, 31*: 107–35.

Interviews

Steven Kennedy, Sue and Catherine Jessup, 26 June 2007
Maria Berger, 27 June 2007
Audrey Gavshon, 28 June 2007
Susie Wiener, 28 June 2007
Jan Wiener, 29 June 2007

For Product Safety Concerns and Information please contact our EU representative GPSR@taylorandfrancis.com
Taylor & Francis Verlag GmbH, Kaufingerstraße 24, 80331 München, Germany

www.ingramcontent.com/pod-product-compliance
Ingram Content Group UK Ltd.
Pitfield, Milton Keynes, MK11 3LW, UK
UKHW021830101126
477531UK00015B/13

* 9 7 8 0 3 6 7 3 2 8 5 7 3 *